THE SECOND STEP

THE SECOND STEP

Baccalaureate Education for Registered Nurses

MARY W. SEARIGHT, R.N., M.S., Editor

California State College, Sonoma
Department of Nursing
Rohnert Park, California

F. A. DAVIS COMPANY
Philadelphia

Library of Congress Cataloging in Publication Data
Main entry under title:

The Second step.

    Includes bibliographies and index.
    1. California State College, Sonoma. School of
Nursing. 2. Nursing—Study and teaching. 3. Nursing—
Study and teaching (Continuing education) I. Searight,
Mary. [DNLM: 1. Curriculum. 2. Education, Nursing,
Baccalaureate. WY18 S439S]
RT80.C22R67   610.73'071   76-3499
ISBN 0-8036-7780-4

Dedicated to

James B. Enochs, Ph.D.
Professor Emeritus
Formerly Executive Vice President
California State College, Sonoma

Yvette M. Fallandy, Ph.D.
Vice President for Academic Affairs
Formerly Dean for Academic Planning
California State College, Sonoma

Joe H. Brumbaugh, Ph.D.
Professor of Biology
Formerly Chairman, Division of Natural Sciences
California State College, Sonoma

Whose courage and mission in supporting an
untried idea in nursing education made the
Second Step Program and this book possible.

Preface

It might be said that closed minds and open curricula are incompatible. In recent years, innovative curriculum models have been developing out of the recognition that most conventional professional education has suffered from the flaws of uniformity, rigidity, and learner passivity. Mandates directed to professional education as a whole to make the system equal, relevant, flexible, and assessible have landed squarely on nursing. Generally nursing curricula are prepackaged and assume a prior knowledge of educational needs. Such prepackaged curricula often depend on faculty consensus, suppression of pluralism, and uniformity of student preparation, interests, and career plans.

One of the most compelling and yet controversial curriculum reforms within nursing is the open curriculum model. An open curriculum in nursing education is a system that takes into account the different purposes of various types of educational programs but recognizes common areas of achievement. It is a move to adapt nursing education to the needs and interests of students who wish to enter and progress in the field of nursing. It operationalizes, for example, the possibility of mobility from preparation at the associate degree or diploma level in nursing to the baccalaureate degree through an interrelated system of achievement with clear articulation rather than quantitative serial steps.

Open curricula in nursing education is a subject of great interest and concern in many quarters. An increasing number of diploma and associate degree nurses are seeking admission to baccalaureate programs. The highly transitory state of nursing education obscures certainty about the direction and methods in programs for registered nurses. Faculties are struggling to solve problems involving the selection and placement of students, to generate curriculum designs that enhance flexibility, and to devise systematic plans for evaluation. Out of the assembled melange of educational programs, a proliferation of apparently unrelatable premises has emerged. The elements of curriculum design, program objectives, learning experiences, and evaluation are *the* questions in an open curriculum. These questions have been answered differently in the Second Step Model than in traditional nursing programs.

This book was conceived during a faculty workshop in the spring of 1974, after full accreditation of the Second Step Program by the National League for Nursing had been received. The faculty felt that this action had validated their own and their students' pioneering commitment. Moreover, numerous requests for information and consultation led us to believe that our experience would have real significance for nurses and nurse educators. We have taken as the task of the book an illumination of the problems, issues, and alternative solutions in the process of devising an open curriculum model— a second step for registered nurses seeking baccalaureate degrees.

The book is directed to administrators, educators, researchers, and students who are engaged in planning, implementing, and evaluating baccalaureate curricula for registered nurses. We have addressed many of the concrete and philosophical problems involved in "opening the curriculum" through the experience and perspective of a nursing faculty that has been on the frontier of this social and educational movement. Included are ideas, tools, criteria, course descriptions, and research findings developed by the California State College, Sonoma nursing faculty in our upper division baccalaureate program built expressly on the base of associate degree or diploma education.

Each of the eleven chapters, organized sequentially, addresses a key dimension of the endeavor. Chapter 1 presents an overview of the pressures in society, education, and nursing to open the curriculum. A conceptual framework, including considerations of learners' needs, characteristics of the setting, and knowledge base, is presented in Chapter 2. In Chapter 3, innovations in organizing learning to enhance flexibility and to meet program goals are discussed. Chapter 4 focuses on the thorny issues surrounding admission and placement of students in the program. Chapters 5 and 6 discuss baccalaureate level contractual study and preparation for family nurse practitioner roles. Chapters 7 and 8 are directed to the human experiences involved in the process—from the point of view of both student and faculty members. Chapter 9 confronts the current issues of the perpetuation of stereotypes of ethnicity and femininity in traditional nursing education. Finally, Chapter 10 presents our evaluation research design and findings in a case study format, and Chapter 11 explores the general subject of curriculum evaluation.

Mary W. Searight, R.N., M.S.

Acknowledgments

It is readily apparent that the Second Step Program developed as it did only with the courage, faith, and cooperation of a large number of people. There were many who served on committees, arranged meetings, sought information, and gave publicity and recognition, to whom we can best express our appreciation by continuing to serve our community and students. We would like to mention here some of the people especially instrumental in the development of the program and this book.

Community pressure to develop a nursing program began shortly after California State College, Sonoma was established in 1960. There was serious discussion among many of the faculty as to whether nursing belonged in its liberal arts setting, until biology professors Kenneth Stocking, Ph.D., and Wesley Ebert, Ph.D., with the support of the Division of Natural Sciences, were successful in carrying the concept through the various committees of the Academic Senate for approval and the inclusion of the nursing department in the master plan. In 1971, funds were allocated for a planning year and a committee, consisting of Wesley Ebert, Ph.D., Joe H. Brumbaugh, Ph.D., Leonard Pearson, Ph.D., and Yvette M. Fallandy, Ph.D., was appointed to search for a chairperson for the new department.

Community support had been mobilized through the efforts of the local unit of the California Nurses' Association, District 15, and its Nursing Education Committee, chaired by Patricia Anderson, R.N., M.S. Committee members, including Beverly Eagan, R.N., M.S., Carla Estabrook, R.N., M.S., Ann Hardin, R.N., B.A., Helen Keefer, R.N., M.N., Mary O'Brien, R.N., Rae Rehn, R.N., M.S., and myself, assessed by means of a questionnaire the needs of the area's nurses, and sought through education and legislation to provide opportunity and strong support for career articulation. Dr. Ebert met frequently with the Nursing Education Committee during this period, serving as liaison between the college's proposed plan and the nursing group.

The District 15 Nursing Education Committee also provided a sounding board to me, as our ideas for baccalaureate degree nursing education for registered nurses continued to grow. As a result of my own educational, professional, and teaching experiences, the Second

Step concept was almost fully formed in my mind by the time I had moved to Santa Rosa, joined that community's active nursing association, and become aware of the local college's plan. Trends in the campus, community, and profession of nursing, staunchly advocated by many mentioned here and others who are not, were at last converging.

Following my appointment as the first chairperson for the new Department of Nursing, administrative support for the experimental program was steadfast. California State College, Sonoma traditionally has sought to question old ways and to experiment with alternative ways of doing things and to encourage self-actualization and social action. It is not, therefore, surprising that a nontraditional nursing program, planned to meet an historically underserved population, would be embraced and strongly supported by the faculty and administration.

During the planning year of the program, the chairpersons of the new department of nursing and of the area's five community college nursing programs met monthly to discuss philosophy and process of the programs' interrelationships. The original group consisted of Lyla Cromer, R.N., M.S., of the College of Marin, Margretta Fortuin, R.N., M.A., of Santa Rosa Junior College, Ellen Gibson, R.N., M.S., of Pacific Union College, Donna Harris, R.N., M.S., of Solano Community College, Doris Zylinski, R.N., M.S., of Napa College, and myself. We were later joined by Marilyn Flood, R.N., M.S., from the graduate program at the University of California, San Francisco, Connie Roth, R.N., M.S., from the graduate program at the University of California, Davis, and, upon the retirement of Miss Fortuin, by Joe Hagerty, R.N., M.S. The group continues to meet periodically to explore areas of mutual concern.

A community-based advisory group also gave generously of their time during the planning year, and continued to meet periodically as the program developed. The chairperson of this group was Sister Mary Esther, C.S.J., of Santa Rosa Memorial Hospital; health providers were represented by Patricia Anderson, R.N., M.S., and Walter Clowers, M.D.; health consumers were represented by Fran Bigelow, bilingual community worker, Kenneth Bubb, Director of the Common Health Club, Robert Sherrill, insurance executive, William Sullivan, bank manager, Walter Zylinski, attorney, Charles Belden, community college administrator, and Barbara Noel, high school counselor. California State College, Sonoma representatives were Mildred Dickeman, Ph.D., Professor of Anthropology, John Dunning, Ph.D., Associate Professor of Physics, Francisco Gaona, Ph.D., Professor of Spanish, Victor Garlin, Ph.D., Associate Professor of Economics, Wyman Hicks, M.A., Professor of Management, Dorothy Overly, Ph.D., Professor of English, and Hobart Thomas, Ph.D., Professor of Psychology and Provost, School of Expressive Arts.

Mary Lou McAthie, Consultant for the Department of Health, Education, and Welfare, Division of Nursing, provided early and continuing assistance in the preparation of two special project grant proposals. The funding of the first grant made possible a more complete and well qualified faculty the first year and the initiation of a longitudinal evaluation study; the second grant provides a valuable research component.

Barbara Lee, Program Director, W.K. Kellogg Foundation, provided counsel and assistance in securing funding through the Kellogg Foundation for the family nurse practitioner preceptorship and its evaluation, extending nursing education for our students and nursing care for the community.

Throughout all of these steps, wise, thoughtful, and challenging guidance was provided by Verle Waters, R.N., M.A., who served as curriculum consultant. Nowhere was her critical assessment and encouragement more important than during our self-evaluation study in preparation for accreditation.

The presentation of our experiences in this book has required a special kind of participation and expertise. Since cooperative teamwork has been a very positive characteristic of the faculty since its inception, the writing and editing of this book were shared. Contributing authors served as editors for each other and sought the assistance of faculty whose names do not appear. As editor of the book and chairperson of the department, I owe a greater debt of gratitude to all of the faculty than does any other contributor. Other colleagues in nursing, by their responses to our program and to this manuscript, have encouraged us to believe that our work has been and will be useful to them in their respective settings. Judith Kim of the F.A. Davis Company has been unfailingly supportive. From California State College, Sonoma, J.J. Wilson, Ph.D., Associate Professor of English, has assisted us editorially; Don Cabrall of Instructional Resources and Carl Campbell of Public Affairs provided graphics and photography. LaVerne Joyce typed all of the manuscript, and our own office staff, consisting of Lucy Kortum, Carol Turner, Betty Gale, Kim Terry, and Sally Cochran, were involved at almost every phase of the project.

We hope the book says for us: We warmly thank you all.

Mary W. Searight, R.N., M.S.

Contributors

Christine H. Beaty-Morton, R.N., M.S., Assistant Professor of Nursing,
California State College, Sonoma
Hannan E. Dean, R.N., M.S., Assistant Professor of Nursing, California
State College, Sonoma
Ruth E. Haskell, R.N., M.S., Assistant Professor of Nursing, California
State College, Sonoma
Janice E. Hitchcock, R.N., M.S., Assistant Professor of Nursing, Cali-
fornia State College, Sonoma
Harriett J. Lionberger, R.N., B.S., candidate for M.S. Degree in Nurs-
ing, University of California, San Francisco
Marilyn J. Little, M.A., Research Associate, Department of Nursing,
California State College, Sonoma; candidate for Ph.D. Degree
in Sociology and Education, University of California,
Berkeley.
Vivian A. Malmstrom, R.N., M.S., Associate Professor of Nursing,
California State College, Sonoma
Leonide L. Martin, R.N., M.S., F.N.P., Assistant Professor of Nursing,
California State College, Sonoma
Virginia Y. Meyer, R.N., M.S., Assistant Professor of Nursing, Cali-
fornia State College, Sonoma
M. Elizabeth Monninger, R.N., M.S., Assistant Professor of Nursing,
Arizona State University, Tempe
Renée Romanko-Keller, R.N., M.A., Assistant Professor of Nursing,
California State College, Sonoma
Mary Jane Sauvé, R.N., M.S., Assistant Professor of Nursing, California
State College, Sonoma
Mary W. Searight, R.N., M.S., Chairperson, Department of Nursing,
California State College, Sonoma
Barbara Reed Tesser, R.N., M.S., Assistant Professor of Nursing,
California State College, Sonoma
Sue A. Thomas, R.N., M.S., Associate Professor of Nursing, California
State College, Sonoma

Haywood C. Vaughan, M.S., Research Associate, Department of
    Nursing, California State College, Sonoma
Verle Waters, R.N., M.A., Curriculum Consultant
Holly Skodol Wilson, R.N., Ph.D., Associate Professor of Nursing,
    California State College, Sonoma

Contents

Chapter 1　Pressures for Opening the Curriculum　　　　　1
　　　　　　Verle Waters, R.N., M.A.

Chapter 2　Developing a Conceptual Framework for Cur-　11
　　　　　　riculum Decisions
　　　　　　Holly Skodol Wilson, R.N., Ph.D., Mary
　　　　　　Jane Sauvé, R.N., M.S., and Mary W.
　　　　　　Searight, R.N., M.S.

Chapter 3　Strategies for Organizing Learning　　　　　33
　　　　　　Hannah Dean, R.N., M.S., Ruth Haskell,
　　　　　　R.N., M.S., and Barbara Reed Tesser,
　　　　　　R.N., M.S.

Chapter 4　Issues and Problems of Articulation and Admis-　59
　　　　　　sion
　　　　　　Vivian Malmstrom, R.N., M.S., and Virginia
　　　　　　Meyer, R.N., M.S.

Chapter 5　Preceptorship Study: Contracting for Learning　82
　　　　　　Mary W. Searight, R.N., M.S.

Chapter 6　Family Nurse Practitioner Preparation at the　105
　　　　　　Baccalaureate Level
　　　　　　Elizabeth Monninger, R.N., M.S., Leonide
　　　　　　L. Martin, R.N., M.S., F.N.P., and Marilyn
　　　　　　Little, M.A.

Chapter 7　Liberating the Curriculum from Stereotypes of　141
　　　　　　Ethnicity and Femininity
　　　　　　Renée Romanko-Keller, R.N., M.A., and
　　　　　　Christine H. Beaty-Morton, R.N., M.S.

Chapter 8   Faculty Group and Interpersonal Processes   170
             Sue A. Thomas, R.N., M.S., and Janice
             Hitchcock, R.N., M.S.

Chapter 9   The Sonoma Experience: A Student's View   187
             Harriet Lionberger, R.N., B.S.

Chapter 10   The Second Step Research Project   206
             Haywood C. Vaughan, M.S.

Chapter 11   Curriculum Evaluation Research   223
             Holly Skodol Wilson, R.N., Ph.D.

Index   249

CHAPTER 1

Pressures for Opening the Curriculum

Verle Waters, R.N., M.A.

Nursing has a history of earnest concern for its educational programs.
Just as American thought from earliest times has placed great value on
the importance of an educational system to the well-being of free men,
in that same spirit nursing has invested in its educational system enor-
mous confidence in the educational program to reform the ills of practice, enhance the stature of the profession, and strengthen the hand
of the practitioner. The proper domain of the educational program
in nursing is the subject of a mountain of literature, and the rhetoric
of program goals reflects the belief that nursing education has a mission to reform inadequacies in health care delivery. Many phrases
commonly used in the objectives of educational programs, such as
"continuity of care," "comprehensive patient care," and "change
agent," express the hope that through learning provided for the neophyte, the work world can be reshaped.

Against this backdrop of strong belief about what education for
nursing should or should not be, any change creates strong responses.
Convictions are expressed by written and spoken word for or against
the development or change. Reactions more passionate than considered were generated in nursing with the provisions of the Cadet
Corps program, the publication of the Brown report, the establishment of the associate degree program, and the issuance of the First
Position Paper on Education.

So-called open curriculum developments in nursing have engendered
similarly strong responses. A program such as the Second Step at
Sonoma State is both heralded and deplored, reported with pride and
viewed with alarm. Bullough characterizes the position of nurse educators toward the open curriculum movement as one of "concerned
ambivalence."[1] The sense that educational programs have been arti-
ficially rigid and unresponsive to students as individuals co-exists
with a fear that to make the programs otherwise will lower standards,

1

dilute quality, and devalue nursing and nursing care. The course of nursing thought regarding educational mobility for registered nurses has not been smooth, and the vagaries in that brief history relate to significant events within nursing itself as well as in the larger arenas of higher education and the health care system. Indications are that a period of growth and expansion of the type of program for R.N.s represented by the Second Step curriculum is underway. Such expansion is not an unexpected outgrowth of nursing's own history as well as an expression of larger trends in higher education. A perspective on the past events and professional policy regarding continued education for R.N.s is useful in understanding the pressures for present expansion. Further, a perspective on the past may direct a course of action within which educational quality and integrity may be assured.

Career mobility has been a topic of concern among nursing educators for the past quarter century. The goal of providing upward mobility for nurses is not new, nor are the techniques for granting credit for past educational achievement. In fact, Katzell notes that the original purpose for development of the National League for Nursing achievement tests was to permit students in Cadet Corps schools to avoid time-wasting duplication of learning experience.[2] Though the goal and methodology for providing career mobility are not new developments, attitudes toward the education of R.N.s seeking a baccalaureate degree have changed sharply. Sanction for the second step has recently emerged, in concert with the open curriculum movement in higher education. The open curriculum, sometimes called "nontraditional study," employs a number of enticing phrases which fit nicely in discussions of nursing education and the R.N. who seeks a baccalaureate degree. In addition to "open curriculum," the terms "diversity by design," "the learning society," and "less time, more options" all suggest a welcoming of the formerly unwelcome by providing more flexibility, more paths, and less repetition.

The literature describing developments in higher education toward open access, lifelong learning, individualized instruction will not be reviewed here; interested readers unfamiliar with those changes will easily find description and documentation of new directions in higher education elsewhere. A review of recent events in higher education reveals that the chief difference between the so-called "closed" and the open curriculum is the approach or point of view regarding the grounds on which curriculum decisions are made. An open curriculum gives greater weight to students goals, characteristics, and motivations in determining content and selecting learning experiences.

A significant shift in nursing's point of view on the acceptability of programs introducing radically different conceptions of the student's influence on the program of learning occurred with the

2

adoption of the open curriculum position statement. In February 1970 the National League for Nursing's board of directors adopted a statement favoring the open curriculum. While the "concerned ambivalence" Bullough speaks of may be read between the lines, the statement set the stage for many variations in educational programs.

An open curriculum in nursing education is a system which takes into account the different purposes of the various types of programs but recognizes common areas of achievement. Such a system permits student mobility in the light of ability, changing career goals, and changing aspirations. It also requires clear delineation of the achievement expectations of nursing programs from practical nursing through graduate education. It recognizes the possibility of mobility from other health-related fields. It is an interrelated system of achievement in nursing education with *open doors*, rather than quantitative serial steps.

The National League for Nursing believes that:

1. Individuals who wish to change career goals should have an opportunity to do so.

2. Educational opportunities should be provided for those who are interested in upward mobility without lowering standards.

3. In any type of nursing program, opportunity should be provided to validate previous education and experience.

4. Sound educational plans must be developed to avoid unsound projects and programs.

5. More effective guidance is urgently needed at all stages of student development.

6. If projects and endeavors in this area are to be successful, nursing must accept the concept of the open curriculum.[3]

One project and endeavor in this area, of great interest to many, has been the reopening of programs designed to meet the educational goals of registered nurse students seeking baccalaureate degrees. Though baccalaureate education in nursing has existed since early 1900, few registered nurses went on for degree study prior to 1950. The value of such study for nurses and nursing was clearly in the thought and voice of nursing leadership, and the great women of the first half of this century, Nutting, Dock, Goodrich, Stewart, and others, attached great importance to the development of a system of nursing education which would lead nurses to the baccalaureate degree, and establish nursing in the mainstream of higher education with the benefits and perquisites attached to it. Early reports and studies reinforced the importance of higher education for nurses. A turning point came with Brown's "Nursing for the Future," published in 1948. Brown asserted that most of what went on in the nursing schools of the period could scarcely be called higher education and urged nursing to move in concerted fashion to strengthen the educational quality of its programs. As had others before her, she emphasized the importance to the profession of establishing educational programs in the colleges and universities. The indictment of the diploma school as it then existed was a strong one, threatening, and undeniably one to which nursing had to listen.

While there were nearly 200 nursing programs leading to a baccalaureate degree in 1950 (another 1,000 led to a diploma) the degree programs were "in" higher education but not "of" it. Nursing instruction no different from that in the diploma school was added to a lower division course of study in general education; where both programs were offered by one school, diploma and degree students customarily had identical experiences in the nursing portion of their programs. Five year programs added a final period of study in administration, teaching, or public health. Later that curriculum would be described as additive in nature, in contrast to the integrative form which developed as baccalaureate educators achieved reorganization of existing baccalaureate programs or developed new programs. The new form was called "basic baccalaureate" or "generic" and the nursing curriculum was conceptualized as a whole, drawing upon a body of knowledge unique to a level of practice at the professional level. Throughout the program academic standards and practices typical of collegiate study prevailed. The new basic baccalaureate program was planned, implemented, and evaluated by the college nursing faculty, and students were assumed to be like other college students, and therefore deserving of schedules and learning activities typical of the academic pattern. Innovative and pioneering leaders in the 1950s included Lulu Wolf Hussenplug and Helen Nahm who established at the University of California campuses in Los Angeles and San Francisco programs which conceptualized learners, the knowledge of nursing, and the environment of nursing as a unified and consistent whole. In the postwar expansion of higher education, provoked by the Brown report, and supported by a newly potent professional accrediting program, nursing achieved the establishment of baccalaureate education, new in format, better in quality, and promising for the future.

That postwar decade was for nursing education and all of education a time of expanding horizons, resources, and social consciousness. Nursing recognized the educational forms of the prewar period would serve neither patients nor their nurses, though the awareness of change may have been greater than the understanding of its implications or meaning. Nursing was moving rapidly into the mainstream of education, and to a new level of social responsibility. The profession faced a choice between focusing energies on the development of the basic baccalaureate program for students entering nursing, or mounting a large scale effort to provide degree education for R.N.s already graduated or enrolled in the 1,000 diploma schools of the time. We know from the events which followed, that the decision was to direct energies toward the establishment of the basic baccalaureate program. To a considerable extent continued education for R.N.s *was* offered, but the hope for the future seemed to lie in the generic baccalaureate program. R.N.s who went on for a degree entered "supplemental" baccalaureate programs—the very term implies a point of view toward the student and her previous education.

The nursing literature of the 1950s and 1960s conveys a growing picture of the search for baccalaureate level content in nursing. Educators and theorists of the time contributed to the definition, explication, and structuring of knowledge for a baccalaureate program in nursing which was unique, distinguishable from the "other" in nursing content. The academic model of lower and upper division to rationalize the arrangement of learning was engaged, and examples were employed from other fields wherein specialized or professional content is built upon a base of liberal arts preparation. The characteristics, then, of the baccalaureate program in nursing, though emergent with regard to the difference in the nursing content, were explicit with regard to the placement of the liberal arts in the program:

> . . .[The] basic premises upon which undergraduate education for professional nursing is founded: first, that liberal education precedes and is basic to professional education; second, that instruction in the nursing major is largely at the upper division level. . . .[4]
>
> Nursing practice in collegiate programs builds on and integrates the liberal arts into the nursing curriculum; to give college credit for nursing courses taken apart from the liberal arts or before acquiring a broad base in the arts and sciences would contradict the entire philosophy and practice of collegiate education.[5]

That strong association between the definition of the true professional curriculum and the placement of liberal arts courses would later become a point of reference for opponents of the Second Step curriculum format. Meanwhile, for a nearly 20 year period after the war, registered nurses went to colleges and universities to obtain a degree. An article by McDonald in a 1964 issue of *Nursing Outlook* reviews the policies and practices of advanced education for R.N.s over that period. She concluded that R.N.s had adequate opportunity to obtain a baccalaureate degree if they wished. Some programs at that time were special B.S. programs for R.N.s, which included special upper division nursing courses. Some were programs in which R.N.s were admitted into the generic program. Many other nurses obtained a B.S. degree in institutions which offered no nursing courses and had no nursing faculty, but provided a two year course of study in general education and awarded the degree upon completion.

The quality of the programs described above ranged from excellent to awful. A number of the leading university schools offered excellent programs for R.N. students. Others awarded a degree after two years of lower division general education. Blanket credit was given: 30 to 60 units of college credit awarded toward the baccalaureate degree simply for the possession of the R.N. license. Even though it was considered an academically unsound practice at the time, it became widely used. Inevitably, such a situation engendered negative reactions, and nursing's status in higher education was second class, at best.

In 1963 the National League for Nursing issued a "Statement of Beliefs and Recommendations Regarding Baccalaureate Nursing Programs Admitting Registered Nurse Students." In a position that was to be swiftly effective, the statement called for the closing of all separate B.S. programs for R.N.s, and the establishment of "one baccalaureate program in nursing . . . for the professional education of all undergraduate students, including registered nurses who are graduates of diploma and associate degree programs."[6]

The educators who accepted and supported the statement felt that quality in nursing education at the baccalaureate level required that there be only one degree for all students; that integrity of baccalaureate education for nursing required that it be one degree, standing for achievement of a single, professionally sanctioned course of study. The additional time required of the registered nurse student to complete all lower division courses required in the generic program, and then complete the nursing requirements was justified as that which was to be expected with a change of educational goal and change of type of educational program.

Within a two year period after the statement of beliefs was issued, all but a few of the special B.S.N. programs for R.N. students closed. The transition was speedy and resulted in increased frustration and anguish on the part of R.N.s at what seemed to them insensitive and insensible barriers to their doing what the profession called for—advancing their educational preparation.

> Most university doors, at that time, were indeed wide open to the diploma graduate—except now these graduates would spend an inordinately long time pursuing what they would see as similar aims, mastering what would seem to be repetitious learnings.[7]

Associate degree graduates were growing in number, and many of them encountered the same experiences in going on for a baccalaureate degree as the diploma R.N.s had had and were having.

> The early graduates of the associate degree program experienced many of the same problems faced by diploma graduates. They were not exactly welcomed with open arms into baccalaureate programs and often had a difficult time if they were admitted. Although this attitude is undergoing change in many parts of the country, acceptance of the associate degree graduate is not yet

universal. Many nursing educators still think that, if nurses graduate from a "terminal" program, they should at least have the good grace to remain terminal.[8]

It is tempting to view the foregoing period in nursing education in black and white terms, to see the closed, restrictive baccalaureate programs as giving no quarter to the poor rejected diploma graduate seeking to improve her educational preparation for the good of her patients and her profession. Such a view is as colorful, and as inaccurate, as seeing the educators all riding the white horses of high standards, quality, and pursuit of excellence, and the diploma graduate as intellectually lazy, seeking an easy and expedient degree. A balanced view must acknowledge that the progress nursing has made in the improvement of its educational programs in the past 25 years is nothing short of remarkable. The overall response on the part of nursing and of higher education to the challenge voiced in the Brown report has been responsible and sound. Out of the experience of the past 25 years, including both the perspective gained on our own previous attempts to solve pressing problems and the way the world around us has gone in that time, there is a basis for sound planning of program which are high in quality and geared to diverse student populations.

The baccalaureate educators involved with selection of curriculum content have been concerned with determining the legitimate domain of content for baccalaureate education. While accusations that baccalaureate content was all the same as that taught in diploma and associate degree programs are unfounded, neither has it been quite true that it was all different. The search for clearly differentiated distinctions between baccalaureate content and the rest has been wordy and inconclusive, and the baccalaureate curriculum has at times seemed to be a program in search of its identity. Bolstered by a dominant practical view of the work of nursing, many R.N.s found it easy to devalue the contribution baccalaureate education could make to the daily work world of being an R.N. On the one hand we have had within the profession a strong surge for educational preparation which will develop in students the ability to think, make decisions, make a difference; on the other hand, there is the suspicion that theory has little to do with practice, and that the ivory tower approach to nursing bears little resemblance to the reality of the work world.

Certainly a great deal of professional attention was paid to the problem of the registered nurse seeking a baccalaureate degree between 1963, when the Statement of Beliefs was adopted, and 1970, the year in which the NLN adopted the statement on open curriculum. Titles of articles appearing in nursing journals in that period include the following: The Registered Nurse Seeks a College; Going on for a Bachelor's Degree; Nurses Caps and Bachelors Gowns; Direction or Dilemma for R.N.'s in Baccalaureate Education? The R.N. Writes Her

Own Transfer Credit; A Nursing Major without Nursing; Artificial
Barriers to Progress in Nursing; Granting College Credit to Registered
Nurse Students; Credit for Competency. In addition, a special conference sponsored by the Department of Baccalaureate and Higher
Degree Programs of the NLN was held in 1966 on baccalaureate
education for the registered nurse student. Still, dissatisfaction and
hostility toward baccalaureate educators grew among registered
nurses who desired a baccalaureate degree, or said they did.

In the discussions surrounding the Position Paper on nursing education, in which the American Nurses Association recommended clear
differentation in nursing between technical and professional levels
of education and practice, nurses and others in health career education began to talk about the career ladder as an educational concept.
Rutgers University had experimented with a modified baccalaureate
program after the establishment of an associate degree program
within its school of nursing. Though the program was described
with enthusiasm at the point of organization, it was closed without
fanfare after a ten year period of operation. A few "two-plus-two"
or career ladder programs were developed in other universities, but
the negative reactions toward such programs, or the concept of such
a program, was widespread among baccalaureate educators. "What
would be the consequences of planning the bachelor's on the base of
an associate degree in nursing? Inevitably, the bachelor's curriculum
would be diluted and thus the base for graduate education weak-
ened."[9]

Not until the emergence in higher education of the open curriculum
movement, about 1970, would the pressures for re-establishing a baccalaureate nursing program expressly for registered nurse students outweigh the forces restraining such a move. Together with pressures
from students, legislative intervention and a changing public attitude
toward the system of higher education and its responsibilities have
forced a re-examination of the ten year position.

Maybe the dilemma is in trying to ensure the universality of the
B.S.N. degree when two distinctly different groups of students
are involved. This course of action emanated directly from the
position statement requiring a single B.S.N. program for basic and
R.N. students accepted by the Council of Baccalaureate and
Higher Degree Programs in 1963. After acceptance of that philosophy and approach, the conflict between R.N. students and
educators seemed more polarized than ever.[10]

The open curriculum point of view asserts that changed assumptions are required for the planning of educational programs. Curriculums have traditionally been developed on the assumption that the
function of the school is to thoughtfully design programs, and then
carefully pick students who will succeed in that program. Certainly

8

such a statement describes the traditional approach to program planning in nursing. Now, however, that assumption is challenged, and it is said that the function of the school is to design programs based on the students, their needs and interests. Many specific population groups have been identified as learners for whom education has a responsibility. For example, in 1973, 31 of the grants announced by the U.S. Office of Education were aimed at noncollege age women, minority women, adult urban residents, veterans, minorities, Indians, Puerto Ricans, Spanish-speaking adults, prison inmates, former inmates, and "underserved clientele or new clientele." Nursing has through its own historical choices created a very large underserved clientele: the registered nurse seeking a baccalaureate degree.

Resolution for the future lies in a broader base of consideration in making our decisions. In education and in society as a whole, the glamor of the baccalaureate degree as the hallmark of distinction has tarnished or, perhaps, been brought down to earth a bit. We are entering or are now in a period of considerably reduced emphasis on the importance of the baccalaureate degree. For nursing in the last analysis this means that future planning of baccalaureate programs must be determined by a sober consideration of what the profession needs in its practitioners. Program planning for baccalaureate nursing education rests not so much on what the lower division has been as on what the upper division is. For such curriculum determinations, the planning model proposed by Chater allows for the development of curricula which incorporate theoretical conceptions of nursing knowledge, yet rest as well on a description of the learners, and are planned within setting reality.[11]

Within that approach, explicated in detail in pages which follow, lies the potential for resolving the ambivalence.

REFERENCES

1. Bullough, Bonnie: Public, Legal and Social Pressure for a Career Ladder in Nursing. *Current Issues in Nursing Education*, New York, 1972. NLN Council of Baccalaureate and Higher Degree Programs.
2. Katzell, Mildred E.: Upward Mobility in Nursing. *Nursing Outlook* 18:36, 1970.
3. NLN: *The Open Curriculum in Nursing Education.* Statement approved by the Board of Directors, National League for Nursing, February 1970.
4. Boyle, Rena, Ren, E., and Paterson, Frances K.: The Registered Nurse Seeks a College. *Nursing Outlook* 10:652, 1962.
5. Kibrick, A.: Why Collegiate Programs for Nurses? *New England Journal of Medicine* 278:765, 1968.
6. NLN: Department of Baccalaureate and Higher Degree Programs Statement of Beliefs and Recommendations Regarding Baccalaureate Nursing Programs Admitting Registered Nurse Students. National League for Nursing, New York, 1964.
7. Sheehan, Sister Dorothy: The Hospital School Graduate—Can the Birthright Be Restored? *Nursing Forum* 12:274, 1973.

8. Matheney, Ruth V.: Open Curriculum—Yes! in *Open Learning and Career Mobility in Nursing*, Carrie B. Lenburg, ed., St. Louis, The C.V. Mosby Co., 1975, p. 85.
9. Anderson, Edith H.: The Associate Degree Program—A Step to the Baccalaureate Degree? *Current Issues in Nursing Education* 1972. Papers presented at the Ninth Conference of the Council of Baccalaureate and Higher Degree Programs, March 1972.
10. Lenburg, Carrie B.: Openness and Mobility in Nursing Education, in *Open Learning and Career Mobility in Nursing*, Carrie Lenburg, ed., St. Louis, The C.V. Mosby Co., 1975, p. 29.
11. Chater, Shirley S.: A Conceptual Framework for Curriculum Development. *Nursing Outlook* 23:428, 1975.

BIBLIOGRAPHY

Bridgman, Margaret: *Collegiate Education for Nursing.* New York, Russell Sage Foundation, 1953.
Brown, Esther Lucile: *Nursing for the Future.* New York, Russell Sage Foundation, 1948.
Bullough, Bonnie, and Bullough, Vern: A Career Ladder in Nursing: Problems and Prospects. *American Journal of Nursing* 71:1938, 1971.
Chater, Shirley S.: Upper Division, Lower Division, the Academic Structure of the Baccalaureate Degree. Unpublished paper.
Harty, Margaret: Trends in Nursing Education. *American Journal of Nursing* 68:767, 1968.
Lenburg, Carrie B. (ed.): *Open Learning and Career Mobility in Nursing.* St. Louis, The C.V. Mosby Co., 1975.
McDonald, Gwendoline: Baccalaureate Education for Graduates of Diploma and Associate Degree Programs. *Nursing Outlook* June 1964, p. 52-56.

CHAPTER 2

Developing a Conceptual Framework for Curriculum Decisions

Holly Skodol Wilson, R.N., Ph.D., Mary Jane Sauvé, R.N., M.S., and Mary W. Searight, R.N., M.S.

The decisions made in designing a nursing curriculum frequently derive from many sources. Political pressures, budgetary exigencies, vested interests of faculty, past experiences, and intuition all constitute forces capable of molding and shaping decisions about what courses to include, what teaching strategies to employ, the ratio of required to elective units of study, and evaluation practices, to name only a few. Quite often the outcome is a curriculum that lacks internal cohesiveness, coherence, and unity. As Chater has pointed out, "Curriculums have become increasingly additive in an attempt to be ameliorative."[1]

A conceptual framework for curriculum decisions offers one means by which to decrease the patchwork approach to designing a curriculum and to bring a logical consistency to the process. Bevis defines a conceptual or theoretical framework as "an interrelated system of premises that provides guidelines or ground rules for making all curricular decisions—objectives, content, implementation, and evaluation."[2]

Such a framework is usually in a dynamic state if it is to keep the curriculum current. A conceptual framework for curriculum decisions is never fully completed but rather continues to become more refined, explicit, and useful. The development of a curriculum framework is a highly complex task involving numerous choices among a variety of alternatives. Chater lists defining, sorting, classifying, patterning, and relationship-seeking as the thinking processes used by faculty in constructing a framework.[3] Because a conceptual framework is constantly in the state of emergence and reformulation, faculties usually experience the process of constructing one as a gradual unfolding of an increasingly explicit set of propositions, facts, and concepts that can explain the "whys" of a nursing curriculum and can be tested and demonstrated empirically.

11

Many possible concepts serve to bring organization and unity to the various events or phenomena basic to curriculum development. For the sake of parsimony as well as scope, Chater has proposed a model that uses only three components: setting, student, and subject.[4] Her model is depicted in Figure 1. Taba suggests similar foci: society, learners, and the knowledge base.[5] Because settings, learners, and faculty hypotheses about the nature of nursing as a discipline and its requisite knowledge base usually combine to create a unique picture, it is unlikely that a curriculum design logically deduced from the conceptual framework of an individual program could reasonably fit the characteristics and conditions of another. Hence the value in the efforts of each program to undertake the task of designing a curriculum by first attempting to bring together data relevant to its unique circumstances. The curriculum ultimately adopted should reflect these areas of uniqueness as synthesized in a conceptual framework.

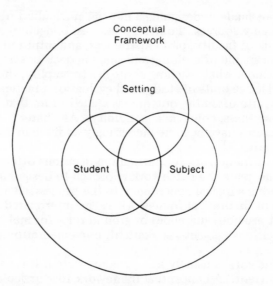

FIGURE 1. Chater model for conceptual framework for curriculum development.

DEVELOPING A CONCEPTUAL FRAMEWORK FOR THE SECOND STEP PROGRAM

Sonoma State College's Second Step Program began with the hypothesis that upper division nursing education leading to a baccalaureate degree could be built upon associate degree or diploma preparation in such a way as to be educationally sound. Such a hypothesis was grounded in the self-reports of nurses originally prepared in diploma programs who subsequently spent years making

12

up deficiencies in the process of finally earning a baccalaureate degree. The experience of the nursing department chairwoman as a teacher at the associate degree level and in the preparation of teachers for associate degree education gave additional support to the germinating idea. The more program goals of the varied nursing programs were studied, the more they looked the same. All stated that they were preparing beginning practitioners. All were preparing nurses to take the same licensure exams. And all claimed to produce a nurse able to give beginning bedside nursing care under supervision. The problems of lack of articulation between various nursing programs, lack of clear differentiation between the graduates, and the barriers and obstacles to career mobility within the conventional educational system all gave impetus to the search for alternative approaches.

Collection of other initial data yielded the following set of propositions which would be tested by the Second Step Program.

1. There is a body of nursing knowledge that is basic to registered nurse preparation. It can be effectively taught at the lower division level and licensure can be acquired based on that preparation.

2. There is a body of knowledge which does not duplicate basic preparation for registered nurses but which builds on that foundation and provides the opportunity to expand and extend nursing competencies.

3. The educational system in California that provides for lower and upper division study is organized in such a manner that direct articulation between the first two and the last two years of collegeate education is feasible.

4. All students deserve the right to progress in their educational endeavors and should not be penalized because of their initial choice of a nursing program.

5. All individuals seek to reach their highest potential. Registered nurses are no exception and should be afforded the opportunity for educational mobility.

6. An upper division nursing major expressly designed for registered nurses could be developed in such a way as to qualify for accreditation by the National League for Nursing.

These propositions gained sufficient interest and support to enable a small coterie of faculty to embark on the demanding task of formulating the specific conceptual framework for the program and its subsequent curriculum design. Making the conceptual framework for the Second Step Program an explicit one has continued to be a developmental process. Data has been synthesized concerning the multifaceted characteristics of the setting, the needs and characteristics of the learners as well as specific relevant learning theories, and finally the cognitive base for the discipline of professional nursing. The collection of this data began during the planning year when a skeleton of the program, a feasibility study, a major proposal for the college Chancellor's Office, and a Health, Education and Welfare special

13

project grant proposal were all developed and submitted to the respective agencies by the program chairwoman. Each of the interlocking components of the conceptual framework will be taken up in detail throughout this chapter.

The Setting

Frank Lloyd Wright once wrote the following paragraph about a "natural house."

> What is needed most in architecture today is the very thing needed most in life—integrity. . . . Integrity is not something to be put on and taken off like a garment. Integrity is a quality within and of man himself. So it is in a building. The Usonian house, then, aims to be a natural performance, one that is integral to site, integral to environment, integral to the life of the inhabitants. . . .[6]

The faculty in the Second Step Program sought to design a curriculum that possessed this kind of integrity with the distinguishing aspects of its setting. The setting needed to be examined and portrayed in the conceptual framework at the levels of: (1) the educational institution, (2) the sociocultural milieu of the community, (3) the dominant health care needs in the college service area, and (4) the nature of the health care delivery system, particularly with regard to nursing's place in it. Analyzing the setting enables a faculty to make decisions in the selection of content for the curriculum that have high relevance for real problems. Such analysis also places the faculty in the position to intelligently assess pressures from the variety of referent groups when making their curricular decisions.

The Educational Institution

This dimension of the setting was defined as not only the specific college in which the Second Step Nursing Program would reside, but also the California system of higher education in general. One of the strongest influences on the development of the Second Step Program was the Master Plan for Higher Education in California. This plan, published in 1960, included proposals for meeting higher education needs in California for a ten year period.[7] One of the recommendations made at that time was to increase enrollment at the junior college level and place greater emphasis on upper division and graduate education in state colleges and universities. By 1966 there was evidence that the ratio of lower division to upper division enrollments in state colleges was gradually decreasing. By 1968, approximately three fourths of all lower division students were enrolled in California's junior college.

14

The Coordinating Council for Higher Education endorsed a Joint Statement of Policy in Respect to the Admission of Eligible Applicants for Transfer from California Public Junior Colleges which insures all students entering public higher education institutions as freshmen who maintain satisfactory academic records the opportunity to progress to the baccalaureate degree without encountering arbitrary barriers.[8] The same year, 1969, the Coordinating Council issued another report titled *The Undergraduate Student and His Higher Education.*[9] Issues raised included the relevance of previous or concurrent nonclassroom experience in the educational process, the circumstances under which external degree programs should be provided, the questionable value of campus residency requirements, and the inadvisability of holding a student to one specific curriculum pattern desired by a single faculty. All of these had particular salience for existing patterns of education for nurses.

In July 1966 with the assistance of a committee composed of health care providers and educators, the Coordinating Council for Higher Education published a statement entitled *Nursing Education in California.* Among their findings were the following:

> Problems of articulation make educational progression difficult and may impede associate degree or diploma school graduates from returning to school to obtain a degree. . . . Policies are not uniform among institutions offering nursing programs, both as to transfer of general education and nursing courses.[10]

It had become apparent that strategies for enhancing articulation between lower and upper division nursing programs were badly needed.

Legislative mandates in California were also forcing nurses to examine the issue of career and educational mobility. Title 15, California Administrative Code, Chapter 14, Nursing Education and Registration (1970) clearly required that schools of nursing give transfer students the opportunity to obtain credit through the use of challenge examinations or other evaluative methods. In the period from 1960 to the present there obviously has been considered interest on the parts of consumers and legislators in the delivery of health care and the educational preparation of the health care givers. California nurse educators continue to thoughtfully scrutinize the education of nurses. The Second Step Program is one response to such scrutiny.

Of the 19 colleges and universities in the California state system of higher education, the Sonoma State College campus provided the specific setting for the Second Step Nursing Program. California State College, Sonoma (C.S.C.S.) opened its doors to the first students in September 1961 and grew at a relatively slow pace from 274 students in 1961 to 1,400 in the Fall of 1966. Since then a dramatic growth has taken place and the student enrollment reached 5,554 by the early

1970s. The original number of faculty has similarly increased. The college offers 31 undergraduate degree programs in the school of arts and sciences, degree programs in three cluster schools, nine masters programs, and four credential programs. The academic year is organized into two semesters plus a summer session.

Despite its recent growth, C.S.C.S. remains a relatively small college, located in a rural setting, near a small town, and just off a freeway. There is limited space for residential students, but the majority commute from the counties that comprise the college service area, six counties north of San Francisco roughly equal in area to the state of New Hampshire. There is limited public transportation and most students must use private cars.

Nursing is the first professional program offered at C.S.C.S. Located in a farming community, the campus holds a pastoral charm and a flexible, informal atmosphere often unusual in traditional nursing programs.

Sonoma State faculty emphasizes the liberal arts and sciences and has developed programs that reflect this emphasis. A considerable amount of flexibility is allowed for creativity and innovation. However, throughout the total college there is a shared concern with three general goals. First, the different disciplines should be related to each other in specific and definite ways so that the student will view his or her education as a unified and unifying experience. Second, there is an attempt to provide maximum opportunity for students and faculty to develop and maintain strong interrelationships, to keep alive the feeling that faculty will assist students on an individualized basis and that faculty are genuinely concerned about them as individuals. Third, there is an effort to develop programs that seek not just the definition of problems, but also the possible solutions. In offering this kind of educational opportunity to students and faculty alike, the college expresses its own definition of relevance in education.

There are several distinguishing features of the college. First, the faculty and administration have continually sought to question old ways of doing things and to experiment with alternatives. There are currently three alternative schools in existence that offer nontraditional routes through the liberal arts and sciences. These schools enroll about 10 per cent of the students.

A second feature of the college is its small size and warm, friendly atmosphere. There is a sense of community and closeness between students and teachers that is rare in essentially commuter institutions.

A third characteristic is a campus climate in which relevance is emphasized. This emphasis takes two forms. One is the widespread concern among students and faculty for the enhancement of self-actualization. This concern receives institutional support through the program in humanistic psychology, the Hutchins School, and the School of Expressive Arts. The other is a concern for social action in the community. This second concern is the focus in the School of Environmental Studies, the campus-wide community involvement projects, and the political activities of many college participants especially in regard to preserving the quality of life in this region. With such an institutional philosophy, it is not surprising that a nontraditional nursing program, designed to meet an underserved population of students, would be embraced and strongly supported by Sonoma State College.

It was in this college setting that negotiations were conducted concerning policies for awarding credit toward upper division majors for work completed by nurses at junior colleges. After considerable debate, opportunities for diploma graduates were also provided by granting associate degree equivalencies through junior colleges. With these structural arrangements settled, the Second Step Program became part of the college's Division of Natural Sciences.

The Sociocultural Milieu

The six county service area of the college contains a wide variety of geographic characteristics and life styles. The very rural county of Mendocino is sparsely populated and dominated by lumber and fishing industries. Napa and Sonoma Counties are in the heart of the wine country. There are many vineyards and orchards and some light industry. There are several cities of 10,000 to 20,000 population with the largest city, Santa Rosa, reporting a population of 65,000. Solano County is supported by industry and refineries and is more densely populated. Marin County is the wealthiest county with 88 per cent of the population residing in bedroom communities and engaged in professional occupations.

Ethnically, Whites predominate, followed by Mexican-Americans. Blacks and Asians are represented in almost equal numbers with higher concentrations of Blacks in Solano County. All six service-area counties have an unusually high percentage of elderly persons. The climate and location in suburban and semirural areas appeal to retired individuals. Table 1 presents some comparative statistics that illustrate both the extent and diversity of the areas.

Although referred to as the "six North Bay counties," it can readily be seen that there are significant differences in the composition of each. Marin County is an area of high income families, with a large number of professionally employed persons, commuter and otherwise. Not so evident are its sizeable public housing facilities and the number of small rural communities in its northwestern area.

Sonoma County, immediately north of Marin on U.S. Highway 101, is undergoing the same pattern of growth Marin has experienced in the past decade. Something of each of the other counties is represented in Sonoma: Bay Area commuters, agricultural emphasis, recreation, and industry, to a lesser degree. In addition, Santa Rosa

17

Table 1. C.S.C.S. Service Area

County	Population 1960[1]	1970[1]	Projected 2000[2]	Area[3] (sq. mi.)	Population[4] (per sq. mi.) 1969	Income[5] (per cap.) 1968
Lake	13,786	18,816	41,000	1,328	15.3	$2,763
Marin	146,820	204,046	400,000	607	391.4	4,345
Mendocino	51,059	50,610	78,700	3,511	15.2	2,919
Napa	65,890	76,819	192,500	794	102.6	3,135
Solano	134,597	165,949	405,100	901	211.7	3,329
Sonoma	147,375	199,360	480,600	1,608	127.3	3,047
				California average	(126.8)	($3,916)

[1]*California Statistical Abstract 1970,* State of California Documents Section, Sacramento, p. 13.
[2]"Provisional Projection of California Counties to 2000", Population Research Unit, Department of Finance, Sacramento, September 15, 1971.
[3]*California County Fact Book 1970,* County Supervisors Association of California, Sacramento, p. 5.
[4]*Ibid.,* p. 20.
[5]*Ibid.,* p. 32.
(From "Feasibility Study" prepared by the Dept. of Nursing in 1971 for the California State Board of Nursing Education and Nurse Registration.)

has developed as a service center and a medical center for the entire north coast area. It is designated as a planning area for health maintenance organizations.

Mendocino County, farther north, has actually decreased in population in the last decade, but population pressures from the south along busy Highway 101, the expansion of the second home subdivision industry and increased recognition of its recreation potential are expected to offset its otherwise vascillating economy.

Lake County, though isolated by mountains through which there are no major highways, is nevertheless visited by increasing numbers of summer and winter vacationers, many of whom have retired and purchased homes there. Industry centers on its natural resources: agriculture, ranching, mining, and lumber.

Napa, like Sonoma, is on the outskirts of the Bay Area and is increasingly feeling its population pressure. A growing Mexican-American population is associated with the important grape industry.

Solano County is also a county of commuters to some degree. With Mare Island Naval Base and the refineries and industry along its San Francisco Bay margin, it supports a large number of blue collar workers and minorities, and extends into large agricultural acreage to the east.

Dominant Health Care Needs

Improved technology and advances in knowledge have raised the level of health for larger numbers of people in the college service

18

area. Sophisticated equipment saves scores who previously died of heart disease, immunizations prevent deaths from communicable diseases, and antibiotics and other drugs treat infections that formerly went uncontrolled. Clients are able to be treated more successfully and in less time than ever before. Hospital stays are shorter. The emphasis in health care is now able to turn more toward prevention of illness and promotion of health. Primary prevention has a greater possibility of succeeding because we are better able to deal with secondary and even tertiary prevention. The emphasis on health care is outside the acute care setting with approximately 95 per cent of those receiving health care services located in the community.

Mass media has alerted the population to the advances in health care. Persons are more aware of the extent to which health and well-being are possible. The public is beginning to demand quality care for all.

Our population continues to grow, at least partially because advances in health care have increased life expectancy. Health problems of the elderly, usually chronic in nature and of long duration, are being treated at home or in extended care facilities.

The advent of a National Health Insurance or the increase in third party payment plans will have a major impact on health care delivery. Facilities must be organized to offer the most care to the largest number of people for the lowest cost. Outpatient facilities will continue to increase and patients will move in and out of acute facilities more rapidly.

In summary, the dominant health care needs in the college service area are those associated with a widely diverse but stable population ranging from urban metropolitan to rural, suffering some growing pains, expecting increased population pressure, especially an increase in the proportion of minority groups, an increase in the very young, and in the very old.

The Health Care Delivery System

The Health Manpower Committee of the California State Health Planning Council studied the health manpower needs of California and estimated that 40,000 additional nurses would be needed between 1968 and 1975.

The Surgeon General's Office recommended that one third of all nurses hold baccalaureate degrees. In 1970, California was graduating only about one half of the nurses needed in the state and despite the fact that registered nurses were demanding more options for baccalaureate education, California schools of nursing were only preparing about one third of the recommended number with baccalaureate degrees.

The need for more nurses prepared at the baccalaureate level is critical. Trends in the delivery of health care indicated a need for

19

nurses able to assume broader clinical responsibility, who have community health experience, and who are able to plan, teach, initiate change, and provide leadership changes in health care delivery. All indications point to a greater emphasis on the prevention of illness and the promotion of health. Agencies are developing to provide more ambulatory care. The whole possibility of nurses functioning as practitioners in expanded roles has become a national trend.

Clearly a paradox exists, students clamor to be nurses, registered nurses ask for more education, yet the health care needs of the state remain underserved.

A parallel pattern exists in the six county service area of Sonoma State College. There is a serious lack of manpower prepared to meet expanding health needs. Within the six counties, there are approximately 100 licensed hospitals and health care facilities. Thirty of these are short-term facilities with approximately 2,000 beds. In contrast there are approximately 5,000 long-term care beds. Each of the six counties has a health department which supplies community health nursing services. The largest of these, located in Santa Rosa, employs 17 community health nurses. Other facilities employing nurses include a 1,000 bed veterans' hospital, two state mental hospitals that are gradually being replaced by community mental health programs, school health programs, outpatient clinics, the Family Practice Clinic at Sonoma Community Hospital, Head Start Programs, senior citizens organizations, regional medical programs, and the Comprehensive Health Planning Organization.

In the Fall of 1971, a moratorium was established on long-term beds in Sonoma County, but several of the acute care hospitals were planning to expand. Acute psychiatric care units are emerging. Mental hygiene clinics are expanding. One hospital recently established an alcohol and drug detoxification unit as well as enlarged its obstetric unit and added an intensive care unit for newborns. Another hospital has enlarged its bed capacity, established an emergency room, and developed an inhalation therapy clinic. The college service area offers a rich combination of clinical facilities.

Clearly a curriculum requiring clinical experience restricted to conventional community health agencies for hospitals would be limited in view of the scope and diversity of alternative clinical placements.

The setting component of the conceptual framework for the curriculum provides important data that yield direction for program development. The educational system in California is structured to facilitate a two year upper division major. Societal pressures are mounting against nursing to provide for career mobility. The health care needs in the community call for more nurses with advanced preparation as leaders who can offer a more community oriented kind of nursing care. Nurses practicing in an extended role are earning a solid place in the health care delivery system and an upper

20

division program for registered nurses can provide preparation for such a role.

Students and Learning Theory

The abilities, background, interests, motivations, expectations, and potential of the students along with faculty hypotheses about how students learn, constitute the second major component of the conceptual framework for curriculum decisions.

The faculty in the Second Step Program views the goal of education as a change in the thinking, feeling, and overt behaviors of learners. Tyler postulates that while educational objectives represent the changes in behavior that faculties or institutions seek to bring about, a study of the learners is necessary to identify the changes in behavior that are needed.[11] The faculty's hypothesis that associate degree or equivalent nurse preparation can form the foundation upon which professional nursing education is built mandated a thorough investigation of our learners as well as an examination of relevant learning theories. The student category of our conceptual framework consists of descriptive characteristics of the student population and concepts about motivation, goals, self-concepts, and identity drawn from learning theory. Both of these dimensions have direct implications for curriculum planning.

The Student

The characteristics of the learners in the C.S.C.S. Department of Nursing vary considerably from the characteristics of model college students and particularly from the generic baccalaureate nursing student.

Age. The average student in our program is older than other students beginning their junior year in college. The average age of juniors in the California State College System in 1972-73 was 23.2 years. The average age of juniors at California State College, Sonoma was 25.1 years for the same period. Our first class of nursing students in 1972 had a mean age of 34.9 years; in 1973 the mean age was 32.8 years; and in 1974 the mean age was 32.3 years.

Ethnic Background. In the past three years 75 per cent of those nursing students who reported on their racial/ethnic backgrounds were Caucasian. Blacks represented 2 per cent of the enrollment in 1972 and by 1974 represented 10 per cent. During this same period, two students reported Mexican-American heritage and four students Oriental heritage, together representing approximately 3 per cent of the total enrollment. Twelve students described themselves as "Other" and 18 students gave no answer.

Residence. Sonoma Second Step nursing students reside primarily in the service area which encompasses Marin, Sonoma, Mendocino,

Lake, Solano, and Napa Counties. This is a large geographic area and approximately 95 per cent of the students commute by car or bus to the campus. Of these, 9 per cent have commuted from Contra Costa and Alameda counties which are located to the south and east of the service area. The range of miles which the students commute one way is from 2.5 miles for those living in the neighboring communities of Cotati and Rohnert Park to 73 miles for a student who commuted from Ukiah, in Southern Mendocino County. The average student in the C.S.C.S. Department of Nursing commutes 26.4 miles from home to campus.

Basic Nursing Education. Of the students in the C.S.C.S. program in nursing, 39 per cent were prepared for licensure in diploma school programs and 61 per cent were prepared in associate degree programs. Some of the students had been enrolled in a major other than nursing or had attended college classes in other majors before entering their basic educational program. Some had enrolled in a college program with a major other than nursing since completing their basic educational program. Some had taken college classes or had enrolled in a program with the aim of acquiring a baccalaureate degree in nursing prior to entering C.S.C.S.

Work Experience. A comparison of years of nursing experience of students prior to entering the nursing program yielded a mean of 7.6 years for students entering in 1972, and a mean of 6.1 in 1973. It should also be noted that the range was from no years to 30 years of nursing experience. In 1972, 10 per cent of the students reported no work experience as a registered nurse upon entrance into the program while in 1973, 14 per cent of the students reported no work experience. An increasing number of students are entering the Second Step Program directly from their basic educational programs.

The majority of students reported that their practice had been in hospital settings with medical-surgical nursing the most frequently reported area of concentration. Only seven students in the first two classes reported any actual nursing experience in the community. These included one student who had spent two years with the VISTA program, one who spent two years as a junior public health nurse, and a student who reported working part time in a health department.

Sex. The student body is primarily female with males representing 9 per cent of the total enrollment over the past three years.

Financial Support. All of the students in the first two years of the program entered as full time students yet over 53 per cent reported they planned to continue to work if only on a part time basis, and 13 per cent of these students reported that they were planning to continue to work full time while attending school. Forty-four per cent reported support through scholarships, student loan funds, or government grants; 9 per cent stated that their husband or parents would be their main source of financial support while attending school.

Marital Status. Of the students who reported on their marital status, 44 per cent were married, 14 per cent were widowed or divorced, 32 per cent were single. Fifty-one per cent of the reporting students had no children. However, 49 per cent reported having children, with two children being the most frequently reported number.

Reasons for Returning to School. The vast majority of students gave more than one reason for returning to school. Their responses have been categorized into six general areas:

1. Career concerns—better pay status, job opportunities, or leadership role.
2. A change in nursing interests (hospital to community) either in work setting or job description.
3. Professional—increase competency.
4. The availability of the program, a continuation of further education. Personal growth and satisfaction.
5. To obtain a baccalaureate degree.
6. Intellectual—to enlarge knowledge base.

This very brief description of the student in the C.S.C.S. Department of Nursing represents part of the information we have gathered to formulate our assumptions about our learners. In summary, the average student is a white female, 32 years of age, who is married and has a high probability of two dependent children in the home. She commutes an average of 26 miles a day to school, has received her basic education in nursing in an associate degree program, and has an average of six years clinical experience in a hospital setting. Her reasons for returning to school are varied and include job promotion, change in work setting, and a desire for professional, personal, and intellectual growth.

Learning Theory

Andragogy is a term introduced by Knowles to describe the art and science of helping the adult to learn.[12]

Implicit in the assumptions of andragogy is that the characteristics of the adult learner are different from the characteristics of the child learner. As a person matures, (1) self-concept moves from one of being a dependent personality toward one of being a self-directing human being; (2) a growing reservoir of experience accumulates that becomes an increasing resource for learning; (3) readiness to learn becomes oriented increasingly to the developmental tasks of social roles; and (4) time perspective changes from one of postponed application of knowledge to immediacy of application, and accordingly orientation toward learning shifts from one of subject-centeredness to one of problem-centeredness.[13]

The self-directing personality of the adult emerges as he or she takes on the status of a doer or producer in society. Each time he or she experiences success in endeavors, the evaluation of self and goals increases. He or she begins to recognize and have confidence in capabilities and self-worth. The registered nurse student has been making decisions and facing the consequences of them in many facets of life; work, marriage, family, friends, and community. He or she may be involved in and responsible for several of these aspects at one time. He or she has become accustomed to receiving respect from family and peers.

Rosendahl points out that this concept of maturity and self-direction has two implications for nursing educators.[14] The relationship or interaction between the faculty and student becomes a primary factor in the establishment of the learning climate. The instructor must convey an interest in and respect for the student in establishing a relationship which is personally warm, open, and understanding. This relationship must facilitate the growth of the learner and communicate to the learner the teacher's respect. Teachers who view themselves as imparters of knowledge and students as the receptors of this transmission will have little success with adult learners. Registered nurse students particularly resist learning situations which negate their self-concepts as experienced practitioners. Having to repeat basic nursing courses is particularly affrontive to them. They view this policy as a negation of their accomplishments in the practice of nursing.

The second implication for nursing educators also requires a break from the traditional method of outlining for the student what he or she needs to learn. Andragogy places a great emphasis on self-diagnosis by the learner of personalized learning needs. Knowles states that this process consists of three phases.[15] 1. The first phase is construction of a model of the competencies or characteristics required to achieve the desired performance. This implies that a clear definition of the characteristics of the professional nurse and professional nursing practice must be given to the students. This model provides the learners with an idea of the faculty's, the institution's, and society's expectations of professional nursing. 2. Provision of diagnostic experiences in which the learners can assess present levels of competencies as compared with those outlined in the models is the second phase. This process, while difficult, is rich with possibilities. Computerized games, simulation exercises, or sociodrama could be utilized to provide registered nurse learners with feedback about their performance. These methods facilitate the objective assessment of their strengths and weaknesses in the nursing process. 3. The final phase of the process is helping the learners measure the gaps in their present performance and those required in the model. Having identified the gaps in their performance and competencies, the students become dissatisfied. They have a clear idea of the goal and coupled with their sense of dissatisfaction are motivated to find means to achieve their goals. Rogers has hypothesized "that significant learning takes place when the subject matter is perceived by students as having relevance for their own purposes. Further, learning is facilitated when students participate in the learning process."[16] In nursing education this means students are involved in the planning and implementation of their own learning experiences. "To be involved is ego-involvement, which stirs interest, awakes enthusiasm, and arouses curiosity."[17]

Most adult learners have accumulated a vast store of experiences that they bring with them to any learning situation. This background of experience provides a broad base which they can relate to new learning and it also makes them a rich resource of learning for their peers. Knowles states, "to an adult, his experience is him."[18] If adults define themselves largely by their experience, then a negation of its worth will be viewed by the adult as a negation of his or her person. The implications of this concept for nursing education are many. It is crucial that the faculty identify and capitalize upon the rich and varied experiences and backgrounds that nursing students bring with them. In this way students learn from their peers as well as from their teachers. Faculty also gain new insights and knowledge from their students. Teaching strategies are directly affected by this concept. Activities which emphasize student involvement such as case studies, role playing, and seminars become the preferred mode for the sharing of and transmission of knowledge. "Learning, involving the whole person of the learner, feelings as well as intellect, is the most pervasive and lasting."[19]

New learning also becomes meaningful for the adult learner when he or she can relate it to past experiences. Lewins' cognitive field theory of learning defines learning as "a dynamic process, whereby, through interactive experience, insights, or cognitive structures, life spaces are changed so as to become more serviceable for future guidance."[20] Insights occur for the adult learner when he or she is able to grasp an idea and actually apply it to everyday life. Learning in the adult is purposeful; it is a reaching out; it is a search for understanding in a constantly expanding world; it is a guide for conduct.

Registered nurse students who come from a wide age range and varied nursing and life experiences have different learning goals and needs. Each student has perceived a personal objective or goal that additional learning will help him or her achieve. The learning environment must then provide for these individual differences. It needs to be creative; it needs to provide options and choices in learning experiences. Learning is an internal process and those teaching strategies which involve the student most deeply in self-directed inquiry will produce the greatest learning.[21] Students must be encouraged to identify their own learning objectives, participate in the selection of meaningful educational experiences, and evaluate the outcomes of their endeavors.

The role of the faculty in this process is that of guide or facilitator. The teacher suppresses the compulsion to teach the students what he or she believes they need to know in favor of helping the students learn for themselves. The teacher expects and encourages the student to be responsible for his or her own learning. The teacher becomes a promotor of individual initiative and independence of thought. The truly creative teacher stimulates learning by communicating enthusiasm for nursing, thirst for intellectual development, and openness to new ideas. There is a willingness to take risks and a constant striving toward more creative and innnovative approaches to teaching.

Learning readiness refers to the fact that a person must learn some things before proceeding to additional material or that one skill must be acquired before others can develop.[22] The concept of learning readiness can also be applied to the adult. Learning readiness in the adult, however, is closely aligned to the evolution of social roles.[23] For example, the new graduate of a basic nursing program is not ready to assume the role of a supervisor. He or she must instead complete the tasks associated with being a staff nurse before assuming additional nursing responsibilities. The adult, like the child, reaches a level of maturity and comprehension in which "he begins differentiating and restructuring himself and his environment, he is gaining or changing insights."[24]

The registered nurse student returns to school for a variety of reasons including job promotion, change in work setting, and a desire for professional, personal, and intellectual growth. Ideas and concepts about self and the practice of nursing are in a state of change. There is a motivation to seek a new identity and place in the nursing arena. However, while the student has reached a point of receptiveness to learning, he or she also brings into the educational settings previous experiences with learning.

Typically the adult expects to be treated like a child. The adult who enters an atmosphere in which he or she is treated with respect, involved in mutual inquiry with instructors, and is given responsibility for personal learning, usually reacts with shock and disorientation.[25] Nurses who have been educated via the cookbook format are not prepared for self-directed learning. They need to have a time of transition—of orientation to the learning process.

At least two implications for nursing education can be drawn from these propositions regarding the registered nurse's readiness to learn:

1. The structure of the curriculum should be developed by building upon the student's previous knowledge and skills.

2. The sequence of courses should provide the learner with increasing opportunities for self-direction.

The adult who enters into an educational program views the experience as a practical means to improve his or her ability to handle life's problems. Unlike the child who learns subjects which can perhaps be applied later in educational experience or life, the adult's perspective is on the immediacy of application.

The very essence of nursing behavior is problem solving. The practice of nursing consists of utilizing and organizing those concepts and principles which provide the rationale for the cognitive, effective, and psychomotor skills constituting the discipline of nursing.[26] The problem-solving approach to nursing consists of an assessment and analysis of each client situation; a definition of the multiple variables which operate to produce the client situation; the generation and initiation of interventive measures; and the application of criteria to explain, justify, predict, and evaluate outcomes of these measures. It provides a systematic methodology for thinking and decision making.

While the emphasis for cognitive field theorists is upon students' growth in seeing the world and themselves differently, they recognize that facts are acquired and used in this process. Facts, however, are best learned "when they are regarded by the learner as instruments for serving purposes which he feels are important—when they are connected with problem solving."[27] The teacher who utilizes the cognitive-field approach to learning interacts with students to help them formulate and solve problems. The teacher promotes an atmosphere of mutual inquiry. The teacher assists the student to discover meaningful relationships, perceive the interconnection of ideas, and to think in a highly generalized way.

Learning is a matter of changing cognitive structures. Cognitive structures are changed by:

1. Differentiating—the process of discerning more and more specifically aspects of oneself and one's environment. Differentiation implies that a person is able to make more sense of what was previously vague or confusing.[28] Nurses frequently interact with patients who are suffering from a sense of loss; a positively valued aspect of the patient's life is no longer available to him.[29] However, in planning a nursing intervention which is designed to relieve current distress, it is necessary for the nurse to differentiate. A sense of loss may be the result of physical, emotional, social, or religious factors.

2. Generalization—"the process whereby one groups a number of particular objects or functions under a single heading."[30] A person generalizes when forming a concept. Physical or mental disorders or distrubances which lead to complaints on the part of the patient, usually at a subjective level, such as headache, palpitations, or pain, are categorized by the nurse into the concept of symptom.

3. Restructurization—the process by which "one defines or redefines directions in his life space; he learns what actions will lead to what results."[31] The nurse restructures cognitive structures when he or she is able to see new relationships and perceive the interconnection of ideas. The prodromal signs of heart failure include pale cool skin, increased heart rate, normal or slightly increased blood pressure.

The nurse can relate these to the body's homeostatic response to stress. Heart failure is a physical stressor, but an emotional or social stress can produce the same signs. It is the body's mechanism to ready the individual to fight or take flight.

Learning is a purposeful dynamic process. It consists of differentiating, generalizing, and restructuring cognitive structures so as to acquire new or changed insights. In other words, it is a change in knowledge, skills, attitudes, values, or beliefs, and may or may not result in a change in overt behavior. Learning occurs through and as a result of experience. Transfer of learning occurs when insights developed in one learning situation can be employed in others. The faculty of the Second Step Program believe that transfer of learning is facilitated when the learner can discover relationships for himself, and if he has opportunities to apply his learning in a variety of tasks.

Motivation in the adult learner is a state of tension resulting from an unsatisfied need; this tension may spring from changes in the evolution of social roles or from identified problems in everyday life. Motivation in learning for the adult is enhanced when the learning climate induces personal or ego involvement and when the learner receives frequent feedback about progression toward goals.

The following statements summarize the learning principles which serve as a basis for curriculum decisions in the Second Step Program.[32]

1. Good teaching takes into account past negative school experience, remoteness of past schooling, and the self-doubts of adults, and provides at the earliest possible time in the class for encouragement and for an experience of success.

2. Good teaching takes into account the relation between a pleasant social atmosphere and a satisfying educational experience.

3. Good teaching takes into account not only the need for an early experience of success, but the need for frequently recurring experiences of success.

4. Good teaching takes into account the loss of speed in performance in academic activity during the mature years.

5. Good teaching recognizes the validity of the principle of involvement.

6. Good teaching recognizes the adults themselves as a prime teaching resource.

7. Good teaching recognizes the concreteness and immediacy of most adult goals.

8. Good teaching takes into account the key place which motivation holds in the learning process.

9. Good teaching recognizes physical and mental fatigue as a deterring factor in adult learning.

10. Good teaching recognizes each teaching experience as an opportunity for professional growth.

The Subject

The subject component of a conceptual framework for curriculum development calls for an explicit definition of nursing and conceptualization of nursing practice. Since the pioneering efforts made by Peplau and Abdellah in the early 1950s, nurses have been actively engaged in research and theory building concerning the nature of the discipline of nursing. The work of Johnson, Roy, Rogers, and others offers nursing faculties examples of theories of nursing which have implication for nursing curriculums. Nursing theory explains what happens to a client when he or she is nursed. Despite differences in focus and emphasis, most conceptualizations of nursing can be dimensionalized into six categories. These are: (1) the goals of nursing, (2) the client(s) served, (3) the nature of problems solved, (4) the interventions used, (5) the practice locale, and (6) the work relationships of the nurse. These dimensions of the concept of nursing serve to organize discussion of the model of nursing constructed by the Second Step nursing faculty.[33]

In Figure 2, the theory of nursing synthesized by the Sonoma State nursing faculty is depicted as a systems model. From this definition of the profession, the faculty has made decisions about the significant concepts, processes, knowledge, and skills to include in the curriculum. As Harms has pointed out:

> If faculty are to proceed logically and soundly to prepare nurses to offer the services society deems essential tomorrow as well as today, they must critically analyze all facets of nursing practice and state their views in terms of assumptions and hypotheses. These will form bases for decisions about the curriculum.[34]

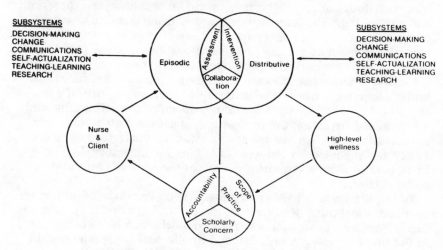

FIGURE 2. Conceptual model of nursing process.

According to the Sonoma model, professional nursing is defined as fundamentally an interpersonal process, the *goal* of which is to assist persons in the achievement of optimum health. Health is conceptualized by Dunn as a dynamic condition of change toward a higher potential of integrated bio-psycho-social functioning within a changing environment.[35] A set of sub-processes comprises the professional nurse's unique repertoire of *interventions* used in his or her practice with clients. These sub-processes include: decision-making, change, communication, self-actualization, teaching-learning, and research or inquiry. According to our model, the nurse-client relationship can be established with individuals of all ages and in all phases of development. The *client* may be an individual, a family, a group, or an entire community. The professional nurse encounters the client under both episodic and distributive *practice locales* and the client may be at any stage of contact with the health care delivery system—including making an initial contact.

In the process of assisting the client toward optimum health, three valued nursing behaviors occur—assessment, intervention, and collaboration with other health team members. The faculty specify accountability, scope of practice, and scholarly concern as three essential properties which characterize the professional. These characteristics serve as criteria for evaluation which act as feedback into the systems model developed. Professional nursing is further differentiated from lower division nursing in terms of the kinds of problems solved by the nurse and the attitude toward practice. These differentiating properties were identified by Waters and associates in their study of professional and technical nursing.[36] The professional nurse solves complex *problems* that are not readily apparent and relies on covert cues. Solution of these problems requires attitudes of creativity, innovation, exploration, self-direction and risk taking. The technical or lower division nurse solves more commonly occurring, readily apparent *problems* that comprise the common domain of nursing practice. Solutions to these problems are more standardized and more likely to have predictable outcomes.

Finally, whereas the associate degree or diploma nurse functions under supervision within the structure of the conventions of a *practice situation* with multiple traditions, specific role definitions, and a formalized structure, the professional, baccalaureate nurse deals in increasingly ambiguous situations, often characterized by uncertainty and the need for independent thinking, ingenuity, and imagination. Her *work relationships* occur at the level of egalitarian collaboration.

To use the words of Wilson in an article on the place of humanities in professional nursing education, the C.S.C.S. Second Step nursing faculty define a professional nurse as one who combines both "sense" in the problem solving, rational, and intellectual approach brought to bear on abstract client problems, and "sensibility" in the capacity to establish sensitive, caring, and effective interpersonal relationships with clients and other health professionals that humanize the delivery of health care services.[37]

The knowledge base emphasized in the preparation of this practitioner is one of process as content. Content is usually thought of as the compendium of information that comprises learning material. Process on the other hand includes all the operations that can be associated with knowledge. The processes included as sub-systems in the Sonoma model of professional nursing are examples.

Clearly such a process oriented definition of the nature of the discipline has different implications for organizing and selecting a knowledge base than would a definition of nursing that emphasizes given sets of facts, principles, and theories to be absorbed by the learner or rote motor skills to be perfected in carrying out nursing procedures. The emphasis in the Second Step Program is on knowledge that produces knowledge and processes that transcend static content.

SUMMARY

This chapter has presented in detail the specific conceptual framework developed by the C.S.C.S. Second Step nursing faculty as a basis for designing an upper division nursing curriculum. Each component of the framework has been taken up in depth and implications for curriculum decisions have been discussed.

REFERENCES

1. Chater, Shirley S.: A Conceptual Framework for Curriculum Development. *Nursing Outlook* 23:428, 1975.
2. Bevis, Em Olivia: *Curriculum Building in Nursing.* C.V. Mosby Co., St. Louis, 1973, p. 18.
3. Chater, *op. cit.*
4. *Ibid.*
5. Taba, Hilda: *Curriculum Development: Theory and Practice.* Harcourt Brace Jovanovick, Inc., New York, 1962.
6. Wright, Frank Lloyd: *The Natural House.* Horizon Press, Inc., New York, 1954.
7. California Department of Education; *A Master Plan for Higher Education in California 1960-1975,* 1960.
8. Coordinating Council for Higher Education: *Annual Report of the Director, 1969.* Sacramento, No. 70-2, February, 1970, p. 18.
9. Coordinating Council for Higher Education Statement. *The Undergraduate Student and His Higher Education: Policies of California Colleges and Universities in the Next Decade.* Sacramento, No. 1034, June, 1969.
10. Coordinating Council for Higher Education. *Nursing Education in California.* Sacramento, No. 1025, July, 1966.
11. Tyler, Ralph W.: *Basic Principles of Curriculum and Instruction.* The University of Chicago Press, Chicago, 1949, p. 6.
12. Knowles, Malcom S.: *The Modern Practice of Adult Education, Andragogy Versus Pedagogy.* Association Press, New York, 1970, p. 38.
13. *Ibid.,* p. 39.

14. Rosendahl, Pearl: Self-Direction for Learners. *Nursing Forum* 13:139, 1974.
15. Knowles, *op. cit.*, p. 42.
16. Ericksen, Sanford C.: *Motivation for Learning, A Guide for the Teacher of the Young Adult.* University of Michigan Press, Ann Arbor, 1974, p. 73.
17. Rosendahl, *op. cit.*, p. 141.
18. Knowles, *op. cit.*, p. 44.
19. Erickson, *op. cit.*, p. 73.
20. Bigge, Morris L.: *Learning Theories for Teachers.* Harper and Row, Publishers, New York, 1964, p. 220.
21. Knowles, *op. cit.*, p. 51.
22. Kuethe, James L.: *The Teaching-Learning Process.* Scott, Foresman and Co., 1968, p. 82.
23. Knowles, *op. cit.*, p. 46.
24. Rosendahl, *op. cit.*, p. 143.
25. Bigge, *op. cit.*, p. 239.
26. *Ibid.*, pp. 224-225.
27. Shontz, Franklin C.: *The Psychological Aspects of Physical Illness and Disability*, Macmillan Publishing Co., Inc., New York, 1975, p. 92.
28. Bigge, *op. cit.*, p. 227.
29. *Ibid.*, p. 227.
30. *Ibid.*, p. 228.
31. *Ibid.*, p. 283.
32. Hendrickson, Andrew: Adult Learning and the Adult Learner. *Adult Leadership.* Vol. 14, No. 8, 1966.
33. Verle H. Waters is gratefully acknowledged for her ideas on the dimensions listed here.
34. Harms, Mary: Development of a Conceptual Framework for a Nursing Curriculum. Paper presented at 12th meeting of Southern Regional Education Board Council on Collegiate Education for Nursing, April 9-10, 1969, Atlanta, p. 2.
35. Dunn, H.L.: *High Level Awareness.* R.W. Beatty Co., Arlington, Va., 1961.
36. Waters, Verle H., et. al.: Technical and Professional Nursing: An Exploratory Study. *Nursing Research* 21:124, 1972.
37. Wilson, Holly S.: A Case for Humanities in Professional Nursing Education. *Nursing Forum* 13:406, 1974.

CHAPTER 3

Strategies for Organizing Learning

Hannah Dean, R.N., M.S., Ruth Haskell, R.N., M.S., and Barbara Tesser, R.N., M.S.

The faculty takes a thoughtful and strategic approach to organizing learning throughout the total curriculum. The philosophy, conceptual framework, program objectives, curriculum design, plus the content and learning experiences constitute an organization for student learning. This chapter will serve to illuminate the strategies that structure the curriculum, provide for active, process oriented content and learning experiences, and meet some of the health and health education needs of the community.

DEVELOPING THE CURRICULUM

In the process of developing the curriculum for this innovative program, the faculty began with a conceptual framework. Information about the setting, the student, and the subject matter of nursing plus the beliefs of the faculty initially provided the basis for the curriculum design. The conceptual framework was developed utilizing characteristics of the setting and the student, the teaching-learning process, and knowledge about the nature of nursing. The authors of Chapter 2 elaborated on specifics that are true for the conceptual framework of the Second Step.

The students are, on the average, in their late 20s and early 30s. They vary in their work experience; some come directly to the program from an associate degree program and some have had more than 20 years of nursing in a variety of settings. Wilson, Sauve, and Searight further state that the knowledge base for the curriculum is a distillation of information available about health promotion, health maintenance, and health teaching in the following areas: man as a bio-psycho-social being, the family, the community, the health-illness continuum, self-actualization, and the nurse as leader and an agent for change. The setting for this program is rural, albeit, within range of a major metropolitan area. While traditional health facilities are adequately staffed and there appears to be no shortage of nursing personnel, there are opportunities for nurses who want to create new roles in nontraditional nursing settings. The conceptual framework provides a basis for a curriculum that allows implementation of one of the recommendations of the Lysaught report on nursing and nursing education.[1] The Lysaught report urged development of a career pattern that would emphasize nursing practice designed for health maintenance and disease prevention.

Chater states that the curricular objectives derive from the conceptual framework. She then suggests that the faculty develop a curriculum design. This she defines as the "overall plan or structure of the curriculum, showing the arrangement of courses and the organization for its operations. It includes the methods and procedures to be used to achieve the objectives."[2] Taba writes that "the design should clearly indicate the bases and provisions for the scope and continuity of learning."[3] By this she is referring to cumulative learning, continuity, integration, and sequence.[4] Cumulative learning refers to building on previously mastered skills and knowledge; continuity refers to vertical organization or reiteration of major curriculum elements within different courses; integration refers to the horizontal relationship between areas of study; and sequence is putting content and learning experiences into order of succession. Also important in curriculum design is the concept of integrative threads, which Bloom describes as "any idea, problem, method, or device by which two or more separate learning experiences are related."[5] He points out further that these integrative threads can be used as a platform for organizing curriculum and instruction. They are effective to the extent that they can be reformulated, altered, and added to as experiences move on. They should provide common elements for comparing and contrasting experiences which would otherwise be unrelated. They should be sufficiently comprehensive to extend over the entire range of subject matter in some area of human experience. These considerations provided means by which to organize the curriculum.

Taba and Chater therefore were important models in the development of the Second Step Program's philosophy, conceptual framework, curricular objectives, and curriculum design. From the curriculum design are drawn strategies for organizing learning. The philosophy and conceptual framework delineated the knowledge base, learner, and setting.

PLANNING ACTIVE LEARNING FOR ADULTS

Not only did the faculty have to consider, in a general sense, how to organize a curriculum, but specifically how to teach adult learners. Knowles has developed the concept of andragogy, the art and science of teaching adults.[6] He identifies four main characteristics of adult learners that differentiate them from child learners. First, the adult's self concept is that of a self-directed individual; second, the adult has a body of experience as well as specific knowledge that serve as resources in learning; third, the adult is motivated to learn by the demands of social roles; and fourth, he is interested in the possibility of immediate application of knowledge and skills being learned. He further mentions that motivation for learning is based on the demands of the various social and/or professional roles in which the adult finds himself and the development tasks with which he is dealing.

The developmental tasks of early adulthood include getting started in an occupation, beginning to take on civic responsibility; in middle age developmental tasks include achieving adult civic and social responsibilities, establishing and maintaining an economic standard of living; in old age the individual redefines his role in relationship to his occupation and civic and social responsibility. Knowles postulates that adult students will be emotionally invested in and motivated toward learning activities that assist them in achieving their particular developmental tasks. However, an adult student in the early years of adulthood may have different priorities and interests than a student in the middle or later years. These differences have an effect on the students' responses to learning experiences and on the experiences students select for themselves.[7]

Because most adults come to a learning situation as a response to pressure from social and professional roles, they tend to be problem-centered and are interested in immediate transfer of knowledge to another situation. The admonition for educators is to be person-centered and problem-oriented rather than subject-centered.

In this day of social change, where women, in general, are either having to support themselves or are actively seeking the opportunity, it is no wonder nurses return to school. It is to be assumed that these students' motivation to learn is high. But *how* to teach them, as well as *what* to teach, concerned the faculty. Most of these adult learners come from rather traditional nursing programs with emphasis on rigid, prescriptive, categorizational, passive-receptive models of learning plus a strong clinical orientation to apply prescribed care to patients in acute care settings. The art was to learn a multitude of facts and procedures. While children tend to tolerate a totally other-directed approach to their learning, adults usually see themselves as self-directed and often resent this approach. Therefore, teaching methods that allow the adult student to feel in control and to be actively involved tend to be more appreciated and more successful.

Furthermore, in planning for adult learning, consideration had also to be given to a definition of nursing practice. Nursing has been described primarily as an applied discipline, an interpersonal process, a helping process, all action-oriented, process-oriented terms.

35

What are action-oriented methods of teaching? What is process-oriented content? Do they exist? Yes. Content refers to "the compendium of information which comprises the learning material for a course of study."[8] Process refers to "all the random and ordered operations which can be associated with knowledge."[9] There are a variety of processes through which knowledge is created, for example, researching a problem or creative writing. There are also processes for utilizing knowledge and for communicating it, for example, operating a television station. Processes are involved in arriving at decisions and in evaluating consequences. Every process, of necessity, must have a "construct—an underlying scheme which provides order and direction."[10]

Parker and Rubin identify the difference between content and process as the difference between passive and active approaches to learning. When process is stressed, greater importance is attached to the methods of acquiring knowledge and its subsequent utilization. If there is a contradiction between process and content it lies in the difference between active and passive approaches to learning. When the primary emphasis is on content, the learner ordinarily functions in the passive mode.[11] Where the stress is on process, the learner functions in the active mode. Active process-oriented learning also involves the student in actual or simulated experiences which enable the learner to integrate and transfer learning. Process teaching, therefore, ensures transfer by making it necessary to use information as it is being learned. Thus, as one learns the information one also learns the system into which it fits. For example, as one drives, one learns the route as well as how the car operates.

A situation was faced in the planning of the Second Step curriculum of defining the *what* as process, and the *how* as giving more control to the learner and providing active learning experiences. DeTornyay writes about two teaching strategies that give the learner more control. One method is teaching for discovery, the other is self-directed learning.[12] Bruner talks about the act of discovery as a form of obtaining knowledge.[13] A method of teaching for discovery is the exposing of the learner to a variety of experiences, facts, events, and phenomena, and expecting that he will find the relationships, categories, and concepts that organize and explain the experience.[14] "The teacher provides the experiences and the student actively makes sense out of them by finding the meaning in the event."[15] Other terms for discovery teaching are inquiry training, heuristics, or experiential learning. Discovery learning is essentially an inductive process, concerned with the development and organization of concepts, ideas, and insights. "The major hypothesis of discovery learning is that cognitive and motivational factors involved in learning by discovery enhance the learning, retention, and transferability of knowledge."[16] This certainly meets the goal of the adult learner—of finding ways for immediate applicability and transfer. Some other teaching issues noted by Wittrock involved in discovery teaching are:

(1) rote versus discovery learning, (2) student control versus teacher control, (3) inductive versus deductive learning, (4) interaction of methods of learning with individual differences among students, and (5) the order of presenting rules, principles and more specific information and problems to students.[17]

It is important to keep in mind, as DeTornyay points out, that discovery favors the well prepared mind.

Another method of allowing students more control and more active learning is the use of individualized instruction. One example, independent study, involves the student in initiating, planning, carrying out, and evaluating a project. Faculty responsibility lies in the careful guidance and support of the student throughout the process of independent study. A student chooses an area of study in which he is particularly interested, develops objectives, identifies the best setting and preceptor, selects supporting courses or activities, does extensive reading, writes papers, and demonstrates a command of the subject matter. Another example of individualized instruction is the self-paced learning which offers a variety of means for achieving the objectives of a given course. The student can choose the mode of learning which best suits his style of learning and may work at his own speed in meeting the objectives at the level he chooses to meet them.

In order to give control to the learner, discovery teaching methods and self-directed study are used whenever feasible. While discovery learning is a very effective strategy, it does require more faculty time and breadth of expertise. Another deterring factor is that there is the possibility of erroneous learning. There is still a place for expository teaching and teaching of concepts and facts to meet the objectives of the program and the exigences of the practice settings. It is the proportion of active learning versus passive learning that marks the difference in the Second Step Program from the basic generic program or the associate degree program.

STRATEGIES AND EXAMPLES

Chater points out a problem, which is: how does one identify the relationships between facts and concepts among the three components of her model—the subject, the setting, and the student?[18] In other words, how do you build links between these floating islands? One concept is that of strategy. Strategy may be thought of as a method by which to teach. For example, DeTornyay identified four major teaching strategies: expository teaching, seminar teaching, teaching for discovery, and self-directed learning. She says that the choice of a strategy is determined by the nature of the content, the objectives, and the teacher's style.[19] Bevis stated that such strategies must be consistent with the theoretical framework, be within the learner's style and rate of assimilation, and be appropriate to the terminal objectives of the program.[20]

The term strategy as used in this chapter, however, refers not only to teaching methods, but also to the larger concept of a "pattern of acts" of a "plan, in a special order, to achieve a definable goal."[21] These are footbridges, if you will, among the three components, the student, the subject, and the setting. The strategies utilized by the faculty serve to interrelate the adult learner, the rural setting, and the nursing knowledge base and to offer a rationale for choosing methods of teaching. Furthermore, these strategies help serve to determine the organization of the curriculum and the arrangement of the courses. One of these strategies was the use of integrative threads.

Integrative Threads

Integrative Threads provide for the repetition of key concepts and principles such that areas of experience can be understood in greater breadth and depth. They provide horizontal organization of the curriculum. They are part of the basic elements of a curriculum design and help an individual create unity of knowledge. Threads of integration can be found in objectives which are common to several courses. These objectives might require relating facts and broad principles or they might require interrelating theory and real life problems. A third possibility is objectives that combine knowledge, feelings, beliefs, and values. Concepts understood after multiple experiences, skills that require practice for mastery, and the gradual development of values and attitudes are reflective of integrative threads in a curriculum.[22] In the Second Step Program the Integrative Threads are: (1) health-illness continuum, (2) diagnosis, intervention, and evalution, (3) leadership and change, (4) professional nursing practice, and (5) self-actualization.

Tables 1 and 2 demonstrate the evolution of the integrative concepts in the program. While the concepts are not developed in every course, each semester of the program deals with building comprehension in a step-like fashion. The emphasis on the health-illness continuum the first year builds upon previous nursing education and nursing experience of the students. The students come from programs providing experience in dealing with individual patients in acute care settings. In the Second Step Program the setting is changed to the community, to families in private homes, health agencies providing out-patient care, or in simulated laboratories. Nursing is seen not only as cure and restoration, but as encompassing prevention of disease and maintenance of health. In the senior year, the students are expected to demonstrate comprehension of the health-illness

38

continuum and its ramifications in a variety of settings and with different groups of patients.

In the junior year the understanding of diagnosis, intervention, and evaluation extends from the students' previous levels of education. Instead of caring for just individuals, they provide services for the family unit. The development of the nursing process is reinforced in the senior year as students are involved in working in settings of their own choice. Students are able to assess clients in multiple ways which include the physical, emotional, and cultural aspects of the client system. They are able to formulate care plans with provisions for extenuating factors, and to implement and evaluate these plans. Students are capable of providing service to clients by utilizing their own resources, clients' resources, and/or community resources. Upon completion of the program, it is expected that students will be able to identify nursing problems and solve them comprehensively.

The next three concepts, leadership and change, professional practice, and self-actualization as values and attitudes as well as theoretical concepts, are built upon over the two years of the program. Preceptorship Study acts as a spring board to experience these concepts and Preceptorship Seminar as a place to discuss the experiences and relate them to theory.

By the end of the senior year each of these concepts has been experienced, discussed, and embraced by each student. The extent to which the experiences have been integrated will vary from student to student. Some illustrations will demonstrate this integration.

Marietta had graduated from a diploma program 17 years before entering the Second Step Program. She had a strong background in intensive care nursing and entered the junior year with some misgivings related to working with families in the community. She did not see that the issues of health maintenance, health teaching, and prevention of illness were the concern of nursing. Her experience in her junior year was to learn to assess psychosocial factors, evaluate family strengths, and become familiar with community resources. She already knew physical assessment skills and used them readily. Her experience demonstrates the interrelatedness of the key concepts and courses in the junior year.

Marietta had a number of clients over the year: an older couple referred because of the wife's congestive heart failure and frequent hospitalizations, a family with three children and the suspicion of child abuse, a young woman with a new ileostomy whose mother referred her because of her difficulty in coping with her changing body image, and several others. Marietta's understanding of the health-illness continuum was influenced by her experience over time with her clients. The woman with congestive heart failure required close supervision until her death at which time the student continued working with the husband who was then at high risk of physical

Table 1. Junior year. Courses that demonstrate development and integration of key concepts within courses of the nursing major of the Second Step Program.

Integrative Threads	Science Principles	Physical Assessment Laboratory	Community Health Lecture-Practicum
Concept of health-illness continuum	Basic physiological processes. Pathological disruptions.	Assessment of physiological and anatomical states of health-illness.	Patterns of psychosocial behavior in individuals, families, and communities. Age and maturational levels. Systems and organizations for health-care delivery. Influence of political factors on this delivery. Optimal functioning during health/illness.
Diagnosis, intervention, and evaluation	Actual/potential disruptions in health status. Physical assessment tools explored. Interrelationship of causational factors studied. Formulate inference and nursing diagnosis of specific clients in simulated case studies. Develop plans of care for these cases.		Use of tools to assess psychosocial, sociocultural as well as physical factors. Systems and organizations available during disruptions. Formulate diagnosis of health needs of individual, family, and community. Develop plans of care. Implement care plan through nursing action, use of resources and involving the clients. Evaluation of implementation.
Leadership and change	Change in levels of functioning due to illness. Leadership behaviors improved through experiences in information processing problem-solving.		Change in nursing care plans after they are implemented. Leadership behaviors improved with numerous experiences in decision-making and problem-solving and designing innovative plans for care.
Professional practice			Indentification of roles of nurses vis-a-vis other health professionals: the dependent, independent, and interdependent roles.
Self-actualization			Emphasis on personal responsibility for nursing practice. Through experience with other health professionals, an application of sexist molding in role expectation and performance in male-dominated society.

40

Interaction and Change	Micro-teaching	Health and Culture
Patterns of psychosocial behavior. Effective communication skills facilitate change in health behavior. Psychosocial commonality of individuals.	Principles of teaching to facilitate changes in health behaviors.	Cultural and ethnic variations and role of values and attitudes on health behavior.
Inner resources available to an individual or family. Assessment of the significance of disruptions on the individual or family. Assessment of communication within the family.	Evaluation and writing critiques of peer performance. Development of teaching skills to increase repertoire of nursing behaviors available for intervention.	Cultural factors that affect the use of health resources.
Change in interpersonal behaviors. Leadership behaviors improved through communication skills, human relations training, and group leading. Experience in goal setting and goal attainment through group work. Begin to explore concept of peer support.	Change in health behaviors as a result of effective teaching. Learn how to give constructive feedback to peers to allow for change in behavior.	
Identification of personal beliefs about self, man, society, and nursing.	Indentification of learning needs of clients and self and skills to teach.	
Interpersonal sensitivities are emphasized. Acknowledging one's own feelings, making clear statements about personal needs and wants, and developing empathetic identification and an openness to new experiences. Through interpersonal experience, development of tolerance and acceptance of difference between individuals, groups, and cultures.		

Table 2. Senior year. Courses that demonstrate development and integration of key concepts within courses of the nursing major of Second Step Program.

Preceptorship Study	*Preceptorship Seminar*
Identify and define physical, psychosocial processes which affect a group and/or system as it moves on health-illness continuum in relation to curative and restorative aspects of care and maintenance of health and prevention of illness. Also, identify health services in the community that are emerging.	Identify potential for change in health care delivery systems based on theoretical analysis of the organization of health delivery agency.
Collaboratively define and establish client or group needs. Determine priorities; predict consequences of priority settings; identify available health personnel and/or community resources; formulate inferences about clients, groups, or communities and make diagnoses. Formulate plans to provide comprehensive and goal-directed care for client or group. Collaborate in evaluation of immediate and long-term consequences of interventions.	Identify areas of dependence, independence, and interdependence in area of preceptorship study. Evaluate patterns of communication and line of command within practice setting.
Make changes as necessary in formulated plan of care or in delivery of health care within an agency. Can formulate a plan of action designed to facilitate and support change within a system. Can identify need for consultation and obtain it.	Theoretical considerations of organization, change, and leadership behavior and style. Emphasis on peer support and team building. Identification of potential for change, strategies of change, inhibitors of change, and consequences of change within health agency of preceptorship. Identify own leadership style. Identify conflicts of nurses assuming leadership roles.
In-depth study in one field of nursing allows the student to be able to define nursing practice to others outside of nursing, understand varying roles of other health professionals, collaborate with peers and other health professionals. Define the area of nursing accountability in that field.	Explore the concept of and develop support systems as a part of professional practice. Identify factors that inhibit or enhance professional practice within institutions of the health care system.
Identification and implementation of personal learning goals and activities. Involved in the "pursuit of potential." Emphasis is on personal responsibility.	Discussion of social role expectations: nuturance vs. decision-making, dependence vs. independence, and submissiveness vs. dominance.

	Current trends in nursing practice. Knowledge of political and legislative development affecting nursing practice and health care delivery.
Plan process applied in real life situations. Utilize systems analysis and decision-making techniques.	Identification of nursing issues in a problem. Search out data defining the issues. Formulate an argument based on data.
Plan a real life situation with innovative alternatives.	Peer group experience in dealing with nursing problems. Build peer support systems and team effort.
	Take controversial issues in nursing and propose alternative solutions.

illness or accidents. Her nursing practice also involved cooperation and collaboration with other health professionals in clarifying and interpreting information about her clients to improve their care.

The young woman with the ileostomy moved through all phases of the health-illness continuum as she was recovering from the first surgery; she began adjusting to the changes in her body and life-style, developed severe pains and had to be readmitted for surgery to relieve adhesions, and returned home for another period of recuperation. The student was involved with the client and her family throughout these phases and was able to observe, first hand, movement on the health-illness continuum.

Each course in the junior year contributes to the students' understanding and use of the concept of the health-illness continuum. Marietta utilized information and skills from each course to understand physiologic processes and disruptions, to observe patterns of psychosocial behavior and their influence on the health of her clients, to effectively communicate with clients, to utilize components of teaching in facilitating change in health behaviors, and to appreciate the influences of cultural differences on the response of her clients to their health or illness and to her offer of a helping relationship.

Marietta began to develop a sensitivity to the effect of feelings and attitudes on a helping relationship. She decided to lead a discussion group for nurses and physicians on a hospital unit which had a high number of terminal patients. The group members were faced daily with the issue of death but had not had a way to discuss and work through their feelings and attitudes. Marietta assumed leadership, initiated a change, and experienced the value of peer support and interdependence.

By the end of her junior year, Marietta was expressing a broad understanding of her role as a nurse in the community working with families and individuals in all phases of the health-illness continuum. She had demonstrated an ability to make use of the concepts of diagnosis, intervention, and evaluation as well as leadership and change. She made clear statements about her own feelings and needs and took responsibility for her own practice.

Rachael had similar experiences in her junior year and was well prepared to begin preceptorship study in a psychiatric out-patient clinic. She chose a setting which had used nurses only as "dispensers of medication" and wrote a contract to include working with groups and couples in collaboration with other helping professionals. She identified her need for supervision and was able to obtain it from several sources in the agency. She also arranged for ongoing peer support with another student with whom she met weekly. In the first semester, Rachael became familiar with the formal and informal lines of communication and power and was even able to arrange for office space for herself in a facility that had little extra space. She co-led a group with a psychologist who reported her to be quite skilled at assessing situations, intervening, and evaluating her effect on clients.

One specific incident in Rachael's experience demonstrates her grasp of the key concepts. The psychiatric clinic had one psychiatrist and one medical officer, the remainder of the personnel were psychologists and social workers, persons unprepared to deal with physical symptoms and problems. One day a group member was very agitated, drooling, and having difficulty with gross motor control. Rachael determined that his behavior was not normal and needed further attention outside the group. The psychologist co-leader suggested that the man be taken to the medicine nurse in the medical clinic for a tranquilizer. Rachael accompanied the man but was ordered away by the medicine nurse who declared that she could handle the situation. Rachael returned to the psychiatric clinic and consulted with the medical officer. She voiced her concern and described the man's symptoms. She and the medical officer determined that the man had probably had too many tranquilizers and needed medication to provide physiological support to counteract the effects of the tranquilizers. The medicine nurse, meanwhile, had found the man "impossible to control" and came to the psychiatric clinic demanding that Rachael do something. The medical officer ordered the medication and Rachael stayed with the man until he was recovered. This situation evidences the student's use of her knowledge of the health-illness continuum, her ability to diagnosis, intervene, evaluate, and change plans as necessary, to assume leadership in a situation, and to understand the role and make use of other health professionals.

Sequence and Continuity

The second strategy to help organize the curriculum is to develop an order of succession and to provide a relationship between parts of that succession. Ordering refers to sequence. What is required is to put content and learning experiences into some sort of succession. Important questions in sequence are: "(1) What should determine the order of succession of materials of instruction, (2) What follows what and why, and (3) What is the most propitious time to acquire certain learnings?"[23]

The curriculum design is the example of ordering and succession of the curriculum. Content is taught first in regards to an individual, next to relation to the family, and finally, in relation to groups and systems.

One reason for developing sequence along an individual-to-systems continuum is because, theoretically, it moves from simple to complex and from concrete to abstract.[24] For example, in developing communication skills, they are generally taught one-to-one, in dyads, then in triads, and then in groups. Each additional person in attendance presents a different communication problem as each individual brings

45

his own perceptions, expectations, and favored modes of expression to the interaction. Consequently, there is step-like learning in going from one-to-one to one-to-group.

Science Principles, Community Health Nursing, Micro-teaching, and Interaction and Change preceed Preceptorship Study, Preceptorship Seminar and Professional Issues. The junior year courses provide expansion of content in unique learning experiences that lay a foundation for students being able to choose varied and complex practice situations for themselves in the senior year. Senior year can thereby become a time for greater development of values, attitudes, and judgement in nursing practice of choice. Generally, depth of understanding and mastery of processes requires time, time available in the senior year. Breadth of content is concentrated in the junior year.

The most propitious time to acquire learning seems, to the faculty, to be when the student returns to school motivated to seek what the program has to offer. For some students it is immediately after finishing the basic nursing program, for others it is after their children finish school and they want to renew their professional careers. It is still questionable which "learning" should be first.

Within a number of courses taken concurrently, certain concepts, skills, and mental processes will be repeated. The deliberate use of these will provide for the student developing greater sophistication and subtlety in knowledge and understanding. One common means is to utilize a learning experience to meet several objectives. For example, second semester of the junior year, students organize and run a nontherapeutic group. They do this as a part of Community Health Nursing Practicum and receive supervision for their experience in Interaction and Change. Multiple objectives are met: community organizations and resources are explored, clients' positions on the health-illness continuum are assessed, communications skills are sharpened in negotiating with the group, leadership skills are built in assuming responsibility for the group, and self-disclosure and problem-solving lead to team building and peer support among classmates.

Another example of continuity are the innovative and exciting Preceptorship Studies which build on ideas and skills developed by previous education and the junior year experience. This type of continuity refers to cumulative learning. The student is able to deal with more demanding situations, more complex materials, and more exact analysis. Such an example is Sarah.

Sarah is a 45-year-old woman, married and a grandmother. She has worked at a State Hospital for the mentally handicapped for 20 years. She originally graduated from a diploma school of nursing and returned to school to obtain her Bachelor of Science and to learn more "in depth" nursing to apply to the care of handicapped patients. She was very familiar with in-patient residential care for retarded children. She taught in-service programs to nonprofessional staff in the state hospital and was a supervisor for a hospital wing. Community Health Nursing Practicum took her out of a hospital setting for the first time in her career. Science Principles and Physical Assessment added depth to her knowledge of patients' health. She had had experience ministering to physical needs of severely developmentally delayed residents. However, she was dealing with a new array of patient problems in homes and in simulated laboratory situations. Although she had taught "in-service education," Sarah said she had not been aware of ways of improving her own techniques and had merely followed a pattern of doing what she had been taught. She said Micro-teaching provided background information for upgrading her teaching skills and for helping her demonstrate to other staff how to impart their special knowledges.

In her senior year, Sarah devised a preceptorship study in the community. She contracted with the supervising nurse at the regional developmental center for the mentally handicapped to learn discharge planning. Each state hospital participates cooperatively with the regional centers in the admission of appropriate patients from the community and the discharge of patients to resources within the community. Sarah set out to learn the state and federal legislation affecting placements and facilities, the role of and organization of the regional centers, the process within the hospitals for assessing patients for placement, formulating plans, and interacting with the community agency. She also examined the role and functions of the regional center in finding placements, assessing them for placement of individuals, and careful follow-up in evaluating on-going placements. She followed two patients through the entire process and analyzed the existing system.

Upon graduation, Sarah said she would be taking a new position at the state hospital, that of discharge coordinator. Sarah is just one example of an adult learner who came to the Second Step Program and has built upon her previous education and experience in such a way as to fit into a new, challenging role in nursing.

The challenge within the program has been to meet the needs of adult learners. One method is to plan learning experience that build on previous learning of students, another way is to teach process as content.

Process as Content

As a discipline, nursing utilizes many processes. These processes characterize professional behavior in nursing. Some of these processes were selected by the faculty to be taught as curriculum content. The processes considered basic to this program are: problem-solving/decision-making, interaction, teaching-learning, change, and research.

When processes are taught as content, progressive development is as important as it is in comprehending key concepts. Theoretical information and specific learning experiences related to a process are emphasized in specific courses. For example, nursing process is emphasized in Community Health Nursing and interactional process in Interaction and Change (Table 3). However, other courses as well contribute to the students' comprehension and mastery of the process. Data collection and assessment are stressed in Physical Assessment. Learning experiences are devised to formulate plans of care based on nurse assessment of case histories in Science Principles. Interaction and Change content is focused on the verbal skills which, in turn, facilitate history taking and interviewing in the process of data collection and assessment in Community Health Practicum.

Table 3. Processes selected for curriculum content and courses through which implemented

Process	Course
Problem-solving/decision-making	Community Health Science Principles Preceptorship Study
Interaction	Interaction and Change Preceptorship Seminar
Teaching-learning	Micro-teaching Preceptorship Study
Change	Interaction and Change Preceptorship Seminar
Research	Research Design Professional Issues Seminar

The progressive development of a process is illustrated well in the development of the teaching-learning process. In Micro-teaching, students learn the microelements of teaching and apply them in the presentation of "teaches" to fellow students. Peers, instructors, and hired student audiences evaluate these "teaches" not only for content and mastery of a particular microelement, but also for style of presentation. Students have five experiences in choosing topics, gathering materials, writing behavioral objectives, and preparing for the "teach." Each student has an opportunity to learn from the process of preparing and presenting a subject to learners.

The teaching-learning process is elaborated as students write their contracts for Preceptorship Study. They must assess what they want to learn and formulate a plan for accomplishing it. They must gather materials, including a preceptor and a practice facility. Students devise means for demonstrating mastery and comprehension within the year of specific study. They also write behavioral objectives and the methods of evaluation.

A third and different way that process is taught is illustrated by the change process. Change is encountered by the student in different orders or levels. In Interaction and Change, the first magnitude is the examination of internal values and attitudes. The second magnitude of change encountered is the interaction between formulating and evaluating actions and plans as in Community Health Nursing. The third magnitude is the realm of personal influence on systems and organiztions as in Preceptorship Study (Fig. 1).

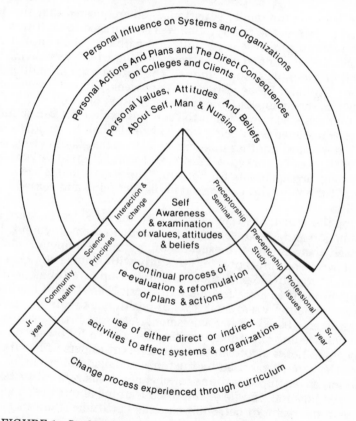

FIGURE 1. Students' experience of change process in three realms.

An example of students' experience with change process is Leslie, age 22. She came to the Second Step Program after working for two years in an out-patient crisis clinic. She stated that of all the patients she saw, she most disliked working with alcoholics. They were, in her words, "unmotivated to change, dependent, and disgusting." In

Interaction and Change she described her awareness of her attitudes and their affect in reducing her helpfulness to this type of patient. She disclosed her numerous disappointments at home with an alcoholic mother who had been institutionalized for drinking.

In Community Health Nursing, Leslie was assigned a family with an alcoholic husband who had recently been laid off from work because of drinking. The wife was referred initially by a local physician because of incapacitating migraine headaches. Mr. and Mrs. G. also had a 13-year-old boy. The wife said her headaches were due to her concern over money, her husband being laid off work, and her on-going dread that her son might steal or be expelled from school.

After assessing the family situation, Leslie requested that she not be asked to follow the family. She was encouraged to continue with the family and to seek consultation with a local alcohol abuse program. Leslie planned alternatives with the wife for involving the husband in Alcoholics Anonymous. The wife started attending AlAnon. Initially, Leslie visited the wife weekly to continue encouraging her to seek support from spouses of other alcoholics.

Another crisis occurred when the son was excluded from school and was threatened with being sent to juvenile hall for vandalism. Mrs. G. developed another migraine headache that kept her in bed for a week. Leslie worked with Mrs. G. to find alternative schooling and housing arrangements for her son. The arrangements seemed to benefit the boy who progressed in his schooling and ceased his vandalism.

During the year that Lesie worked with the G's, Mrs. G. started a part-time job and Mr. G. returned to his previous employment. Leslie expressed amazement at the success of anything helping Mr. G.

Leslie wrote her preceptorship to study with a nurse clinician who had a grant to provide placement and follow-up care for alcoholic patients brought to a metropolitan hospital. The student learned to interview patients, assess their level of health, make referrals to treatment programs based on her assessment, lead supportive groups for alcoholics needing extended hospital care, and to follow-up on placements. Leslie wrote an evaluation report as part of her final paper. Her report was used by the nurse clinician in her yearly evaluation as recommendations for changes in the referral system within the hospital. Leslie exemplified learning about the change process in the realm of personal values and attitudes. She also experienced change in reformulating and evaluating her plans of care for the family with the alcoholic father. And she further participated in effecting change in the hospital system of providing care for alcoholic patients through her preceptorship study. Various courses throughout the two year program contributed directly to her experiencing change in these different levels or realms.

50

She indicated in her final interview that the change in her personal values about caring for persons with addiction problems had evolved from one of digust to one of positive belief that people and systems can change and that nursing has a role in facilitating the change.

Process as content has proved to be a successful approach to curriculum planning in the Second Step Program. The adult learners in the program report satisfaction with the skills and knowledge they acquire. Preceptorship Seminar students freely discuss their application of these processes in analyzing their performance and that of their peers.

Another strategy for organizing learning is to choose teaching methods to be utilized in presenting selected content to particular students. The faculty of the Second Step Program uses all four teaching methods: discovery teaching, self-directed learning, expository teaching, variation in modes of learning, and their faculty-student relationship in the education of their adult learners.

Discovery Teaching

The faculty believes that adult students' learning is facilitated by involving them in an active, process-oriented, discovery-type curriculum. This teaching strategy is used extensively throughout the program. Community Health Nursing Practicum presents discovery learning through care for a case-load of families, the use of role playing, and simulation games. Role playing is introduced by demonstrating an initial visit between a community nurse and a client. The student group receives an hypothetical referral. They employ discovery learning as they plan the initial visit, role play the first encounter between the nurse and client, and then evaluate the effectiveness of their plan. This and other similar experiences involve the students in an active process of discovery within the safety of a peer group where they can work out a variety of solutions to problems and determine their effectiveness. This is done before being faced with a similar situation in a reality setting.

Another example of the use of role play occurs in the seminar section of the Community Health course and relates to the theoretical presentation of crisis intervention. Students are presented with a background script of a client whose current life circumstance is indicative of crisis and who is expressing doubt as to the value of life. Students role play the situation between hypothetical client and a community health nurse, analyze the interaction between the players, devise a plan for proceeding, role play the devised plan of action, and evaluate the result.

Late in the second semester of Community Health Nursing, by which time the expectation for level of involvement includes the relationship of self to the community, a simulation game is utilized. The game consists of a situation in which a mock board of supervisors (county governing body) is conducting hearings to receive requests for revenue sharing funds to be distributed throughout the county. Students select different roles, such as board of supervisors, spokesmen for various agencies asking for funds, consumer leaders, or perhaps representatives from official agencies also asking for funds. Those students representing agencies must carefully build their case for the need for and proposed use of funds while those students serving as the board of supervisors hear all requests for funding and then come to a decision as to distribution. The simulation game continues for three seminar sessions. Two are devoted to requesting funding and a final one for the results. It is a learning activity that requires that students make use of all the processes identified in the curriculum design.

Another discovery activity utilized as a learning experience is the preparation of a community analysis, a requirement for the Community Health Nursing Practicum. The students are provided with a framework to study and analyze a community. They must then "discover" the resources which they will need in order that they may work with families. Students then further their practice in discovery by using the same technique with families as they assist their clients in solving problems.

Discovery learning is also evidenced as students carry a case load of families, lead a health related group, and work cooperatively and collaboratively with other helping professionals in the community.

The course, Interaction and Change, provides a fertile climate for discovery learning. For example, students discover the effect of various communication techniques which facilitate development of trust and understanding, such as perception checking, giving and receiving feedback, and expressing feelings by participating in structured experiences. One such exercise sets students in groups of three. Student One spends five minutes describing himself to Student Two with Student Three acting as an observer. Student Two paraphrases and restates what Student One has said about himself until Student One is satisfied that Student Two has heard accurately. Student Three describes and evaluates the interaction. The exercise is repeated until each student has acted as the observer. The exercise gives students an expeience in attempting to communicate clearly, in listening carefully and openly, and in evaluating an interaction. They discover techniques that hinder or facilitate interaction.

Another example of discovery learning occurs in Interaction and Change as students experience group dynamics, such as phases of group and roles of members. In the second semester of the course they gain further insight into group dynamics as they are members of a peer support group as well as being leader of a health related group.

Action, feedback, and videotape replay are the process/discovery methods utilized in Micro-teaching for Nurses. After having heard a lecture/discussion of a particular micro-element, such as, reinforcement, questioning, or set induction, each student develops a five minute "teach" on any subject to be presented and is videotaped demonstrating the micro-elements. The peer group evaluates the method and gives written feedback after each teach. A hired student audience is used as another, more objective, source of feedback. Students discover by seeing and hearing themselves as the videotape is replayed immediately and each can critique his own presentation and get reinforcement for the feedback received from his peers and the hired student audience. Another form of active learning utilized is self-directed study.

Self-Directed Study

Another method of allowing the student to get actively involved in his learning is through self-directed study. Integral to it is the discovery process, however, in this case the student either picks his own learning experiences and/or his timing and sequencing. The senior year preceptorship, described in Chapter 5, is an example of the student choosing his own learning experiences.

Independent study is a teaching strategy offered through student selected community involvement projects and special studies. Through independent study, the student may elect to fulfill one to four units of academic credit. The student determines an area of investigation he wishes to pursue and approaches a faculty member to agree to act as a sponsor for the independent study. The requirements for the project and unit value are agreed upon by the student and instructor. The instructor is responsible for giving guidance, evaluating, and assigning a grade to the student. Community involvement projects and special studies serve only as elective credit and are not a part of the program requirements.

The Physical Assessment course at Sonoma is a self-pacing laboratory course. Modules have been developed to teach aspects of physical assessment such as examination of the eye, the ear, or cardiovascular system. If a student passes the pretest, he or she is considered to have passed the module successfully. If he does not pass the pre-test at a level of proficiency, he chooses a method for completing the module, either videotape lecture/demonstration, audiotape lecture, or reading from selected resource texts. Anatomic models of eyes, breasts, and genitals, and instruments, stethoscopes, otoscopes and opthalmoscopes, are available for practicing the skills presented in the module. Students determine when they are ready to take the post-test and when they pass at a level of proficiency, they demonstrate this newly acquired skill on laboratory partners with a faculty member evaluating and assisting. Students complete three response sheets indicating use of each physical assessment skill outside the laboratory setting. Modules are completed at each student's own speed and according to the mode he chooses.

Self-direction is utilized in Community Health Nursing Practicum, within the limitations set by the course objectives, as students collaborate with the faculty in determining the profile of cases which they follow clinically. As registered nurses, students are responsible for their own practice, they use faculty as consultants and resources in their work with families in the community. Some students pursue particular interests in community health such as working with aged clients, working with unwed mothers, working with particular cultural groups, and so forth. This is possible in conjunction with the caseload required to fulfill the course objectives. Another teaching method, expository, is not active learning centered, but developed for different reasons.

Expository Teaching

Lecture/discussion as a teaching method is useful for presenting concepts, processes, and issues to a large group of students so that they all have a common base. DeTornyay suggests the expository teaching strategy as one of the most efficient means of "conveying material in an organized way so that all students receive the same information." [25]

Two courses in the Second Step Program are organized in lectures or lecture/discussion entirely. They are Science Principles Applied to Human Phenomena and Community Health Nursing Theory. The student is taught, in both courses, to look for ideas, rules, principles, and concepts that organize and correlate theory with experience. The material is presented deductively, that is, the principles and concepts are presented and then the implications are discussed. Each course has a small group discussion section to allow students to question, seek clarification, and further explore the lecture material. Students' evaluations indicate dissatisfaction with these courses, possibly due to factors related to adult learners as well as the faculties' discomfort with this mode.

Another use of expository teaching utilized is that of mini-workshops. These are six-hour lecture/discussion sessions which may utilize multiple visual aides, guest lecturers, and small group discussion for questions, reactions, and feedback. They are planned to deal explicitly with a particular topic such as death and dying or human sexuality. The faculty decided that these topics could not adequately be dealt with in a one hour lecture. In the first semester of Community Health Nursing Practicum, the students have a six hour workshop on human sexuality as expressed in well individuals, couples, and families. In the second semester, the workshop on human sexuality deals with various dysfunctions that affect sexual response. Films, discussion groups, and panel presentations are used for both workshops on human sexuality as a means of presenting all students with a framework within which to examine their own understanding and misunderstanding of human sexuality and its expression.

DeTornyay suggests that one of the few good reasons to select the expository mode is to provide students an opportunity to hear particularly stimulating guest lecturers.[26] The mini-workshop method was selected as a means of presenting one of the national leaders in death education who agreed to speak to our students about his experience with cancer. We were also able to invite several other persons who were involved in exciting projects having to do with death and dying in our area. The presentations were informal enough to allow for give and take between the students and the guests. An excellent film, "How Can I Not Be Among You," was also used to stimulate thought and discussion.

All three mini-workshops were extremely well received by the students and some of the best course evaluations referred to the mini-workshops. The positive reception may have been due to the increased amount of time allowed to develop the topic, to the use of varying stimuli, to the opportunity to hear particularly stimulating guest lecturers. Several other workshops are being planned to present such topics as Problem-Oriented Records, History Taking, and Assessment of the Family.

A third example of the use of expository teaching in the Second Step Program is the lecture/discussion section of Micro-teaching. In this course, the faculty member uses videotapes to illustrate the micro-element of teaching that she presents in the lecture.

It is important to consider the weighting of the curriculum with discovery and self-directed learning versus expository teaching. Discovery and self-directed learning are utilized more extensively if appropriate to the adult learners and the knowledge and skills that are expected to be gained. An unorthodox teaching method rapidly gaining popularity in many nursing programs, including the Second Step Program, is the use of variety and choice in the mode of learning.

Variations of Modes of Learning

The faculty believes that if the student is offered options and choices in his learning experiences, learning is more readily internalized. Therefore, students are encouraged to identify their learning needs, participate in the selection of meaningful educational activities, and learn their own best style of learning.

The Physical Assessment Self-Pacing Laboratory is probably the best example presently offered. In this instance, the student is not only able to sequence and pace his own learning, but he can also choose from several modalities, auditory, visual, or a combination of the two.

The instruction and experience in the first year provide students with experience in nursing practice which is different from nursing in institutional settings. For example, two semesters devoted to nursing in the community places emphasis where the majority of health problems are found and where students have little or no experience practicing. The junior year includes clinical learning experiences in a variety of settings, thus encouraging a much broader understanding of the many variables which influence health and may contribute to illness. Self-awareness, group dynamics, and interpersonal relationships in groups and health service organizations are stressed. The first year provides a firm base for contractual study in the senior year. The preceptorship is a flexible approach to learning and allows the student an opportunity to explore, in depth, a chosen area of study and/or to develop expertise in a selected area of practice. This approach allows opportunities to practice self-assessment, identify individual needs, develop behavioral objectives, select learning experiences and work cooperatively and collaboratively with others. Preceptorship study affords the opportunity to practice autonomous and responsible behavior as an active agent for change.

The development of a peer-colleague relationship between faculty member and student is the basis of the final teaching method.

Faculty-Student Relationship

It is important for the adult learner to have confidence in his capabilities and self-worth; therefore, a faculty-student relationship of support and mutual respect is considered an essential ingredient in the Second Step Program. Self-disclosure and the development of self-awareness is modeled by the faculty throughout the curriculum and especially in Interaction and Change where the establishment of open communication is an objective of the course. Students are encouraged to seek clarification of unclear communications and to make their needs known to faculty. Much of the work in Community Health Nursing Practicum occurs in small group discussion where honesty and self examination are encouraged. The senior year preceptorship builds a one-to-one relationship between student and faculty in the faculty's role as advisor for the student. The climate for creativity and innovation relies heavily on a trust relationship between students and faculty.

An on-going problem in the maintenance of such a climate of trust and support is the faculty's role in evaluation and responsibility in assigning grades to student performance. Faculty members consistently work with each other and with students in the effort to reconcile this dichotomy.

CONCLUSION

As the faculty continues to evaluate the strategies involved in organizing learning, some of the outstanding strengths and weaknesses of the program become apparent. Strengths identified include the development of the integrative threads, the extensive and effective use of discovery and self-directed learning, and the identification of a curriculum significantly different from the students' basic nursing education.

The integrative threads of the curriculum have been clearly spelled out and analyzed so that they are evident throughout the curriculum and are supported and dealt with in several courses and from various points of view. This has facilitated the sequential development of the processes, concepts, and principles from the first semester through the fourth semester.

Students experience the identified skills and knowledge base first-hand through the use of discovery and self-directed learning. They appropriate and internalize values and attitudes related to their professional practice.

The curriculum significantly differs from the students' basic nursing curriculum. Registered nurse students previously have had to fit into generic baccalaureate programs which were ill-prepared to accept them and to offer them meaningful educational experiences.

Problems or weaknesses identified lie particularly in the area of individualizing the curriculum. The philosophy of the Second Step Program states a goal of working toward a flexible, individualized curriculum which will build on previous knowledge and skills. This has been difficult to operationalize. The ability to identify the cognitive styles of students in the Second Step Program is limited as are alternate modes for acquiring knowledge. A faculty project involves developing a means to identify which students learn best by lecture, which by reading, which by seminar/discussion, and so forth, and then to develop a variety of modes by which students can fulfill the requirements and objectives of the courses. This effort has been started in the Physical Assessment course and will be expanded to be available in other courses.

Another difficulty in individualizing the curriculum is in the identification and evaluation of educational and life experience and their applicability to the students' experience in the program. Ways are being developed for students to challenge portions of the curriculum but the process is in its prodromal stage.

The Educational Taxonomies identify levels of skill in the cognitive and affective domains. Nursing programs often have trouble identifying what level of skill is appropriate to expect of students in associate degree, diploma, and baccalaureate programs. The Second Step is not exception. The faculty and students work together continuously in an attempt to solve this dilemma.

The Second Step Program is young and dynamic. It is developing, self-evaluating, and changing. The potential for educating people who are preparing to deal with new needs, new roles, and new directions in health care is real and exciting.

REFERENCES

1. Lysaught, Jerome: *An Abstract for Action.* McGraw-Hill, New York, 1970.
2. Chater, Shirley: A Conceptual Framework for Curriculum Development. *Nursing Outlook* 23:432, 1975.
3. Taba, Hilda: *Curriculum Development: Theory and Practice.* Harcourt, Brace Jovanovich, New York, 1962, p. 428.
4. Tyler, Ralph: *Basic Principles of Curriculum and Instruction.* University of Chicago Press, Chicago, 1950.
5. Bloom, B.S.: Ideas, Problems and Methods of Inquiry. National Society for Study of Education, Integration of Educational Experiences. 57th Yearbook, University of Chicago Press, Chicago, 1958.
6. Knowles, Malcolm: *The Modern Practice of Adult Education: Andragogy vs. Pedagogy.* Association Press, New York, 1970.
7. *Ibid.*
8. Parker, Cecil, and Rubin, Louis: *Process as Content: Curriculum Design and the Application of Knowledge.* Rand McNally, Chicago, 1966, p. 1.
9. *Ibid.*
10. *Ibid.*
11. *Ibid.*
12. DeTornyay, Rheba: *Strategies for Teaching Nursing.* John Wiley and Sons, New York, 1971.
13. Bruner, Jerome S.: The Act of Discovery. *Harvard Educational Review,* 31:21, 1961.
14. Harrison, R.: Classroom Innovation: A Design Primer, in Runkel, P., et al. (eds.): *The Changing College Classroom.* Jossey-Bass, San Francisco, 1969.
15. DeTornyay, *op. cit.*
16. *Ibid.*
17. Wittrock, M.C.: Verbal Stimuli in Concept Formation: Learning by Discovery. *Journal of Educational Psychology,* 64:183, 1963.
18. Chater, *op. cit.*
19. DeTornyay, *op. cit.*
20. Bevis, Em Olivia: *Curriculum Building in Nursing: A Process.* C.V. Mosby, St. Louis, 1973.
21. Smith, B. Othanel: Toward a Theory of Teaching, in Bellach, Arna: *Theory and Research in Teaching.* Teachers College, Columbia University, New York, 1963, p. 4.
22. Taba, *op. cit.*
23. Leonard, J.P.: Some Reflections on the Meaning of Sequence, in Herrick, V.E., Tyler, R.W.: *Toward Improved Curriculum Theory.* Supplementary Educational Monograph No. 71. University of Chicago Press, Chicago, 1950, p. 70.
24. Taba, *op. cit.*
25. DeTornyay, *op. cit.*
26. *Ibid.*

CHAPTER 4

Issues and Problems of Articulation and Admission

Vivian Malmstrom, R.N., M.S., and Virginia Meyer, R.N., M.S.

Discussion of admission practices and policies which characterize the nursing program at California State College, Sonoma, coalesces with imposing influences emanating from contemporary issues in higher education, societal trends, and nursing education. While it remains the function of the policies governing admission criteria and practices to select those students who, in all probability, will successfully complete a specified course of study, the measurements reflect society's values and education's response to those values.

In higher education today, the topic of enrollment is creating concerns of great proportion, resulting in new definitions of educational systems, in all of which nursing education is an integral part. Formalized in 1972, the Higher Education Amendments broadened the base of higher education to include public and new private institutions (proprietary, nonprofit, and sectarian) which are both within and outside the traditional college sector, thereby redefining "higher" education to mean "post-secondary" education. Such a movement was, in part, a response to societal pressures that called for increased mobility for students which would allow for shifts in career goals and accessibility to a variety of institutions with credit for all academic endeavors, all without penalty. Concommittant with these trends has been the gradual movement toward easier access into the post-secondary system by removal of arbitrary barriers, such as prior educational achievement.

Nursing educators, sensitive to these changing trends in post-secondary education, have also listened to the stirrings within the nursing community. They have recognized the confusion of nursing service personnel who grapple with determination of assignments for graduates from the various programs in nursing. They have also recognized the difficulties that graduates from diploma and associate degree programs in nursing have experienced in their attempts to re-enter the educational

59

system in order to improve their practice and expand career possibilities. Legislators are challenging existing nursing education patterns and are engaged in legislating what they believe to be a more equitable system designed to increase mobility within nursing, as well as in the various health occupations. In California, bills have been voted into law which mandate that credit be given for previously acquired knowledge and skill.

Nursing's response to these growing pressures is most loudly heard through the proposals of curriculum reform. Core curriculum, career ladder, and open curriculum promise intriguing challenges for traditional admission policies and practices through which student mobility is most clearly manifested.

ADMISSION PRACTICES OF THE SECOND STEP PROGRAM

Faculty of the nursing program at California State College, Sonoma, were acutely aware that the admission requirements for acceptance into the nursing major of the Second Step Program represented sharp deviations from established practices sanctioned by their profession. Any validity the requirements might claim was based on policies which all student entering California State College, Sonoma, were required to meet and on educated assumptions about quality of nursing preparation in the community colleges.

Requirements and Procedures

The admission criteria and practices of the Department of Nursing meet California State University and College admission requirements and are approved by the state licensing board. Criteria and practices are described as follows:

All applicants to the Department of Nursing must satisfy the admission requirements as prescribed by Title V, Chapter 5, subchapter 2 of the California Administrative Code. In addition to the basic criteria for admission to junior standing, students must satisfy the following criteria for acceptance to the nursing major:

1. Complete 60 semester units of transferrable credit as certified by the community college.

2. Of the above, 30 semester units of California State University and College general education requirements must be certified by the transfer college.

3. Hold a current California license as a registered nurse.

4. Credit for high school or college chemistry with a grade of C or better.

5. College credit for human anatomy and physiology with a grade of C or better.

Students who are candidates for the bachelor of science degree in nursing must have earned an associate of arts degree in nursing or its equivalent.

Diploma school graduates meet the minimum requirements by completing course work in the natural and social sciences and accumulating a minimum of 30 units of general education as certified by the community college. Equivalency for lower division nursing course work is established by the community college and the diploma school graduate whose prior course work meets the equivalency criteria may matricalate with 30 units of ungraded nursing credit. As with all other students, course work recognized as part of the curriculum offered by an accredited college is accepted for full credit.

The admission process for entrance to the college follows the State College Common Admission's Program. Admission is granted to qualified students on the basis of space available within their chosen college and of space available within their chosen or designated major at the college.

Students applying for junior standing in the nursing major who meet the admission requirements are considered equally eligible. If the number of acceptable applicants exceeds the quota established by the resources of the Department of Nursing, a random selection of applicants is made.

Applicants not recommended are notified of the reason for rejection and are invited to have their application redirected to another California State University or College, or designate an alternate major. Lower division nursing units are accepted as elective units by all majors leading to a baccalaureate degree at California State College, Sonoma.

All applications received during the initial filing period receive equal consideration within established enrollment categories and quotas, irrespective of the time and date they are received. Students who are enrolled in the college and wish entrance into the nursing program are required to petition for a change of major. Those who meet the established eligibility criteria are given equal consideration within the final pool of candidates.

RATIONALE FOR ADMISSION CRITERIA AND PROCEDURE

The rationale for the admission criteria and procedures used by the Nursing Department at California State College, Sonoma derive, primarily, from directions for change emerging from The Master Plan for Higher Education in California (1960), the report of the Coordinating Council for Higher Education and Nursing Education in California (1966), reports from the National Commission Studies for Nursing and the movement of the professional organizations supporting experimental approaches through curriculi designed to increase mobility within nursing education.

Of specific import was the establishment of policies regarding transfer from junior colleges. In 1970 the Coordinating Council for Higher Education, an advisory body appointed to work with governing boards of junior colleges, state colleges, and universities, endorsed the "Joint Statement of Policy in Respect to the Admission of Eligible Applicants for Transfer from California Public Junior Colleges." The endorsement statement insures *all students who enter public higher education institutions in California, and who maintain satisfactory academic records, the opportunity to progress to the baccalaureate degree without encountering arbitrary barriers.*

Direct Articulation

Even though educational policies in higher education encourage direct articulation, the argument remains controversial. In fact, a question most frequently posed to the Sonoma State faculty by other nurse educators queries the procedure and measurements used for establishing achievement or mastery of prerequisite content and experience.

The faculty views the argument as arranging itself around these two pivotal positions: (1) carte blanche acceptance of prior preparation with minimum achievement standards vs. (2) course by course evaluation of prerequisite requirements.

Reliance on prior course work to establish prerequisite eligibility implies that entering students begin their course of study with similar backgrounds and achievement characteristics. A more literal interpretation speaks to a standardization of prerequisite education and experience, which is not defensible in view of the diversity of educational patterns in nursing which presently exist. Implicit in the argument is that all students who qualify for entry into the program have an "equal" opportunity to learn the course work that comprises the nursing major.

The seemingly opposing argument lies in the pragmatic properties of the mobility concept. The pattern which characterizes the Second Step Program, delegates to the community college programs prerequisite preparation for articulation with the upper division nursing course and validates this preparation by reliance on the licensure tests granting registration for practice in nursing. While the faculty believes that "education for nursing belongs within the total framework of general education" and "that associate degree or equivalent nurse preparation can be an integral part of and does form the foundation upon which professional nursing can be built," the argument for the current practices at California State College, Sonoma is not, at the present time, founded upon strong evidence. The onus for support of the argument rests with the framework and implementation of the Second Step curriculum. The curriculum is vested in ordering the program pattern in such a way that what the

62

student has learned at one stage has relevance and academic value at the next stage. This arrangement supports the notion that the student shares in the responsibility for demonstrating mobility qualifications and the promise is not implicit that all qualified students will successfully complete the course of study.

While faculty believe that the articulation practices for entrance into the nursing major are sound, the on-going evaluation study of the Second Step Program will provide the data for ordering the argument into a more rational framework from which logical decisions regarding admission practices can be made.

Student Selections: Best Qualified vs. Fully Qualified

The selection process is accountable for estimating the probability of success for the individual applicant. Traditionally, the search for best qualified has not been uncommon. In these days, nursing education finds itself in the incongruent position of responding to higher education trends of liberalizing articulation practices and admission policies and, yet, is forced to select from an applicant pool which numbers far more than its educational resources can absorb. Each school faces this dilemma and answers for itself whether the best qualified student or the fully qualified student is consistent with the philosophy, goals, and objectives of their institution and of their nursing program.

The decision to define admission criteria in tems of "fully qualified" expressed the faculty's best interpretation of the purposes and goals of the Second Step Program. The principle goal, "to prepare a baccalaureate nurse to meet the present and future nursing needs of society," and the faculty's philosophical belief that "each learner has the right to as much education as he is capable of pursuing," mandated that eligible applicants be considered fully qualified and provided equal opportunity for admission.

Random Selection vs. Discriminating Selector Indicators

Random selection of fully qualified applicants for admission to a course of study lacks substance as a method for selection, even though it was the procedure utilized in the California State University and College System during the period when the system was hard pressed to accomodate all of the students seeking entrance. The best that can be said for random selection is that it provides equal access for the fully qualified applicant and disposes of admission committee judgments which accompany discriminating selection procedures. The system does not recognize student attributes such as diligence, determination, and motivation toward career goals. This practice is viewed as unfair and unrewarding by students who are high achievers, but is seen as a most "fair" system by students whose chances for admission would be lessened in a discriminating selection system.

The faculty was cognizant of the problems inherent in formulating success predictors for a student population entering a largely untested pattern of education. In spite of the many studies which have attempted to define accurate predictors of success in generic baccalaureate programs, little progress toward improving prediction can be found. While the faculty was certain that the self-selected student group applying to the Second Step Program would reflect different characteristics from applicants to more traditional programs, assumptions could only be postulated as to the characteristics of this group.

The decision to randomly select did serve the purpose of providing a cross sampling of the pool of applicants qualified for admission to the program. The opportunity to study this randomly selected group from entry to exit promised data for developing rational selection measures predicated on tested predictors of student success. The faculty is striving toward establishment of admission criteria through the application of proven selection measures which can assure not only effective utilization of talent but also equity in the admission of students.

CONCEPTUAL FRAMEWORK FOR ADMISSIONS

In order to test out and affirm the extent to which the admission criteria and practices were substantial and predicted with accuracy the student's potential for successfully completing the Second Step Program, a framework was constructed which could be utilized to systematically collect student and program data. It allows for examination of relationships between entry and exit data within the context of the student's educational experience and constitutes a logical basis upon which decisions about admission criteria and practices can be made.

Validation of current admission standards and procedures is vital if the program is to provide the best educational service to the nurse population requesting admission to the Second Step Program. Of primary import will be to determine if entry data about this select group is, in fact, a profile of a student whose potential for successfully completing the program can be affirmed.

The conceptual framework for admission (Fig. 1) is an open systems model which follows enrollees through their experiences in the Second Step Program to their route of exit. It is designed to capture data which define the entering characteristics of the enrollee, his progress and exit pattern, and quantifying data about his position within the success indicator criteria. The framework allows for analysis of entry data in relation to the multiple variables which overtly or covertly influence the student's experience during his emersion in and exit from the program and correlation with the success indicator criteria.

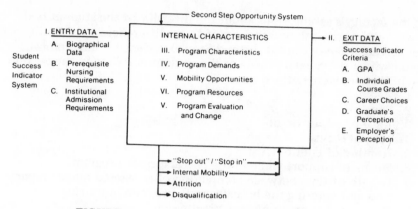

FIGURE 1. Conceptual framework for admissions.

Assignment of the success indicator system as the dependent variable provides the constant from which explanations of student success as it relates to admission criteria and practices can be derived. The entry data are the assigned independent variables and the internal characteristics express the active independent variable. Manipulation of the variable positions within the framework can allow for assessment of the education program in multiple ways. However, the search, in the context presented in this chapter, is for admission criteria and practices which predict success, provide equal access, and increase career mobility.

Entry Data

Entry data are reported only on those students who actually enrolled in the Second Step Program. Recognizing this group represents self-selection from the large pool of registered nurses in the population who have not earned a baccalaureate degree, the faculty were intrigued with comparing their preformed assumptions about the characteristics of the enrolling student with reality.

Items which could best describe the student who had established eligibility to the program defined the entry data. Biographical data that would define the characteristics of the enrollee, prerequisite nursing requirements for admission to the program, and institutional requirements for establishing eligibility to the college were categorically selected to describe the fully qualified student entering the Second Step Program.

Biographical Data

It was assumed that the student group would represent wide diversity as to personal characteristics, life demands, and career experience.

If the faculty's assumptions about the diversity of the student body were, in fact, true, they wondered if these differences would influence success achievement in the Second Step experience. Biographical items which provided a profile of the student enrolling in the Second Step Program were defined as:

1. Age
2. Sex
3. Race or ethnic origin
4. Marital status
5. Number of children
6. Means of support while in the baccalaureate program
7. Length of time between completion of registered nurse preparation and entering the baccalaureate program in nursing
8. Number of years of nursing practice
9. Area of nursing practice where major portion of career time was spent
10. Description of nursing practice in community setting

Prerequisite Nursing Requirements

The major screening of applicants was done through placement of the Second Step Program within the student's career projectile. Completion of an associate degree nursing program or its equivalent established a preselected group in terms of academic success and preparation for nursing practice as established by State Board requirements for licensure.

Admission to the nursing major at California State College, Sonoma stipulated grade achievement in chemistry, physiology, and anatomy of a "C" or better and served to screen out a minimal number of otherwise qualified applicants.

Institutional Requirements

The admission policies at California State College, Sonoma for undergraduate transfers state that eligibility is based on transferable college units attempted. An applicant in good standing at the college attended may be admitted as an undergraduate transfer if he or she meets either of the following requirements:

1. He or she is eligible for admission in freshman standing and has earned an average grade of "C" (2.0 on a scale where A = 4.0) or better in all transferable college units attempted.

2. He or she has completed at least 56 transferable semester units or 84 transferable quarter units with an average grade of "C" (2.0 on a scale where A = 4.0) or better if a California resident. Nonresidents must have a grade point average of 2.4 or better.

The number of transferable semester units for defining junior standing was changed from 60 semester units to 56 semester units in 1974.

In view of the present nursing curriculum and the rigors of completing the program in four semesters of full time study, the Department of Nursing has maintained their requirement of 60 transferable units as prerequisite to the major.

While college policy determines eligibility for all transferable college units attempted at a grade point average of 2.0, the Department of Nursing, in addition, requires a grade of "C" or better in chemistry, physiology, and anatomy. The Department of Nursing can petition the office of admission for acceptance of a student whose grade point average does not meet the minimum institutional requirements.

Although one category of entry data is defined by the institution, the Department of Nursing has the prerogative to determine prerequisite subjects and minimum grade standards for those courses. However, the faculty remains philosophically in agreement with the articulation and admission practices of the state college system.

Exit Data

In programs whose goals are career preparation, faculty responsibly believe success is defined not only in terms of satisfactory completion of the program, but, also, in terms of the practice of the graduate as he interprets his academic experiences into the real world of work. The search for success criterion has developed quantifying exit data in two dimensions.

One dimension defines academic success as graduation from the program, overall grade point average, and grades received in each of the courses required in the major. Faculty use operationalized course objectives for evaluating student progress and assigning grades which provide definitions of academic success, both quantifying and qualifying.

A second dimension is concerned with collection and examination of data about the career parameters of the graduate following completion of the program. Success indicators were derived from the goals and objectives of the program and included: (1) mobility demonstrated in the choices of career following graduation; (2) the graduate's self-reported perception of the relationship of his educational experience and his post-graduate practice; (3) the employer's perception of the graduate as a professional practitioner. Other indicators will, no doubt, emerge as the data are collected and analyzed. This portion of the study began as the first graduates of the Second Step Program neared the one year exit period.

Internal Characteristics

The internal characteristics represent the multiple factors operating within a dynamic system which are fluid and have covert and overt implications for defining successful program completion. By delineating these factors, a continual monitoring of the changes that occur within the system provides a basis for the assessment of facilitating and deterring components which influence the educational experience of the individual student.

Program Characteristics

The philosophy, purposes, and objectives of the program, as well as the individual courses which constitute the major, define the program characteristics. This measurement, largely, became an assessment of "fit" between qualified students as defined by the admission criteria and the student's readiness to begin and master a particular course of study.

The index for program readiness and fit has been assigned to: (1) the final grade for individual courses in the nursing major; (2) times the student repeated particular courses; and (3) grade earned when course was repeated. Correlations between entry data items, program fit, and success criteria indicators should provide definitions for lower division preparation, career experience, and personal characteristics which describe the successful student.

Program Demands

The difficulty or nondifficulty the student experienced in his progression through the program constituted the indices for this category. The cost to the student in terms of money, time, energy, and personal forfeiture had important implications for evaluation of admission criteria and access equality. California State College, Sonoma is a commuter college and students often travel considerable distances to reach campus and clinical placements. The age of the student increases the probability that the student's time was vested in family responsibilities, financial support during their educational time, and other such variables which could generate difficulties or obstacles in achieving educational goals.

Mobility Opportunities

This category evidences the opportunities for mobility within the program which allow students to demonstrate mastery of program components derived from prior educational or career experience. Institutional policy provided that a student may earn unit credit for a course which he successfully challenged by examinations, rather than pursue the usual arrangements.

The concept of challenge examination as a means for increasing mobility is embraced by the faculty. Arrangements for alteration in patterns of progression through the program to meet individual student needs provided yet another route for maximizing the success potential for the student.

Program Resources

Program resources have a direct relationship to the number of students who can be accomodated in each admission period. The number of faculty and their assigned work load determine the degree of assistance that is available for students on an individual basis.

Institutional resources which describe the learning milieu such as learning laboratories, tutoring centers, library facilities, availability of course offerings from other departments on campus, and field experience placements are important considerations when defining predictors for success.

Program Evaluation and Change

The fluidity of internal characteristics is most clearly defined through the continuous evaluation of individual courses and overall curriculum. Semester-by-semester changes are marks of a newly developing curriculum and creative faculty. Short and long range planning in terms of incorporating contemporary trends, restructuring courses, adding new ones and effecting future plans are all major considerations in the assessment of admission criteria and practices.

MOBILIZATION OF THE DATA

Entry data have been tabulated on students who enrolled in the program in September 1972 and September 1973 and a profile of the enrollee is beginning to emerge. Indices which describe the internal characteristics and can generate measurable data are presently being defined. The success indicator criteria remains to be operationalized.

Entry Data

Biographical Data

Biographical data accrues from the student's self-report on items in the initial survey conducted by the research team. One hundred per cent of the students in Class I, students entering September 1972, completed the entering survey while only 85 per cent of the students in Class II, students entering September 1973, elected to participate. All statistics appearing in the biographical description describe those students who participated in the survey.

Age

As was predicted upon initiation of the program, the ages of students enrolling in 1972 and 1973 described a student older than the average college student. Range of ages and average age for each class appears in Table 1.

Table 1. Range of ages of enrollees for Class I and Class II and the average age for each class

Class	Total no.	Age range	Average age
1972	44	22-51	33.9
1973	61	22-57	32.8

Students between 20 and 25 years of age represented approximately 35 per cent of Class II's student body as compared with 35 per cent of Class I who clustered between 31 and 35 years of age. Both classes drew 50 per cent of their student body from the 20 to 35 year age group, but the shift toward a younger aged enrollee is demonstrated by the age distribution of each class in Figure 2.

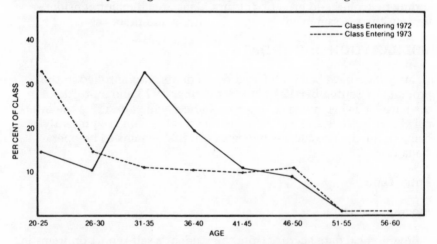

FIGURE 2. Comparison of ages of students entering the nursing program in 1972 and 1973. Average age 1972: 34.7 years; average age 1973: 32.9 years.

Sex

There seems to have been no differences in establishing eligibility to the program between males and females. Twelve men met eligibility requirements and received space reservations for admission to

70

the program in Class II, but only three men actually enrolled as compared with all eligible males enrolling in Class I. Factors other than admission requirements accounted for the loss of men to the program in Class II. Table 2 represents the enrollment of males and females in both classes.

Table 2. Number and per cent of males and females in
Class I and II

Class	Males		Females		Total	
	No.	%	No.	%	No.	%
1972	10	23	34	77	44	100
1973	3	5	58	95	61	100

Race or Ethnic Origin

The data on race or ethnic origin are based entirely on self-reports in the Evaluation Research project. Some students declined to participate and other students omitted various items of information such as race. The totals in Table 3 represent the minimum number of ethnic minority students enrolling in Class I and Class II.

Table 3. Number of students and per cent of class who identified
their race or ethnic origin

Class	Black		Caucasian		Mexican-American		Oriental		Other		No Answer		Total	
	No.	%	No.	%	No.	%	No.	%	No.	%	No.	%	No.	%
1972	1	2	40	91	1	2	0	0	2	5	0	0	44	100
1973	3	5	38	62	0	0	2	3	0	0	18	30	61	100

Marital Status

Students represented all of the categories describing marital status. Table 4 indicates a higher per cent of married students were representative of both classes. While 28 per cent of the students in Class II did not respond to this item, one fourth of those who did respond indicated they were single, representing an 8 per cent increase of single students in Class II.

Table 4. Marital status as reported by students enrolled in
Class I and Class II

	1972		1973	
Marital status	*No.*	*%*	*No.*	*%*
Single	8	18	16	26
Married	27	62	21	34
Divorced	7	16	7	12
Widowed	1	2	0	0
No answer	1	2	17	28
TOTAL	44	100	61	100

Number of Children

Class I and Class II are dissimilar as to the number of children in each student's family. Seventy-five per cent of the students in Class II reported they had no children as compared with 64 per cent of Class I who reported having one or more children. Distribution of the number of children the students in Class I and Class II reported as having is depicted in Table 5.

Table 5. Number of children of the students in
Class I and Class II

	1972		1973	
No. of children	*No.*	*%*	*No.*	*%*
No children	16	36	45	74
One child	6	14	3	5
Two children	12	27	5	8
Three children	5	11	4	6
Four children	2	5	3	5
More than four children	3	7	1	2
TOTAL	44	100	61	100

Means of Support While Studying for B.S. Degree

Students reported they utilized a variety of resources to support themselves financially while attending school. Table 6 indicates that the 44 respondents in Class I received support from a total of 82 sources of funding and 89 sources were reported by the 61 students in Class II.

Table 6. Means of support while studying for B.S. degree reported
by Class I and Class II

Source of financial support	1972	1973
Parents or spouse pay expenses	5	5
Parents or spouse will help	13	13
Funds from part-time summer work	19	23
Funds from full-time employment	13	12
Scholarship	9	9
Borrow funds on loan	12	13
Government grant	3	5
Other ways	8	9
TOTAL	82	89

Length of Time Between Completion of Registered Nurse Prepration
and Entering Baccalaureate Program in Nursing

Approximately 70 per cent of the students in both classes reported
they had completed registered nurse programs within 11 years prior
to entering the Second Step Program. Table 7 shows an increase in
the number of students in Class II who chose to continue their nursing education within one year or less following completion of their
registered nurse preparation.

Table 7. Number of years between completion of registered nurse
preparation and entrance into the baccalaureate program
for students in Class I and Class II

No. of years	1972		1973	
	No.	%	No.	%
0 - 1	5	11	14	23
2 - 6	15	35	21	34
7 - 11	11	25	8	13
12 - 16	5	11	6	10
17 - 21	3	7	6	10
22 - 26	5	11	5	8
37	0	0	1	2
TOTAL	44	100	61	100

Number of Years of Nursing Practice

The majority of students in both classes reported they had practiced
as registered nurses for one or more years prior to entering the Second

73

Step Program. An average 7.6 years of career experience was tabulated for Class I with a slight decrease to 6.1 years for students who entered in Class II. Table 8 represents the variations in the number of years of nursing experience which characterized the students in Class I and Class II.

Table 8. Years of nursing experience of students in Class I and Class II, prior to entering the Second Step Program

Years of nursing experience	1972		1973	
	No.	%	No.	%
0	4	9	5	8
1 - 5	18	41	30	49
6 - 10	12	27	11	18
11 - 15	3	7	9	15
16 - 20	5	12	4	7
21 - 25	1	2	2	3
26 - 30	1	2	0	0
TOTAL	44	100	61	100

Area of Nursing Practice Where Major Portion of Career Time Was Spent

Consistently students in both classes reported their years of nursing experience prior to entering the Second Step Program had been in the acute care setting. The majority described their experience as, primarily, in the care of patients assigned to medical-surgical units. The few students who had practiced outside of institutions had been employed in a physician's office. While many students reported a variety of career experiences, only those areas where students had concentrated their major career efforts were tablulated and appear in Table 9.

Description of Nursing Practice in Community Setting

Two students in Class I reported experience in community settings prior to entering the Second Step Program. One had spent two years with the Vista program and a second had worked on a part time basis in a health department. Five students reported limited work experience in community settings prior to entering the program in September 1973. They reported their experiences as:
1. One year as visiting nurse working in a home care agency
2. Two years as a junior public health nurse
3. Participation in teaching parent classes
4. Nurse in a community health nursing project
5. Six months teaching in a family planning clinic

74

Table 9. Major area of nursing experience background of students in Class I and Class II

Area of experience	1972 No.	%	1973 No.	%
Medical-surgical	10	22	24	39
Psychiatric	8	18	6	10
Mental retardation	3	7	2	3
ICU - CCU	6	14	8	13
Operating room	0	0	4	7
Obstetrics - pediatrics	0	0	5	8
General duty	6	14	4	7
Physician's office	3	7	3	5
No area of experience reported	8	18	5	8
TOTAL	44	100	61	100

Prerequisite Nursing Requirements

All students who enrolled in the program completed nursing preparation either in an associate degree or diploma nursing program and held valid licenses for the practice of nursing in the State of California. Tabulation of the number of students and the programs from which they graduated is shown in Table 10.

Table 10. Number and per cent of Class I and Class II graduating from diploma and associate degree nursing programs

Class	Diploma program No.	%	Associate degree program No.	%	Total No.	%
1972	18	41	26	59	44	100
1973	26	43	35	57	61	100

National League for Nursing achievement tests were given to both classes as one means of determining the student's knowledge base in nursing as he or she entered the Second Step Program. Test results indicated that students entering the Second Step Program had nursing knowledge that closely approximated the knowledge base demonstrated by all other baccalaureate students who had taken the examinations. Comparison of the test scores for diploma school graduates and associate degree graduates yielded no important differences.

All students entered having achieved a grade of "C" or better in lower division course work in physiology and anatomy and in high school or college chemistry. Instructional patterns and unit requirements for the science courses differ widely between institutions. No

75

attempt at this point has been made to stipulate required units or to qualify the science course prerequisites for entry to the Second Step Program.

Institutional Requirements for Admission

Essentially all students who were residents of California met eligibility requirements for admission to California State College, Sonoma for junior standing by accumulating 60 lower division units with a grade point average of 2.0 or better. In the total number of students admitted in Class I and Class II, only one student entered with a grade point average of less than the required 2.0. Table 11 shows the distribution and range of the cummulative grade point averages earned by students in Class I and Class II prior to entering the Second Step Program. The average entering grade points for Class I and Class II were 2.8 and 2.9 respectively.

Table 11. Entering grade point average of students in Class I and Class II

Entering G.P.A.	1972		1973	
	No.	%	No.	%
1.5 - 1.9	1	2	0	0
2.0 - 2.4	8	18	7	11
2.5 - 2.9	19	44	28	46
3.0 - 3.4	12	27	17	28
3.5 - 4.0	4	9	9	15
TOTAL	44	100	61	100

Exit Data

Exit data was accumulated on all students who exited from the program. For students who chose a route other than completion of the program and graduation, time of exit was tabulated and reasons for leaving were probed in terminal interviews. Collection of data which interpret the success indicator criteria began as students who received baccalaureate degrees by completing the nursing program in Class I approached the one year post-exit period.

In general, students exit the Second Step Program through one of the following routes:
1. Complete the program and graduate
2. Change major from nursing to another major in the college
3. Drop from college
4. Disqualify because of academic failure

While the majority of students who enter the nursing program follow regular progression and exit by graduating, some students elect to drop from college for varied periods of time and return to re-enter the program. Progression patterns for Class I and Class II describe students who "stop out" and "stop in" as follows:

1. Drop courses in the major and re-enroll in a following semester
2. Change from the nursing major and re-enter the nursing major in a different semester
3. Drop from college and return in a different semester

Attrition from the program for Class I and Class II followed patterns described in Table 12.

Table 12. Route of exit and number of students who dropped from the program without graduating in Class I and Class II

Route of exit	1972 No.	1973 No.
Drop from college shortly after first semester enrollment	2	4
Change major course of study	3	0
Drop from college at the end of one semester's work	0	2
Disqualify because of academic failure at the end of the third semester	2	2
TOTAL	7	8

Approximately 10 per cent of the 115 students entering in Class I and Class II left the program by dropping from the college, or changing their major course of study. Four per cent were disqualified because of academic failure. Four per cent altered progression patterns and are continuing toward graduation.

Students who changed their college major from nursing to a different major believed their career interest could best be served by study in a field other than nursing. Students who dropped from the program consistently reported personal demands such as finances, family, geographical move, or personal upset as reasons for dropping the program. All but two students expressed continued interest in completing the baccalaureate degree at some future date.

Success Indicator Criteria Data

To date, the grade point average earned by students in Class I and Class II completing the program and grades assigned for individual course work in the nursing major are available. The post-graduate survey, presently underway, will provide data as to career choice, the graduate's perception of his success, and the employer's perception of the graduate as a professional practitioner. These data will allow placement of the graduate within the success indicator system which will permit analysis of the admission criteria and practices of the Second Step Program to emerge.

Exit Grade Point Average

Students who completed the program in regular progression, on the whole, increased their grade point average during their Second Step experience. The average grade point average earned by both classes while completing the baccalaureate requirements for graduation was tabulated at 3.5.

Individual Course Grades

Tabulation of grades earned by the graduates in required course work for the nursing major is underway. Course grade patterns are treated in detail in the discussion of data mobilization on program characteristics in the section on internal characteristics which follows.

Internal Characteristics

The indices which describe the internal characteristics have not been tabulated to yield a statistical basis for analysis. At this point, faculty and student reports serve to focus on those program components which are perceived as potential barriers to student achievement. Data emerging from the evaluation research study will describe the experience of the student in interplay with the defined internal characteristics.

Program Characteristics

One attempt to determine program "fit" has been to examine grades assigned for individual course work. This analysis yielded an index as to the degree of difficulty students experienced in achieving certain knowledge components of the curriculum.

Course grade patterns for failure and disqualification clearly indicated that students experienced the most difficulty in achieving the objectives of the science course in the nursing major. Comparison of grade patterns for all required nursing courses demonstrated that a wider dispersion of grades and a greater number of "D" and "F" grades were recorded in the science course than in other courses. While most students who failed the science course in one semester, repeated it successfully in another semester, one student in Class I and one student in Class II were unable to achieve a passing grade upon a second attempt and were disqualified from the program.

In an effort to assign meaning to the grade statistic as it related to prerequisite preparation, faculty searched for measures which could predict student preparation fit for beginning the science course. Scores received on the National League for Nursing Natural Science Achievement Test, administered to students upon entrance to the program, correlated with the final grades assigned to those students who completed the science course at +.550. Grades earned in lower division courses in anatomy and physiology and final grades earned in the upper division science course correlated at +.348.

An endeavor to establish correlations between items on the entry data such as clinical nursing experience and time lapse between completion of course work in anatomy and physiology in lower division and beginning the upper division science course, with grades received in the nursing science course, continues in an effort to establish reliable data upon which admission decisions can be made.

Program Demands

The cost of full time study for the student in terms of time, energy, and financial sacrifice becomes most apparent in interviews with students who alter progression patterns or drop out of the program. The majority of students explain their reasons for change in educational direction as incompatibility between program expectations and life demands.

Program Resources

The extent to which students need and ask for individual assistance marks an important index of program "fit" for the fully qualified student. Tutoring sessions for the science course were requested by students in Class I and Class II and made available by faculty each semester the course was offered. The initiation of the multimedia learning laboratory has permitted students to achieve at their own pace, thereby minimizing time as a competing factor in learning.

Drawing from their experiences with the first two classes, faculty believes students optimally meet clinical course objectives when faculty-student ratio is maintained at 1 to 9. Similarly, a faculty ratio of 1 to 15 in the group process course, Interaction and Change, has been established and maintained as a means of maximizing the student's growth experience.

Program Change

The curriculum offered to Class I and Class II remained essentially unchanged in terms of course descriptions, course sequence, and requirements. Modifications in course content, teaching strategies, and other internal changes which are common to a dynamic curriculum have essentially been based upon student and faculty evaluations of curriculum components. Definition of the success profile for the graduate of the Second Step Program will allow for system analysis in determining approaches to curriculum change which can be executed and controlled efficiently.

SUMMARY

The faculty's attempt to validate and reaffirm that the present admission criteria and practices do, in fact, predict success, provide equal access, and increase mobility provides a continuous flow of data. Examination of entry data, internal characteristics of the Second Step Program, and available exit data defining Class I and Class II have generated the following statements:

1. The average age enrollee in the Second Step Program is older than the average age college student.

2. Each enrollment group includes both men and students who identify themselves as members of ethnic minorities.

3. The majority of students enter the program, continue in regular progression, and exit by graduating from the program.

4. No differences have been identified in academic achievement and program progression based on the type of nursing program in which the student received his preparation.

5. On the average, the student's GPA increases as he progresses through the program.

6. Students experience the most difficulty achieving academically in the Science Principles course.

7. The majority of students who have failed to meet program objectives have been disqualified during the third semester of study.

8. None of the students have elected to increase internal mobility by petitioning to challenge course work by examination.

9. Reasons students have given for dropping from the program have been: 1) shift in career goals; 2) personal problems; 3) competing life demands.

10. Students have been able to "step out" and "step in" with ease.

Testing out admission criteria and practices through a system which allows for analysis of cluster variables is expected to provide data upon which logical decisions about admission practices can be made. As interpretation of the data from the evaluation study accumulates, the conceptual framework can account for its placement within this decision-making system. Results of the longitudinal study of entry, exit, and post-exit data are expected to provide the means for determining the validity of the admission criteria and practices of the Second Step Program.

REFERENCES

1. Bloom, Benjamin S., and Peters, Frank R.: *The Use of Academic Prediction Scales for Counseling and Selecting College Entrants.* The Free Press of Glencoe, Inc., New York, 1961.
2. Bullough, Bonnie and Vern: A Career Ladder in Nursing: Problems and Prospects. *American Journal of Nursing* 71:1938, 1971.
3. California Department of Education: *A Master Plan for Higher Education in California 1960-1975,* 1960.
4. California State College, Sonoma 1974-1975 Catalog. State of California Printing Office, 1974.
5. Coordinating Council for Higher Education: *Nursing Education in California.* Sacramento, Number 1025, July, 1966.
6. Educational Preparation for Nursing - 1972. *Nursing Outlook* 21:586, 1973.
7. Lysaught, Jerome, and National Commission for the Study of Nursing and Nursing Education: *An Abstract for Action.* McGraw-Hill, New York, 1970.
8. McAshan, H. H.: *The Goals Approach to Performance Objectives.* W. B. Saunders, Philadelphia, 1974.
9. Meleis, Afaf Ibrahim, and Farrell, Kathleen McDonald: Operational Concern: a Study of Senior Nursing Students in Three Nursing Programs. *Nursing Research* 23:461, 1974.
10. National Center for Higher Education Management Systems at WICHE: *Post-Secondary Education Issues: Visible Questions — Invisible Answers.* Proceedings of the Fifth NCHEM National Invitational Seminar, Boulder, Colorado, WICHE, 1974.
11. *Report to the National League for Nursing, a Self Evaluation Study.* California State College, Sonoma, Spring, 1974. (An unpublished report prepared for the National League for Nursing Accreditation Board by the Faculty of the Department of Nursing, California State College, Sonoma.)
12. Runyon, Richard P. and Haber, Audrey: *Fundamentals of Behavioral Statistics.* Addison-Wesley Publishing Company, 1971.
13. *Second Step: Career Mobility for Associate Degree Nursing.* Department of Health, Education and Welfare Special Project, Grant Number 1 D10 NU00920-01, June 1, 1972.

CHAPTER 5

Preceptorship Study: Contracting for Learning

Mary W. Searight, R.N., M.S.

A two semester preceptorship formalized by a student-prepared study contract comprises the senior year of the California State College, Sonoma Second Step Nursing Program. This approach designed especially to meet the learning needs of adult students offers an opportunity to practice skills which are integral to professional nursing. Preceptorship Study is also flexible enough to accommodate a very diverse student population. Furthermore, it allows for the development of expertise in a selected area of nursing content.

BACKGROUND AND RATIONALE

During initial program planning, content for the junior year presented minimal problems. It was relatively easy to identify differences between associate degree and diploma prelicensure education and nursing education in baccalaureate programs. The need for community health nursing, advanced pathophysiology, group dynamics, and communication knowledge and skills was quite obvious. Addressing a wide variety of student interests and challenging the student while providing practice in making a change in role identity were the really perplexing tasks.

Traditionally, the goals of baccalaureate nursing education and successful orientation to the work system have been markedly opposed. Following a study of 220 collegiate graduate nurses working in 37 medical center hospitals, Kramer[1] recommended that nursing faculty study behavior patterns of successful professional nurses and teach these behaviors to nursing students. The California State College, Sonoma nursing faculty decided to take a slightly different approach to the role conception-work setting dichotomy. Our approach is to teach behaviors identified by nursing educators and nursing practitioners as characterizing professional performance in an actual work setting of the student's choice.

For years, literature has abounded with descriptions of professional nursing, attitudes toward practice, problems solved, and relationships with other health team members. Questions about what was technical and what was professional nursing then arose.

In a study of technical and professional nursing by Waters and associates,[2] three major areas were used to differentiate between the two groups of nurses. These areas included the nature of the problems solved, the scope of practice, and attitudes toward practice. When solving problems, the professional nurse uses a broad knowledge base which allows for alternative explanations and predictions.[3,4] The professional nurse identifies abstract, complex problems, not as yet clearly defined or understood.[5] Solutions to these problems may be innovative and probabilistic.[6,7,8] Approaches to patient care may be innovative and individualized.[9]

The professional nurse's scope of practice implies a collegial relationship in planning patient care with the physician.[10,11] The professional nurse is described as one who supplements and complements the physician's role. Other characteristics include increased responsibility for patient welfare[12] and leadership for those team members who are less well prepared.

Attitudes toward practice for the professional nurse include utilization of the scientific method, self-direction, and the ability to act independently. Further, the professional nurse requires consultation but not supervision.

If the purpose of professional nursing is to prepare practitioners with the qualities previously described, then nursing educators must be able to provide learning experiences so that the student will be able to demonstrate the described behaviors. This reasoning is fundamental and yet, as Kramer's study indicated, while most of the above behaviors are mentioned in baccalaureate program goals, graduates of these programs consistently have problems in applying knowledge and skills learned as a student to the actual work situation.

Fearsome battles are fought between nursing educators and nursing service personnel. The nursing educators describe what practice "should be" and nursing service describes "how it is." Caught in the middle is the neophyte baccalaureate graduate nurse. Motivated to succeed and to make a difference in the health care delivery system, the nurse often rushes forth with firm knowledge and a positive attitude but with little or no practice in dealing with the system. Once employed, the security and support of faculty and peers are gone. The nurse must then either adjust to the system, usually with some compromise to identity, consider herself a misfit and find employment elsewhere, or simply become disenchanted with nursing entirely and seek another vocation. Learning to solve complex problems, to behave in an autonomous and self-directed manner, to provide leadership, and create change are skills that must be practiced in order to be learned. This opportunity should be provided while the learner has the safety and security of the student role.

Students entering the junior year of traditional baccalaureate programs are usually much more homogeneous than those entering the Second Step Program. They generally start from a common educational base, are all about the same age, and have had no work experience in nursing, except possibly as LVNs or nurses' aides. These students are able to move ahead in an orderly progression. A structured course in advanced clinical nursing in the senior year planned to offer several areas of interest could challenge the student and meet the basic students' learning needs.

Sonoma students have been described as an unusually diverse group. Ages range from 21 to over 50. Some have completed basic nursing preparation in associate degree programs and others in diploma nursing schools. Some have had no work experience as registered nurses, while others have practiced 25 years or more. Some students are single, others are married or divorced. Many have children. Some live in the immediate community while others commute over 100 miles each day. A number of the students have achieved positions of leadership as head nurses or supervisors. Some have taught nurses' aides and Licensed Vocational Nurses. Several students are experts in ICU, CCU, operating room, or recovery room nursing.

Sutdent motivations for entering the Second Step Program include meeting a requirement for promotion, the need for a refresher, hopes for personal and professional growth, and expressed intent to subsequently enter graduate school. Others view baccalaureate education as leading to certification in community health nursing and therefore an opportunity to try a new role. For such a heterogeneous group of adult students, an approach to learning was needed which could provide for a wide range of abilities, interests, and educational goals as well as individualized immediate involvement in learning.

Due to changes in the health care delivery system, increasing emphasis is being placed on an area of clinical concentration or preparation as a nurse practitioner.[16,17,18,19,20] Costs of hospitalization are soaring, care is becoming highly specialized, and the patients' stays are shorter. Extended care facilities are flourishing both for ambulatory care of those recently discharged from an acute care setting, and also as repositories for the elderly. Mass media is educating clients about the need for preventive care. The government is increasing its support for screening programs and medical care for children and their mothers. And yet, shortages, maldistribution, and inadequate preparation to meet client needs continue to plague those responsible for health care. As increasing numbers of well prepared nurses graduate from associate degree programs, nursing service personnel expect something more from the baccalaureate graduate. Basic preparation for associate degree and diploma nurses includes the ability to provide direct patient care to clients with well defined health problems while working under the direction of a professional nurse.[21] For years, except for the science and general education base, the baccalaureate degree curriculum for nursing was more similar to that of associate degree and diploma programs than it was different. All programs stated that they were preparing beginning bedside nurses. However, with a population of registered nurse students who had demonstrated a knowledge of basic nursing through licensure and practice, the faculty felt that traditional goals were not reasonable and that an area of expertise could and must be developed.

Based upon faculty beliefs that all of the Sonoma students should have practice in professional nursing role identification, that a wide variety of choice in practice should be available to meet the needs of a very diverse group, and that an area of concentration was vital, two curricular patterns were selected for the senior year. A student either prepared a contract for a two semester preceptorship in the clinical area of his or her choice, or the student opted for a two semester program for preparation as a family nurse practitioner. (The latter is discussed in Chap. 6.) The faculty believed that Sonoma students had the potential and the movitvation to learn, given a suitable climate. They firmly believed that students entering the Second Step were mature and goal directed adults capable of making responsible decisions about their future. Further, they believed that the student had enough knowledge about the field of nursing to make choices. The faculty were confident that preceptorship study of two semesters, formalized through a student contract, would provide this climate and at the same time require student behaviors described as those characterizing professional nursing.

CHARACTERISTICS OF PRECEPTORSHIP STUDY

The preceptorship in the senior year is a flexible approach to learning that allows the student to explore in depth a chosen area of study and/or to develop expertise in a selected area of practice. This approach provides opportunities to practice self-assessment, to identify individual needs, to develop behavioral objectives, to select learning experiences, and to work cooperatively and collaboratively with preceptor, instructor, agencies, and families in initiating the plan. Preceptorship study affords the opportunity to practice autonomous and responsible behavior, and to practive as an active agent for change. Preceptorship study occurs under the supervision of a preceptor and a faculty advisor. It is designed by the student to fulfill a self-defined learning goal. Every student is required to register for four units each semester of the senior year. One of these units is earned in a weekly seminar and the other three are earned in nine hours of clinical practice or other professional activity. It is possible to register for more units if more time if needed to complete a particular piece of work. Seldom, however, does a student register for more than six units of preceptorship study.

Activities may include investigating in-service education needs and formulating a plan to meet these needs. Or a questionnaire may be developed to determine the extent to which registered nurses are prepared in biologic sciences and to what degree they utilize this knowledge in their nursing care. A student may wish to master a skill or set of skills such as those involved in the intensive care of newborns or a kidney dialysis center. Attacking a set of problems, such as those presented by clients in a specified ethnic culture, may appeal to other students. Occasionally students become involved in developing a community education program or providing a new service such as health care for families of prison inmates which may ultimately result in a manuscript for publication or a project proposal for funding. Other students may be interested in a preceptorship dealing with a specific body of subject matter such as school health, family planning, in-service education, or nursing supervision. Whatever the choice, preceptorship study provides a clearly defined avenue for an individual or group which will meet individual needs and match interests in attainment of identified professional goals.

PARTICIPANTS IN A PRECEPTORSHIP

The Preceptor

A preceptor is defined by this faculty as a highly competent person in a specific area of expertise who can teach and guide the student and with whom the student wishes to work. The following criteria for the selection of a preceptor are discussed with the students. The preceptor should be an expert in his or her field as determined by his or her peers and his or her agency. The student is encouraged to select a preceptor qualified to provide assistance in meeting the student's educational goals. The faculty advisor serves as a consultant to the student and ultimately shares the responsibility for selection of a preceptor. The advisor may review the preceptor's credentials to determine the adequacy of the preceptor's expertise. The student's goals are also examined to assess their fit with the preceptor's competencies. The preceptor must have the endorsement of his or her agency to participate in the study arrangement. Thus the process of selecting a preceptor becomes a collaborative effort between students, faculty, and agencies.

In developing an initial plan for preceptorship study, the student defines as clearly as possible a problem area or focus for a project. He then outlines broad objectives and proposes several alternative ways in which these may be met. Possible agencies and preceptors are identified and the student makes appointments with individuals to discuss his plan and explore the feasibility of his proposal.

Because nursing draws from a wide variety of disciplines, it is not necessary that the preceptor be a nurse. Physicians, social workers, counselors, hospital administrators, psychologists, nutritionists, or faculty from other departments at the college involved in management, research, or environmental studies may assist the nursing student. The preceptor acts as a resource person, consultant, and teacher to the student. Each student outlines the support required to the preceptor during the semester. For example, if a teacher is serving as preceptor, the student may request the opportunity to attend classes, observe classroom presentation, prepare a unit, and teach. The preceptor may also be asked to observe and critique the student's presentations. If a physician is serving as a preceptor to a student wishing to become expert in inserting intrauterine devices as part of preparation as a family planning practitioner, the physician may serve as clinical teacher and coworker. More commonly, however, the person selected is an expert in some particular area of nursing. Before contacting the preceptor, the student should have a pretty clear idea of what he or she wants to accomplish and by what means. The preceptor will want to know what help the student expects and what the student will do. What will be the role of the faculty advisor and what will be the nature of their relationship? Negotiations by the student progress from sharing a basic idea with the preceptor and gaining initial commitment to a finalized specific study contract. As discussion and planning progress, the student becomes more aware of what the cooperative relationship may be and more explicit about individual roles.

Initially, the preceptor may acquaint the student with the setting and suggest possible learning experiences which are available as well as what learning experience might be particularly appropriate to the student's objectives. Once the contract is initiated, the student and preceptor usually plan to meet at least weekly for on-going conferences to evaluate learning experiences. The preceptor, student, and faculty advisor always have an initial meeting to discuss terms of the proposed preceptorship. It is important that all agree upon the student's stated goals, objectives, activities, proposed evaluation criteria, and responsibilities of each individual. The student, preceptor, and faculty advisor work closely and collaboratively for each particular educational experience. A plan for on-going supervision by the faculty member and preceptor is established. This may include periodic on-site visits, conferences with student and preceptor, telephone calls, or other correspondence. The preceptor is perhaps the most important person to the student. As an expert in his field, the preceptor serves as a role model for the student in the clinical setting.

The Advisor

The faculty advisor is a member of the nursing faculty, and is selected by the student to lend a special interest or expertise to the
preceptorship study. Early in the spring semester, a list of all
nursing faculty is circulated to the students. Included is information about faculty member's educational and experiential background and special interests they may have. Current faculty offer
a wide variety of expertise to the students. Psychiatric nursing
faculty, some with post-master's work in adult psychiatry, community mental health, behavioral modification, family and marriage counseling, and group work, have special interests in crisis
intervention, healing communities like Synanon, rape-victim
counseling, and research in nontraditional treatment for schizo-
phrenics. Faculty educated in maternal-child nursing have additional preparation as nurse midwives, pediatric practitioners, and
family planning and La Maze teachers. Their special interests extend into human sexuality and family life education and many
facets of child health and school nursing. Faculty with preparation
related to medical and surgical nursing offer extended experience,
expertise, and interest in such areas as coronary care, intensive
care, gerontology, in-service education, disaster nursing, and emergency room nursing. The interests of community health faculty
are similarly rich and diverse. Those who hold a master's degree
in community health may also have had experience working in
clinics or communities where the care of the elderly, pregnancy
testing and counseling of adolescents, or health care for disad-
vantaged groups and ethnic minorities provided a significant case
load.

An experienced faculty such as Sonoma's, may have been involved
in drug abuse clinics, parenting groups, child abuse, women's movement nursing, alternative modes of healing, folk medicine and health
care, health care for homosexuals, Peace Corps, armed forces, or
suicide and suicide prevention, to name a few. With such a diversity
and smorgasbord to choose from, it is little wonder that students
are inspired to develop unique and different preceptorships.

Early in the development of the study contract, the faculty advisor
plans to meet the agency administrator and confirm that an appropriate agency agreement has been initated with the college. The
format for these agreements ranges from a formal contract signed
by the agency's board of directors and the Chancellor's Office of
the State Colleges and University to a simple letter of agreement by
the administrator of the agency. The terms and length of the agreement depend in part on the practices common within the particular
agency. All Sonoma students are practicing under their license and
are required to carry malpractice insurance.

The faculty advisor is responsible for keeping records about work with each preceptorship student. These records include a copy of the student's contract, notes made on individual conferences, and clinical visitations, journals, papers, or other work submitted by the student. Upon completion of a preceptorship, a summary or abstract of the work completed is prepared by the student. This summary and the preceptorship contract are kept as permanent records of the student's accomplishments during the senior year. These materials provide a very helpful resource when the student later requests a reference.

An important role for the faculty advisor is that of a liaison between student, preceptor, agency, and community. While most of the preceptorships run very smoothly, at times disagreement, misinterpretation, or disruption may occur. Contractual arrangements may have to be changed, an addendum added or, on a rare occasion, a new preceptor and/or agency found. If such a problem occurs, the faculty advisor serves as an advocate for the student and provides guidance during the crisis. Every effort is made to transform the disruption into a significant learning experience.

The faculty member also has primary responsibility for the student's grade. While the student sets up criteria and conditions, and the preceptor contributes his expertise and judgment, the faculty member gathers together all evidence and is responsible for assigning a grade to the project.

The following preceptorship objectives serve as a guide to students, preceptors, and faculty as they move through the semester.

Within a self-selected area of nursing practice the student will:

1. Utilize the problem solving approach in planning, implementing, and evaluating preceptorship contract.

2. Describe the biopsychosocial characteristics of the client population for which the selected area of nursing practice is tailored.

3. Formulate a knowledge base for the specialized practice area from related and nursing sciences.

4. Demonstrate skill in the techniques and procedures which are essential to the defined area of nursing practice.

5. Demonstrate knowledge of the organization of the practice setting and its impact on the scope of nursing practice.

6. Utilize documented theories of change and leadership to promote change within the practice setting.

7. Demonstrate interdependent, dependent, and independent nursing actions within the framework of the preceptorship.

8. Demonstrate, through the preceptorship, behavior which is indicative of progression toward self-actualization.

These objectives are further delineated with behaviors descriptive of A, B, C, and D level work. The leveled objectives are used by faculty and student in arriving at a semester grade.

The Student

Through careful selection of preceptors and advisors and negotiation of the preceptorship contract, each nursing student has a great deal of independence in planning his or her own senior year. During the planning period, the student should use the advice of current teachers and other resource persons. The student should take a hard look at past experience and his or her future goals. Faculty strongly suggests that students develop a contract, with the assistance of a faculty advisor, by completion of the junior year. Toward this end, the student may be asked to do some reading or otherwise sample the kinds of activity which the new contract may entail. The student is encouraged to critically examine personal motives since it is important not to waste opportunities for learning by proposing a project that will present no challenge. More of the same should not be confused with depth nor should aimless wandering be mistaken for breadth.

The student is responsible for developing and outlining behavioral objectives, learning experiences, evaluation, and other details of the study contract. He or she is responsible for planning and negotiating learning experiences and for carrying out what has been agreed upon. Identifying personal goals, planning one or two semesters of study, finding and negotiating with a preceptor, agency, and faculty advisor are not easy tasks for most students. Many find it a very difficult assignment, but once achieved most feel that it was one of their most valuable learning experiences.

ARTICULATION WITH TOTAL CURRICULUM

Student learning experiences which provide the student with basic skills needed to plan the senior year through a study contract are introduced in the junior year. Nursing 311: Community Health Nursing, teaches the utilization of the problem solving and the decision making process as a framework for assessment, nursing intervention, and evaluation. The student also uses assessment tools to establish a data base which consists of a synthesis of physical and psychosocial components of patient care. The data base is used to identify and define problems at the individual and family level, to formulate plans, identify problems, implement plans, and evaluate outcomes. The same processes of assessment are required in contract preparation, except that the student is dealing with personal goals and plans instead of those of a client. Nursing 367 A and B: Interaction and Change, prepare the student for the senior year by working toward a better understanding of self as a person and as a member of a group. A course requirement for the second semester is the planning, initiation, and leading of a health related group. A group contract is necessary to achieve this goal. As the student learns to utilize new understandings and perceptions of self to promote actualization within the group, he or she moves toward personal analysis of goals to be achieved as a professional. Further the student has some practice in applying these skills within a group.

Mirco-teaching, another junior year course, assists the student in elementary preparation of behavioral objectives. Each micro-teaching course requires at least one objective stated in behavioral terms which can be evaluated by the student audience.

Additional assistance is given half way through the junior year. Mimeographed descriptions of contractual study, details for preparing the contract, and contract forms are distributed. Informal coffee meetings are held and senior students involved in contractual study are also invited. The seniors share their contracts and offer advice to the juniors.

THE STUDY CONTRACT

Study contracts have been in use for several years and remain the major approach to study at schools such as Evergreen College in Washington and Empire College in New York. This method of teaching and learning has been described by a variety of terms such as work-study, internship, or preceptorship. The faculty member may be called a mentor or advisor. Terms of the contract may vary from a brief verbal or written description of a proposed project to a formal contract with objectives stated in behavioral terms. The central theme, however, is that the student identifies a goal he or she wants to achieve and is assisted by faculty and usually a third person and/or agency in describing how the goal will be attained.

Learning contracts serve as flexible yet demanding methods for satisfying the students' interests and needs. Independence in pursuit of inquiries that interest and motivate the student are encouraged. This method is proposed to provide maximum flexibility and independence for students with a wide variety of backgrounds and learning styles which fit this particular strategy.

Components and Ways of Proceeding

The study contract as used at Sonoma is a formal document made in quadruplicate. The form includes the student's name and social security number. A short title for the project and the number of units of credit for which the contract is drawn, the name of the preceptor, the faculty advisor, the name and address of the agency being used and the name of the administrator to be contacted for negotiation of the agency contract are also specified. A beginning date and approximate date of completion are included. These dates usually coincide with final exam dates since the evidence produced for final evaluation and a semester grade must be determined by that date.

Purpose

The purpose of the project is stated. This sometimes includes a rationale for the particular piece of work or is stated as an overall aim. For example, the purpose may be stated as follows:

The overall purpose of this contractual study is to give the student an opportunity to participate in the planning, implementation, and evaluation of a staff development program to increase staff knowledge in assessment and developmental intervention for the severely or profoundly retarded child.[22]

Previous Experience

A summary of previous experience is required. This information gives the advisor, preceptor, and agency an indication of the experiential and educational background which will serve as a foundation for the student's further growth. It gives clues to preceptor and advisor about the feasibility of proposed objectives and indicates whether a realistic appraisal has been made by the student regarding his or her ability to undertake the proposed project. At other times, looking at the work and educational experience may reveal that the student is preparing to do more of the same and that the project proposed would provide little, if any, challenge.

Work experience, classes taken, projects completed, surveys done, interviews completed, data collected, all serve as indicators of the student's preparation to undertake a particular project. The student whose purpose is stated above had the following experience to support her preceptorship contract.

1. Atypical Infant Theory & Field, 6
2. Exceptional Child, 3 units, 1974, (CSCS)
3. Child Development, 4 units, 1974, (CSCS)
4. Behavior Modification, Theory & Practice, 6 weeks, Pacific State Hospital, 1970
5. Developmental Specialist Training, 1 year, Sonoma State Hospital, 1972-73
6. Clinical Experience, Sonoma State Hospital, 1968-74
7. Field experience as a student with families of the atypical child through Community Health and Atypical Infant, 1973-74

Without information about the student's experiential and educational background, the advisor and preceptor might feel that her stated purpose was overly ambitious.

Objectives

Except for the rather limited experience in micro-teaching, most students have had minimal, if any, previous exposure to the preparation of behavioral objectives. This component seems to be one of the most difficult aspects of contract preparation. *Preparing Behavioral Objectives* by Major serves as a helpful reference. Generally, students start with statements about what they want to do and work toward refining these statements until they are stated in measurable behaviors. Some students need a considerable amount of assistance from their faculty advisor while others do an amazing job right off.

Our example student who was planning to assist in the organization of a staff development program for those working with retarded children listed the following objectives:

1. Increase knowledge base related to the care and development of the handicapped severely or profoundly retarded child through recognition of the biopsychosocial characteristics of the client population.

2. Utilize the problem solving, decision making process as a framework for identifying staff educational needs related to developmental assessment and intervention of the target population.

3. Participate in the formulation and execution of a program for staff development in areas where educational needs have been identified.

4. Develop and demonstrate skill in the area of staff development through participating in the teaching-learning process.

5. Develop leadership and appreciation of the change process by assuming leadership to bring about change in staff behavior by participating in a program to increase staff knowledge and improve client care.

6. Participate in an evaluation process to measure if expected outcomes were met by plan.

The faculty advisor discusses the stated objectives with advisees to determine if they are obtainable and measureable. The student's objectives are further evaluated to determine if they reflect the faculty prepared objectives for the senior year.

Support from Advisor and Preceptor

Through self-assessment and analysis of individual needs, the student is asked to state in the study contract the kind and extent of assistance expected from advisor and preceptor. Essentially the student contracts for a certain amount of each person's time and expertise. This portion of the contract is somewhat flexible, but serves as a commitment on the part of those involved to meet and discuss, observe, direct, or give whatever assistance the student needs. On the other hand, it is a commitment on the student's part to keep in touch, to consult, collaborate, and continually validate his learning experiences. The student whose contract we are following, asks for the following assistance from faculty advisor and preceptor:

Support of Advisor: The advisor will have weekly conferences with the student for the purpose of consultation and evaluation. The advisor will meet with the preceptor initially, midpoint, and at the end of the project to assess and evaluate the student's progress.

Support of the Preceptor: Mary Ann Smith, R.N.*, the primary preceptor, will have weekly conferences with the student for the purpose of supervision and consultation. She will also provide the opportunity for the student to participate with the Hospital In-Service Training Program teaching team. The student will also meet with Fred Jones and Clara Brown* throughout the semester when appropriate for supervision purposes.

Results Projected

The next item on the contract form deals with results projected. This component requires the student to take a long view of the end results of his project and make a statement about how the proposed project or study will make a difference. Usually this statement speaks to the attainment of new knowledge and skills and how the student expects to use these. If a tangible product is to be produced, this is often mentioned. The above student submitted the following:

Results Projected: The student will have a greater appreciation for strategies involved in the development of a program for staff development. Through participation in this contractual study, the student will demonstrate utilization of the problem solving, decision making process as a framework for diagnosis, implementation, and evaluation of a program for staff development. The student will assume leadership for making change when appropriate and gain a greater appreciation of the change process. The student will increase her knowledge base related to the teaching-learning process and participate effectively with the HIST teaching team.

Activities

Activities the student has planned are listed next in the contract. Here the faculty advisor looks for a close correlation between the stated objectives and the manner in which the student plans to achieve them. The purpose of the project and the results projected

---

*Actual names not used.

should also be reflected in the activities. Furthermore, the amount of time spent should fit within the general framework of the number of clinical hours to which the student is committed. The student whose contract is being followed submitted these activities:

1. The student will attend HIST classes on Tuesdays 1-3 and Thursdays 9-3. The student will teach at least 3 classes and develop 4 lesson plans.

2. In the clinical setting, the student will work with 6 staff members who have completed HIST classes. Two (2) hours will be spent Monday, Tuesday, and Wednesday implementing a staff development program. The student will assist staff to develop new techniques and integrate theory with practice.

3. Intially the student will develop an assessment tool to identify staff educational needs. This total should be complete by October 18th.

4. Each participant will be interviewed. Staff needs will be identified through analysis of the data collected. The student will then formulate a plan for staff development to be submitted by October 25th.

5. At the completion of the project the student shall submit a summary of the contractual study including an evaluation of its effectiveness.

6. The student shall keep an annotated bibliography of readings done to increase knowledge base.

7. A journal of activities shall be kept by the student.

Evaluation

Methods of evaluation have presented problems for students, preceptors, and advisors. Next to preparing objectives, the student has the most difficulty with determining how he or she will be evaluated and upon what evidence a grade will be given. By far the majority of students are content to simply make a statement of willingness to be evaluated and have a grade assigned by their advisor, or the evaluation can be a cooperative endeavor among the three, student, advisor, and preceptor. This solution omits any specification of what exactly will be evaluated. Objectives may be stated and appropriate activities selected but it appears to be difficult to overcome the practice of avoiding self-critique, preferring instead to place oneself at the mercy of a faculty member when it comes to evaluation. Contracts are more often returned to the student to be rewritten because of an inadequate evaluation section than for any other reason. Frustrated and irate students who have worked very hard on their contracts only to have them returned find their way to the department chairperson's office. Second thoughts emerge when the student is asked, "Are you really willing to commit yourself to all of the work you have outlined in this contract and then leave your final evaluation totally to the discretion of your preceptor and advisor?" Further discussion of the evidence to be produced and what the student considers quality work is helpful in developing the evaluation component. While many students are very creative in thinking of ways in which they can demonstrate their knowledge and skill, others have difficulty in connecting what they want to do with evaluation.

An example of the problem with evaluation is evident in this otherwise excellent contract we have used as an example. The student made the following statement under the topic entitled "Method of Evaluation":

> Clinical Experience: Clinical experience shall comprise 60 per cent of the semester grade. The grade will be given by the advisor from data collected from student, preceptor, and journal.

While it is implicit from the student's activities that specific behaviors will be demonstrated and products produced, these were not included in the evaluation.

The contract was returned for a more definitive evaluation plan. The faculty advisor assisted the student in identifying a variety of kinds of evidence which could be used for evaluation. These included observing classroom teaching, lesson plans, peer review of student's performance in staff development, evaluation of assessment tool to be produced, process recordings of interviews, analysis of data collected through interview, the student's self-evaluation, and her journal.

Contract Closure

The study contract is formalized and evidence of agreement by student, preceptor, advisor, and the nursing department is indicated by signatures of all of the above. The department chairperson signs all contracts. Once all signatures have been secured, on four copies of the contract, the student is eligible to register for Nursing 424 A or B: Preceptorship in Nursing. A copy of the contract is kept by the student, one by the preceptor, and one by the advisor. The original copy is retained in the student's record file in the department office.

EXAMPLES OF CONTRACTS

During the 1974-75 academic year, 52 students utilized study contracts to fulfill the requirements for their senior year. A wide variety of activities were undertaken. The faculty is continually amazed at the creativity exhibited by the students. The following examples of contracts recently initiated demonstrate the versatility of the preceptorship approach:

A student who wanted to become expert at family planning began her preparation during the summer prior to initiating her study contract. She enrolled in an extension course offered through the University of California and completed a 7 week course which led to certification as a family planning nurse practioner. This past year, her preceptorship study has included working in a Women's Need Center Clinic doing history taking, breast examinations, pelvic exams, birth control counseling and prescribing, IUD removal and/or insertion, and physician collaboration or referral upon recognition of a deviation from normal. She attends conferences, lectures, and seminars related to family planning. She also does selected reading and prepares an annotated bibliography. She is compiling a clinical diary of her learning progress at the clinic by recording all referrals to the physician, by recording collaborations and/or his follow-up notes, and by recording collaborations with the family planning nurse practitioner-preceptor. Her perceptor observes and comparatively evaluates her history taking and physical examination technique. This student has the cooperation and assistance of both a physician and a nurse preceptor.

Another student has as her goal employment at a state hospital for mentally disturbed children. She has had work experience in acute pediatrics and in psychiatric nursing and is now combining these interests with new knowledge about school health. Her particular focus is play therapy. Last fall, she spent her preceptorship working with a school nurse to identify and incorporate the role of professional practice of a school nurse through involvement by observation and participation in the school system. During that time, she devoted one day to play learning sessions each week. Presently, she is further developing her expertise in play therapy through the following objectives: (1) Identify and incorporate the role of professional practice as a play therapist through involvement performing play learning. (2) Identify at least one child's psychological and/or social problem(s) and make appropriate decisions. (3) Serve as a resource person for school personnel who need help in identifying children's psychological problems in relation to play therapy. (4) Identify within the school community children with social/psychological or physical problems and work with school personnel to help promote solutions to these problems using the problem solving method. (5) Identify resources available concerning children's mental health problems and make appropriate referrals when necessary. (6) Provide for and make change where necessary.

A third student started her project pursuing her area of interest, the health care of families of inmates of San Quentin prison. She began working in a church supported "house" located outside the prison gates. Her objectives included developing a knowledge of the health and psychosocial needs of an underserved population, namely family and friends of prison inmates. She is increasing her knowledge of poor families, disorganized families, and different minority groups, especially Black and Spanish-speaking people. She is also increasing her knowledge and skills in health teaching. She is identifying and implementing screening services when appropriate, such as blood pressure, urine tests for diabetes, etc., updating her knowledge, skills, and analysis of counseling abilities, and furthering the developing of her skills in planning and leadership by direct experience in establishing her project. Finally, she is increasing her ability to function as an interdependent and collaborative health professional.

THE PRECEPTORSHIP SEMINAR

The preceptorship seminar expands the learning potential by focusing on factors common to the experiences of all the students. It serves as a unifying vehicle by integrating theory related to change, leadership self-awareness, self-actualization, and professional practice. Discussions, guided by the instructor, assist the students in the application of theory to practice in a wide variety of settings. Sharing of student experiences which are constructive and rewarding as well as those in which there are problems or discontent is encouraged. The reality of initiating change and providing leadership as students work through their contracts is a strong force for learning how to cope.

Preceptorship Seminar objectives are as follows:

1. Analyze the factors which inhibit or facilitate planned change within the health care system.

2. Demonstrate in the group the ability to optimize one's own performance and to help others optimize their performance.

3. Identify the conflicts, problems, and resistances of nurses assuming leadership roles and positions in nursing.

4. Recognize in the group the relationship between one's own self-awareness and insight and one's effectiveness in working with others.

5. Explore the concept of and develop support systems as part of professional self-actualization.

6. Continue to strive toward personal self-actualization.

7. Identify the factors that inhibit or enhance professional practice within institutions of the health care system.

8. Identify areas of dependence, independence, and interdependence for nursing action within chosen area of study and practice.

EVALUATION OF PRECEPTORSHIP STUDY

Evaluation data of preceptorship study through a study contract has been received from 31 of the 32 seniors who graduated in June 1974. In response to the question, "How important for your own educational development has your senior preceptorship been?" the responses were: No answer - 1; Not important - 1; Somewhat important - 1; Very important - 28.

Another question asked was: "If you were to single out the most stimulating course you have taken at this institution — what is the most exciting in terms of subject matter, perspective, or set of ideas?" Having named the preceptorship, the following are examples of comments made:

1. Offered the chance to be creative while learning.
2. I got into an area that I wanted.
3. I was allowed to develop the course to fit my needs and interests including bibliography.
4. The course was designed by me in an area I wanted to learn more about.
5. Increased awareness and involvement in an actual research study.

The faculty believe that preceptorship through study contract provides an excellent means for teaching the behaviors which characterize professional nursing, provides a learning mode which appeals to adults, and assists in the development of an area of expertise. They are excited about the ingenuity and creativity of many of the contracts and the excellence of student achievements. Most faculty are also involved in teaching juniors and find their responsibilities as senior advisor a rewarding opportunity to follow individual student progress.

Although faculty are enthusiastic about this approach to the teaching-learning process, a number of problems can still be identified. Driving time to visit students and preceptors located miles away is one of them. Also, weekly conferences with each student are time consuming, especially at the beginning of the school year when students need considerable support in their new venture.

The 1975 graduating class is the second senior class, the second class to utilize contractual study. The first year could only be described as chaotic. Thirty-two of the first graduating class of 39 were involved in preceptorships, the remaining seven were enrolled in the family nurse practitioner preceptorship. Descriptions of contractual study were distributed to the students. Lists of faculty with their interests and expertise were distributed. Many individual and group discussions were held to assist students with contract preparation. Because of the demands on faculty for curriculum development associated with a new program, the department chairperson assumed responsibility for advising all of the students. Each contract required individual conferences and all during the first summer students were dropping in to ask for contract review or critique.

At that time, senior year objectives were the only guidelines available. Preceptorship objectives and seminar objectives had not yet been decided upon by the faculty. Orientation of preceptors and agencies involved hours of one-to-one contact and telephone conversations. Amazingly the idea was well received by the community. The students did a most effective job of selling themselves and their proposals. Agency contracts presented another problem. Although eager to cooperate, agencies required contracts which were acceptable to them as well as to the California State College and University System. Devising such mutually acceptable contracts required time and ingenuity. Technicalities regarding liability, space, staff, student, and faculty had to be dealt with. A preceptorship contract was drafted based on those used by junior students placed in community health agencies and hospitals. Once the contract was duly executed, a follow-up letter was sent to the agency giving the names of the student, instructor, and preceptor. A copy of the planned preceptorship contract written by the student was also enclosed.

The time factor continues to be another problem in dealing with agencies. Since most of the students complete their contracts late in the spring or during the summer, the nursing department is hampered in their negotiations by the absence of administrators on vacation. Further, the absence of faculty during the summer limits student progress unless a fairly firm agreement has been reached prior to the end of the spring semester.

This year the third class of seniors found the faculty better prepared. All faculty will have served as advisor to one or more students and will have gained experience in the process. With 32 students the first year and 52 the second year, more agencies within the community are aware of the preceptorship study option and less orientation is required. For many of the agencies, initial contracts were executed which are automatically renewable and thus less work is required. Preceptorship and seminar objectives are much better refined. A preceptorship handbook was prepared for the fall 1974 semester and was given to each new preceptor. This handbook includes the program philosophy, purposes, and objectives. There is a section which describes preceptorship study. Another section describes the role of the preceptor, the student, and the faculty advisor. A final section describes, in general, how contract evaluation is negotiated between student, preceptor, and advisor. There is also a contract form to be used as a sample in reviewing the student's project.

Perhaps the most helpful addition is the one unit course preceptorship. This course was developed and offered as an elective first during the spring 1975 semester. Although it is not required, almost all of the students enrolled in the class. The class was divided into four seminar sections of approximately 20 students. The faculty responsible for teaching the class guided the students through the entire contract preparation process. Students selected a faculty advisor, as

100

in previous years, but the faculty believes that many hours of one-to-one advising would be eliminated through group discussion in the seminars and that all students would move ahead with a clearer understanding of what was to be done. The phases of contract development which serve as the organizing framework for the course include knowledge and skills generalizable to the planning process in curriculum, research, and project proposal development.

RECOMMENDATIONS FOR PLANNING

Based on the evaluation of our experience with preceptorship study, the California State College, Sonoma nursing faculty recommend that adequate planning time be arranged. In most instances, the use of preceptorship study for nursing is unfamiliar to the institution, the community, the student, and to some degree, the faculty. It is not unreasonable to begin planning one year in advance of preceptorship placement.

1. Gain Acceptance from the College

Investigate college policies regarding field work, independent study, internships, and similar modes of teaching. If guidelines are established which are compatible, use them. Preceptorship study at Sonoma most nearly fits supervised field work done by student teachers. The student-faculty ratio used by the education department is the same as that used by the nursing department. Registration procedures may need to be altered to provide class cards in such a manner that a student may enroll for a range of units as indicated by the individual contracts.

2. Orient the Community

Off campus, clinical agencies and possible preceptors must be oriented. Use every opportunity to describe preceptorship study when speaking to community groups. Be prepared to answer questions about whether the student will be employed, whether the preceptor will be paid, and what is the responsibility of the agency. Questions related to malpractice insurance and workman's compensation are often raised.

3. Develop and Initiate Contracts

Particular attention should be devoted to arranging agency contracts. Official institutions usually request a formal contract. Individuals and nonofficial agencies may be content with a letter from the department of nursing outlining the conditions under which the preceptorship will be conducted. At Sonoma, some standardized contracts were in use but nursing presents some unique problems because of the practice component and liability factor. We now use two forms, one intended

101

for groups of students scheduled on a regular basis for community health, and the other designed especially for preceptorships. The same preceptorship contract form can be used for all preceptorship students without alteration. Each contract is initiated for one year with the condition that it will be automatically renewed for our additional years. Once contracts are established, the task of renewing for successive students presents a minimal task.

4. Develop Guidelines for Faculty

Early in the program it was decided that as many of the faculty as possible would be involved in the preceptorships. Fundamentally, two reasons supported this decision. First, we felt that by making many faculty available for preceptorship advising, the students would be offered a wider choice of educational backgrounds, work experiences, and special interests. Second, we believed that having faculty involved in some way in both first and second year course work promotes cohesiveness in the curriculum. Faculty teaching assignments at Sonoma consists of 12 weighted teaching units and this usually includes responsibility for two or more senior preceptorship students.

Another decision which the department had to make was in regard to the distance to be traveled by faculty advisors. The Sonoma service area covers approximately 9,000 square miles. Not only is the cost of mileage a concern, but time spent traveling can also be costly when students select agencies located in the far corners of the area. This problem is further complicated when students want to establish their preceptorships outside the service area. This year the department endorsed a policy stating that students must select an agency located within the service area. Requests for agencies outside the service area are received through petition and considered when evidence is presented by the student that the particular experience sought cannot be obtained within the service area of the college. These requests are discussed with the faculty advisor. If a compromise cannot be worked out, the student may need to write a new contract.

General guidelines are helpful to faculty as they establish their relationships and responsibility to students. Faculty deal with Second Step students in genuinely collaborative relationships. They tend to work together in a manner which relects the uniqueness of the individual faculty member involved and the particular goals the student is attempting to achieve. Our guidelines to faculty include the recommendation that faculty visit with the preceptor at least at the beginning, mid-semester, and the end of the semester for the final evaluation.

102

5. Formulate Objectives and Evaluation Tools

With such a wide variety of contracts and diversity among the learning experiences, it is necessary to formulate clearly defined objectives for preceptorship study which are compatible with program objectives. These serve as guidelines to faculty, students, and preceptors not only for contract development but also for evaluation. The preceptorship objectives stated earlier reflect the program goals. They are further developed with subobjectives which indicate levels of competencies and thus serve as guides for contract evaluation. Each subobjective is given a percentage weight.

Evaluation is a cooperative venture between student, preceptor, and faculty advisor. It is difficult at best, but is made much easier if leveled objectives have been prepared.

6. Plan a Contract Preparation Seminar

We highly recommend that a class, a series of workshops, or some planned presentations be offered to students to assist in contract preparation. Course evaluations reported the contract preparation seminar to be extremely helpful. Some students felt that the time devoted to the seminar was excessive, others could have used more. Starting with the fall 1975 semester, the Second Step Program will have 65 seniors involved in preceptorships. Without the preceptorship seminar, the task would have been insurmountable. A possible alternative to a regularly scheduled class would be a series of mini-workshops for the large group and drop-in conferences scheduled weekly.

SUMMARY

This chapter has presented a unique method of meeting the highly diverse learning needs of registered nurses working toward baccalaureate degrees in a second step program. The approach, called Preceptorship Study by the nursing faculty at California State College, Sonoma, has been discussed in terms of its background and rationale and its mode of operation. In short, we have attempted to offer the kind of analysis suggested in the following statement by Christian Bay:

> If individual behavior normally is a series of compromises between what the person would most want to do and what appears socially expected of him, then it may be said that an analysis of the relevant roles and incentives is the most powerful approach.[23]

Hopefully, the story of our solutions and our errors will be of value to other teachers interested in a similar approach.

REFERENCES

1. Kramer, Marlene: Role Conceptions of Baccalaureate Nurses and Success in Hospital Nursing. *Nursing Research* 19:428, 1970.
2. Waters, Verle, et al.: Technical and Professional Nursing: An Exploratory Study. *Nursing Research* 21:124, 1972.
3. Johnson, Dorothy E.: Professional Practice in Nursing, in *The Shifting Scene—Directions for Practice*. Papers presented at 23rd conference of Council of Member Agencies of Department of Baccalaureate and Higher Degree Programs held in New York, May 5-7, 1967. New York, Department of Baccalaureate and Higher Degree Programs, National League for Nursing, 1967, pp. 26-34.
4. Bailey, June, et al.: A New Approach to Curriculum Development. University of California School of Nursing, San Francisco. *Nursing Outlook* 14:33, 1966.
5. Johnson, Dorothy E.: Competence in Practice: Technical and Professional. *Nursing Outlook* 14:30, 1966.
6. *Ibid.*
7. Bailey, *op. cit.*
8. Tschudin, Mary S.: Educational Preparation Needed by the Nurse in the Future. *Nursing Outlook* 12:32, 1964.
9. Johnson, Dorothy E.: Professional Practice and Specialization in Nursing. *Image* Vol. 2, No. 3, 1968.
10. Tschudin, *op. cit.*
11. Quint, Jeanne C.: Role Models and the Professional Nurse Indentity. *Journal of Nursing Education* 6:11, 1967.
12. Johnson, *op. cit.*, citation #3.
13. Tschudin, *op. cit.*
14. Rogers, Martha: *Educational Revolution in Nursing*. Macmillan, New York, 1961.
15. Waters, *op. cit.*
16. California Nurses' Association: *Nursing Practice* I/S, 1971.
17. Waters, *op. cit.*
18. Johnson, *op. cit.*, citation #9.
19. Lysaught, Jerome P.: National Commission for the Study of Nursing and Nursing Education. *An Abstract for Action.* McGraw-Hill, New York, 1970.
20. National League for Nursing: *Position on Nursing Education*, 1970.
21. Matheney, Ruth: Technical Nursing Practice, in *The Shifting Scene—Directions for Practice*. Papers presented at 23rd conference of Council of Member Agencies of Department of Baccalaureate and Higher Degree Programs held in New York, May 5-7, 1967. New York, Department of Baccalaureate and Higher Degree Programs, National League for Nursing, 1967, pp. 17-25.
22. Excerpts from a preceptorship contract in staff development, prepared by Rosemary Schmidt, R.N., CSCS class of 1975.
23. Sanford, Nevitt: *The American College.* John Wiley and Sons, Inc. New York, 1966, p. 983.

CHAPTER 6

Family Nurse Practitioner Preparation at the Baccalaureate Level

Elizabeth Monninger, R.N., M.S., Leonide L. Martin, R.N., M.S., F.N.P., and Marilyn Little, M.A.

The concept of the nurse practitioner emerged in the 1960s as a result of a number of related forces. A shortage of health care personnel, particularly physicians, created an increasing gap in meeting health needs of a growing population. Increased concern about inequities in the social system focused attention on the maldistribution of health care services to the poor and to minority groups. Increasing awareness of social responsibility fostered the attitude that health care was a right of the people, not a privilege for the few who could afford it. The great groundswell for racial and sexual equality created a climate for change in which relationships between various groups could be re-examined and opportunity for growth and fuller realization of potentials could be pursued.

The need for more health workers and for better utilization of those already in the field was clearly apparent. The idea of expanding the roles of various types of health workers began to gain advocates in nursing, medicine, pharmacy, dentistry, psychology, and others. In the mid-1960s, physicians and nurses in several locations began formally exploring ways in which nurses could assume more direct responsibility and decision-making in providing care to certain types of patients. The basic reasons for this was to improve the quality and availability of care, a concern which both nurses and physicians shared. Widespread dissatisfaction with health care among consumers and professionals led to research and demonstration programs by Lewis and Resnick,[1] Connelly,[2] Ford,[3] Silver,[4] and their coworkers, designed to test the acceptability, feasibility, and consequences of this new approach for the quality of care. These studies and others in the late 1960s[5,6] supported the concept that the expanded role of the nurse contributed to an increased level of satisfaction with care, was of comparable quality medically, was acceptable to patients, and promised to be less costly.

The report by Jerome Lysaught in 1970[7] and that of the Department of Health, Education and Welfare in 1971[8] also recommended extending the scope of nursing practice. Definitions of primary care, functions, knowledge, and skills of nurses assuming responsibility for primary cares, the articulation between medicine and nursing, and the need for legislative action to change health practice acts were discussed in these reports. The HEW report also gave impetus to a variety of programs which prepared nurses for extended role practice. Initially most of these programs were based in service institutions or continuing education departments of colleges and universities, and they varied greatly in type, length, and content. Most early programs were initiated and conducted by physicians, a necessity because of the absence of nurses prepared to instruct in areas of medical knowledge. As more nurses became prepared for extended role practice, and as this practice became more accepted within nursing, there was increasing involvement of nurse educators and nursing programs in the preparation of nurse practitioners.

In the mid-1970s, there is a strong trend toward incorporation of nurse practitioner programs into collegiate based nursing departments. Also, standardization of education through accreditation of programs and certification of graduates is occurring. The nurse practice acts of many states have been broadened to include extended nursing functions. Although there is some variation in the definition of nurse practitioner, a common acceptance of this term seems to have spread nation-wide. The California Nurses' Association *Glossary of Terms* provides this definition:

Nurse practitioners are registered nurses with additional skills in physical diagnosis, psychosocial assessment, and management of health-illness needs in primary care; who have been prepared in formalized programs affiliated with institutions of higher learning. The extended role of the nurse practitioner integrates health maintenance, disease prevention, physical diagnosis, and treatment of common episodic and chronic problems in primary care with equal empahsis on health teaching and disease management.[9]

Primary care generally refers to a person's first contact with the health care system in any given episode of illness and longitudinal responsibility for continuance of care, and includes maintenance of health, evaluation and management of illness, and appropriate referrals. Nurse practitioners work in a colleague relationship with physicians, providing care within the health care system as part of a team. The nurse practitioner can safely and effectively function in a variety of settings, such as clinics, health centers, physicians' offices, industries, homes, schools, and acute care settings.[10]

106

THE SECOND STEP PROGRAM AND NURSE PRACTITIONER PREPARATION

The philosophy of nurse practitioner education held by this faculty is that nurse practitioner preparation should be within an organized and accredited nursing program. A career ladder program such as the Second Step Program is a natural setting for the preparation of extended role nurses. The purpose of the program is to build upon basic nursing education, enabling the student to broaden and deepen knowledge and skills, pursue individualized areas of interest, and develop greater professionalism. Nurse practitioner preparation has generally been viewed as post-basic education, requiring prior licensure as an RN. A baccalaureate program enrolling only RNs is preferable to the generic program for Family Nurse Practitioner (FNP) preparation. As RN students have already had basic nursing preparation, as well as nursing experience, this background helps them identify themselves as nurses and operate effectively within the health care system. Generic students not only need to acquire their basic nursing education, but also need role models to begin to build their professional self-concept. In other nursing practice many role models are available and contribute to the building of this process. However, the scarcity of FNPs in the community at this time, we believe, would make the professional developmental process a difficult one for the basic student.

Although the initial nurse practitioner pilot programs were developed in other types of settings, it seems that it is now time for nurse practitioner preparation to become related to the mainstream of nursing education. A new role such as FNP is more quickly accepted by the nursing profession if knowledge and experiences can be shared with other students who will be involved in nursing practice. Students matriculated in a college have the advantage of general college resources and activities; college credit can be transferred to other schools. In addition, there are more available related courses that help students transfer knowledge, make relationships, and offer support to the FNP curriculum. Because all Sonoma nursing students are enrolled in junior year courses, the cost factor in preparing a small group of FNP students is reduced. Only one year of specialized preparation with specially trained instructors is needed.

The Family Nurse Practitioner (FNP) Preceptorship

The FNP preceptorship is a senior year option to prepare nurses for expanded role practice within the Second Step Program. It is a two semester, 16 unit planned curriculum in the senior year which offers concurrent classroom study and supervised clinical practice. The goal of the course is to prepare a registered nurse to collaborate with other health care professionals in providing primary care for clients of all ages. Students are given special preparation in health maintenance, physical diagnosis, and treatment of common acute and chronic health problems; this specialized preparation overlaps some responsibilities usually assumed by physicians but maintains a nursing approach with emphasis on teaching and counseling of individuals and families.

Within the Second Step Program, several junior year courses provide support which makes FNP preparation within a two semester sequence possible. Science Principles Applied to Human Phenomena, a three unit required course, promotes the integration and application of physiologic and pathophysiologic concepts to cross-clinical nursing. The focus of the course is upon basic scientific considerations; examination of the patient, integration of concepts, and diagnosis. Experience is provided in applying this knowledge to clients' health problems. Therefore, students come to the FNP preceptorship with a fresh understanding of pathologic processes to use in their study of diagnosis and treatment of health problems. In addition, all junior students acquire physical examination skills in a one credit course taken concurrently with Science Principles. These skills help the student understand normal physiology and disease processes; for example, listening to the sound of a heart murmur helps one understand the anatomy, physiology, and pathology involved. When the student enters the FNP preceptorship, he or she has already learned to relate physical findings to physiology, and curiosity has been aroused about the relationship of skills and scientific rationale to medical treatment.

Community Health constitutes a large segment of the junior year and forms a broad base for primary care practice. When students enroll in CSCS, most have little or no experience outside the hospital setting. By learning to plan and give care to families, assess community services, and become involved in developing community resources, students have already begun expanding their nursing roles. More specifically, the problem-oriented recording process is introduced in community health, in addition to the gathering and analysis of patient histories. All these knowledges and skills provide a firm basis for FNP practice, reduce time needed for the FNP preceptorship, as well as relate the new FNP role to other areas of nursing. Other courses also contribute specific preparation which enhances FNP practice. Interaction and Change, a course in communications, helps students build a repertoire of skills needed for relating to individuals and groups. Also, by developing a better understanding of self, the nurse is able to give support to clients and counsel more effectively. Group work is introduced in the second semester of the junior year; this experience helps develop ideas for FNPs to introduce into primary care. For example, if an FNP is comfortable relating to a group or is proficient in leading a group discussion, then experimentation with such primary care methods as a cluster visit is more likely.[11]

The course on Health and Culture explores beliefs and practices which are related to health behaviors in a variety of subcultural and ethnic groups. Clients of several different cultures may live in one community and seek service at the same health care institution, thus an understanding of unique attitudes toward health and illness and factors influencing health behavior is essential for the nurse. Such understanding allows health care planning according to individual needs.

The goal of the FNP preceptorship is to prepare a registered nurse student to function at a beginning level as a family nurse practitioner. The student is also expected to integrate professional attitudes and gain an appreciation of leadership and the change process (see Table 1). The baccalaureate degree can then serve as a basis for postgraduate study in teaching, research, administration, or further clinical specialization.

FAMILY NURSE PRACTITIONER CURRICULUM DEVELOPMENT

Establishment of the Program

The inception of the FNP project grew out of a recognition of health needs of the area. The six North Bay counties served by the college were expected to experience great population and economic growth in the years ahead. Shortages and maldistributions of health care personnel were predicted. CSCS, as the only state college serving this region, was in a position to contribute along with other health disciplines to the solution of these problems by preparing nurses as FNPs.

The basic relief of the faculty about future directions of nursing practice was compatible with the desire to experiment with a project for FNP preparation at the baccalaureate level, and funding was sought which would provide this opportunity. Preparation of a proposal to W.K. Kellogg Foundation for support in establishing the FNP preceptoship within the Second Step baccalaureate curriculum was begun in 1972. The Department of Nursing worked closely with the medical staff of the Family Practice Residency Program at Sonoma County Community Hospital during the planning period. Established to provide a three year family practice residency for physicians interested in rural practice, the Family Practice Center is organized to resemble private group practice. It is divided into three modules, in which several residents develop their own practices consisting of individuals and families who are seen regularly by the same physician. As in

Table 1. Family nurse practitioner terminal objectives

Upon completion of this course the FNP graduate will:

I. In physical diagnosis and the nurse practitioner assessment process:
 A. Perform thorough screening physical examination on clients of all age groups and both sexes.
 B. Utilize the instruments and techniques of physical diagnosis correctly to obtain pertinent data from all systems.
 C. Interpret findings from the physical examination accurately, identifying normal, normal variant, and pathologic findings.
 D. Utilize a systematic approach for collection of complete and appropriate historic data from physiologic, psychological and social parameters.
 E. Interpret correctly the significance of common laboratory tests and other diagnostic aids.
 F. Obtain appropriate episodic history and perform indicated examination of pertinent systems relative to the problem identified.
 G. Order appropriate laboratory tests and other diagnostic aids as indicated for the problem identified.

II. In management of health/illness conditions:
 A. Undertake health maintenance actions whenever feasible in the care of clients.
 B. Promote health maintenance and illness prevention through identification of health hazards and education of clients, including counseling and preventive treatment for potential or actual problems identified.
 C. Perform pertinent examinations and tests for health maintenance of different ages and sexes.
 D. Manage the care of acute minor illnesses and injuries, stabilized chronic illnesses, common episodic conditions, prenatal, postnatal and well child care, family planning, and other primary care for all types of clients seen in family practice.
 E. Participate in the management of complex problems although not assuming primary responsibility.
 F. Record accurately and pertinently using problem oriented recording.

III. In role identify and professional relationships:
 A. Identify self as a Family Nurse Practitioner with confidence in ability to carry out this role on a beginning level.
 B. Interpret the Family Practitioner role to clients, professional colleagues, other related groups, and the public.
 C. Identify own level of comfort with independent functions and when these are appropriate.
 D. Consult appropriately with other professionals for good management of the client's problems, presenting cases clearly and succinctly.
 E. Practice in interdependent relationship with physician in the management of complex problems.

110

IV. Integrate professional attitudes:
   A. Be committed to the need for life-long learning and assume responsibility for own learning needs.
   B. Accept responsibility for own professional decisions and be accountable for actions taken.
   C. Expect authority within the practice setting concomitant with responsibilities.
   D. Participate in definition and refinement of nurse practitioner role and standard setting for quality health care through special groups, professional organizations, or committees both in and outside the practice setting.
   E. Identify the personal meaning of self-actualization and pursue this partly through professional practice.

V. Recognize the importance of change and her or his role in leadership:
   A. Identify the need for change.
   B. Use theories of change and leadership to assess readiness, support systems, timing, and possible consequences or outcomes.
   C. Implement change when possible and evaluate results.

---

group practice, residents cover each others' patients when the primary physician is on a special service or on vacation. The residents assume full responsibility for primary and secondary (hospitalization) care for their patients, with the medical teaching staff and community specialists available for consultation.

Joint projects were funded by Kellogg to the Department of Nursing and the Family Practice Residency Program. Beginning in 1973, the grants were for a three year period. The major objective of the two projects was to demonstrate preparation of family nurse practitioners and family physicians in congruent roles. Grant funds provided support for a project coordinator and two instructors to function in dual roles as instructor at CSCS and clinician at the Family Practice Center. The FNP faculty were to work with two to three family practice residents, teaching the physicians about the nurse practitioner role and jointly developing a team approach to primary health care. FNP faculty also were responsible for developing and implementing the FNP preceptorship at CSCS, and the third year residents served as preceptors for students enrolled in the FNP courses.

Funds from the Kellogg grant also helped provide materials, hardware, and software for the FNP curriculum. In addition, a physical assessment laboratory and self-paced multimedia learning laboratory were developed from grant funds, and are utilized by junior as well as FNP students.

Student Selection

At the end of the junior year students are selected to participate in the FNP preceptorship. A selection process which is necessary because of limited clinical placement enables the faculty to assess the students' abilities and needs. Junior year faculty submit information regarding students' abilities to collect data, plan, intervene, and evaluate nursing care. An evaluation of level of autonomy and self-direction is also made. Information is considered relating to the students' abilities in applying physiologic concepts to nursing problems in Science-Principles. In addition, written, verbal, and nonverbal communication skills are evaluated. Therefore, areas considered important for a successful FNP student are: application of the nursing process, application of physiologic concepts, interpersonal relationships, and autonomy and self-direction.

While the evaluation of the junior year performance is crucial, other data about the applicant is also relevant. The students are asked to submit information about their past nursing experience, describe their self-concept as a health professional, and as an FNP, in addition to formulating their future nursing plans. This gives the faculty a concept of the student's educational needs and plans for using their FNP preparation.

Two interviewers, usually an instructor and senior student, meet with each student to review the background material in more detail; the student may then offer additional information or clarify. Following the interview, the interviewers formulate their impressions, which are submitted to the full selection committee.

The final step in the selection process is the consideration of all collected data by the selection committee, composed of students and faculty. Both FNP and non-FNP senior students and faculty members are involved, allowing input into the FNP preceptorship from other areas within the nursing department. This selection process permits limiting the number of FNP students to the clinical facilities available to train them, and identifying students most likely to successfully complete the program.

Characteristics of FNP Students

The first step toward selection is made by the student. By indicating interest in the program, the selection process is initiated. Since the nurse practitioner role is still rather new and different from other nursing roles, the question arises whether or not the student who selects this program differs in any way from other student peers.

Earlier research by Martha Sturm White at the University of California at San Francisco has shown that nurse practitioner students differ from other nursing students on a number of variables as measured by several different instruments, including the Edwards Personal Preference Schedule, the Personal Orientation Inventory, and the California Psychological Inventory.[12] According to her studies, nurse practitioner students are more autonomous, dominant, outgoing, and higher in achievement orientation.

Upon entrance to our program, however, no significant differences were found between the nurse practitioner students and the other students in the class, as measured by the Omnibus Presonality Inventory. Some interesting differences were found in responses to the Inventory of Professional Nursing Values, a scale developed by Fred Davis and Virginia L. Olesen.[13] This scale contains items describing stereotyped nursing ideals, traditional views, contemporary views, and characteristics of nursing as an occupation. It contrasts the image which the student has formed of the nursing profession with the characteristics of nursing which are important to the student personally. The image a nurse may form of the profession is normally built upon personal experiences with physicians and nurses, as well as perceptions of feedback from family, friends, and health care personnel. The characteristics of the profession chosen as important to the self personally may be those qualities of the profession which are felt to be important for personal needs. It is possible, of course, for a student's image of nursing to be quite different from pesonal values held. Large differences, however, may indicate dissonance and may point to areas of conflict within the student.

As shown by Table 2, there are many similarities between the practitioner students and their classmates at the time of entry to the program. On all items in the stereotyped and traditional categories both groups of students revealed their image of nursing as more traditional than their personal ideals. The large differences between these scores, for example on such items as "clear-cut lines of authority" and "hard work," show that the nursing students are rejecting what they consider to be the socially accepted image of nursing. Perhaps part of their motivation for returning to school is this rejection of nursing as it is normally expected to be practiced and their search for an expression of the profession which may be more satisfying to them personally. Further dissatisfaction is implied in their discrepancy scores on items indicating contemporary views of nursing work. In this category they indicate nursing has not traditionally been regarded as a profession requiring originality, creativity, imagination, or innovation. These qualities are, however, most important to them personally as students. Clearly, both groups of student nurses feel they are seeking work satisfactions which are quite different from those traditionally expected in nursing.

Although both groups of student nurses indicate a desire to move from the more traditional values to contemporary values, there are several rather revealing differences between the groups in their responses to specific items. Differences in scores for those students

Table 2. Professional values of nursing students: Family nurse practitioner students and other nursing students who upon entry to the baccalaureate program attributed items to nursing compared with those who said items were important to self*

Characteristics	Family nurse practitioner students (N = 18) (nos. in percent)			Other nursing students (N = 87) (nos. in percent)		
	Nursing	Self	Difference	Nursing	Self	Difference
Stereotyped nursing ideals						
Dedicated service to humanity	78	50	-28	74	54	-20
Moving ritual and ceremony	22	0	-22	21	1	-20
Religious inspiration and calling	33	17	-16	15	10	-5
Traditional views of nursing work						
High technical skill	83	67	-16	75	52	-23
Emotional control and restraint	78	56	-22	74	40	-24
Human drama and excitement	72	22	-50	54	43	-11
Clear-cut lines of authority	89	17	-72	72	21	-51
Order and routine	89	44	-45	84	32	-52
Hard work	94	28	-66	82	33	-49
Meticulousness	50	34	-16	57	23	-34
Close supervision and direction	72	11	-61	47	13	-34
Clearly defined work tasks—each person responsible for her job and her job alone	44	22	-22	41	6	-35

Contemporary views of nursing work

Demonstrating care and concern for others in an immediate and tangible way†	83	78	− 5	82	78	− 4
Originality and creativity	34	67	+33	34	74	+40
Exercise of imagination and insight	56	67	+11	41	87	+46
Solid intellectual content	44	56	+12	41	52	+11
Frequent innovation in the solution of problems	78	72	− 6	61	85	+24

Characteristics of nursing as an occupation

An occupation highly respected in the community	89	39	−50	68	34	−34
Job security	83	61	−22	68	37	−31

*This scale was originally developed and used in a study of nursing students at the University of California, San Francisco. Results from this study were published in *The Silent Dialogue, A Study in the Social Psychology of Professional Socialization*, by Virginia L. Olesen and Elvi W. Whittaker. Jossey-Bass Inc., San Francisco, 1968, pp. 123-131.
†In the original scale this item was included under *Stereotyped nursing ideals.*

who are not nurse practitioners are highest on those items describing the skills or tasks required of nurses, i.e., high technical skill, order and routine, meticulousness, and clearly defined work tasks. These students may be reacting to a view of nursing which emphasizes the nurse as a skilled technician, meticulous, precise, and careful in following orders on specified tasks. It is possible they have been quite frustrated with the regimentation of their work; they are now seeking preparation for a work experience which will hopefully allow them greater freedom and opportunity to be imaginative and innovative.

The nurse practitioner students, however, are somewhat more tolerant of the regimentation of the task and the emotional control and restraint needed to maintain the discipline of their work. For them the difficulty lies in their acceptance of the authority and supervision which they feel is normally required of nurses. Perhaps for these students it is the social structure within the profession which is most objectionable. They are frustrated with the limits placed upon them by authority and desire to be more independent and free of these social constraints. The nurse practitioner role may, therefore, be appealing to them as they perceive it offers an opportunity to work more directly and independently with the patient and to relate to the physician as a colleague or peer rather than as a subordinate. For these nurses, changes, if there are to be any, must come within the social structure of the profession.

Curriculum Content

The FNP preceptorship is a structured two semester course, consisting of three units of didactic with five units (15 hours per week) of clinical experience per semester taken concurrently. In keeping with the preceptorship requirements of all seniors, students develop a contract which proposes objectives, learning experiences, and evaluation for an area of interest or need which is not met through the course objectives. For instance, a student may propose to spend part of the clinical time in the care of elderly persons or in an emergency room setting. Students will develop their own objective for the experience and plan with the faculty how they will be evaluated for that portion of the experience. A part of the student's time and grade will be allotted to the contractual experience.

The goal of the beginning portion of the FNP course is preparation of the student for basic practice before beginning experience with her or his preceptor. This portion is referred to as "core curriculum" and is felt by the faculty to be basic knowledge for all FNP practice. The core curriculum provides such knowledge and skills as physical assessment, history taking, and health maintenance for the FNP. Initially, junior year physical assessment skills are reviewed and refined, along with the introduction of additional skills such as the abdominal, joint, and pelvic examinations. This is done with

116

extensive use of videotapes and laboratory sessions in which faculty demonstrates skills and students practice with one another and the faculty. Three hour laboratory sessions are held twice weekly for the first two weeks in the semester. Previously learned techniques are recalled quickly, leaving more time for students to practice new skills. After mastering the performance of an examination, the variety of normal findings and the identification of abnormal findings are taught. For instance, the tympanic membrane has a variety of normal appearances and the FNP must be cognizant of the variations.[14] Therefore, one goal of the core curriculum in relation to physical assessment is to differentiate between normal and abnormal physical findings. In addition the student is expected to be able to organize and perform a complete physical examination.

After the first two weeks, clinics are sponsored by the Department of Nursing and physical examinations are offered free of charge to college students and their families. Nursing students then may practice on an essentially normal population in order to gain self-confidence and increased proficiency. During both the laboratory sessions and physical examination clinics, faculty closely observes and supervises students along with a physician consultant. We are able to provide immediate feedback to help students improve rapidly.

In the following weeks a variety of regular laboratory experiences are scheduled. Students do physical examinations for employees of the County Administration and State Hospitals. Physical examinations are given in nursery schools and pediatric clinics sponsored by the nursing department. Hospital rounds with a physician consultant enable students to identify abnormal physical findings.

In conjunction with review and practice of physical examination skills, the students learn to collect an accurate, appropriate, and comprehensive history. Students who have had some nursing experience may tend to focus upon new skills of physical assessment and underestimate the correlation of these skills with collection of the patient's history. The importance of this correlation cannot be overestimated because it is essential to the treatment of health problems. Like Sherlock Holmes, the FNP needs skills in eliciting information and the ability to deduce, analyze, and decide what is and what is not relevant.

In seminar discussions, communication skills are reviewed to help the student use previously learned skills in patient interviews. In addition, organization of material in a problem oriented format is reviewed and applied to the primary care setting. Students are then required to obtain at least one complete history per week from peers, family, and friends. These histories are reviewed by faculty and discussed in seminars. As the semester continues, episodic histories are emphasized, since they are more difficult to develop. In episodic histories, students must demonstrate an understanding of pertinent physiologic and pathologic processes, as well as show continuity or flow of reasoning in collection of data.

Another portion of the core curriculum essential to all FNP practice is that of health maintenance. It is introduced after the student has mastered physical examinations and is gaining skill in obtaining histories. Again, past experience and knowledge are related, and the student transfers this experience. Nurses are traditionally oriented to help clients cope with health problems. Therefore health maintenance in primary care is an area where FNPs can use their basic nursing preparation to the best advantage. Health risks can be identified from information elicited by history and physical examination. The FNP must learn to assume responsibility for the initiation of a plan of teaching about prevention along with a plan for preventing which is related to that specific patient's health risks. For example, information about eating habits, exercise, smoking and alcohol consumption habits, family history, and blood pressure are obtained by history and physical examination. The FNP needs to be aware of the predominent health hazards of the population with corresponding characteristics to identify each patient's particular health hazards, and to develop and carry out a plan of prevention with the patient.

In addition, classes and seminars include discussions related to the management of normal pregnancies and postpartum patients, well-child care, family planning, and family counseling. Models and multimedia materials, including modules, are available in the physical assessment lab for practice.

The core curriculum is completed by the middle of the first semester at which time the student begins limited clinical experience and curriculum shifts to health problems. These basic skills and knowledge form a framework for assessing and treating health problems.

During the second semester classroom discussion focuses on common acute and chronic health problems of adults and children. Faculty and students exchange examples from their experiences with patients in the discussion of such problems as hypertension, anemia, arteriosclerotic heart disease, and diabetes.

During this semester students also work with preceptors who help operationalize theoretical knowledge and provide clinical experiences. Practicing FNPs and family physicians act as role models and teachers and share patients with the student. Since there are very few nurse practitioners working in the community, preceptors are primarily physicians.

In an effort to identify the most supportive learning situations, we seek physicians who are interested in teaching, who believe in the team concept of delivering health care, and who express interest in the development of the nurse practitioner role. Family physicians whose practice includes all age groups and a variety of health problems offer better learning situations. An established family practice situated in a heterogeneous neighborhood provides an ideal opportunity for learning primary care. Sometimes, however, these situations are not available. Combining several specialized experiences such as a pediatrics clinic, an obstetric office experience, and a Veteran's Administration out-patient department provides an alternative solution. This latter combination of clinical opportunities makes it necessary for the student to extract skills and experiences from each setting. The faculty supervisor in this situation needs to help the students synthesize these varied experiences into a coherent role. Of great importance, too, is the interest and attitude of the preceptor in creating a positive experience for the student.

Locating interested preceptors can be a time consuming but interesting experience for faculty. We believe that faculty and students should work together in identifying preceptors. This procedure is different from many nurse practitioner programs which require students to have a commitment from preceptors before being accepted to the program. This latter arrangement may lead to future employment of the nurse practitioner student which is an advantage. It may also create a situation in which the objectives and needs of the office supercede learning needs. As an employee, the FNP is more obligated to adapt to the situation and provide those services considered useful by the physician employer. She is then not as free to seek those experiences which may possess optimal learning value. In addition, those nurses who begin working in an office as an RN may find it more difficult to accomplish a role change and assume the new responsibilities of a nurse practitioner. Expectations have not been established for the new student practitioner who is, therefore, more free to create her or his own role. Physicians who are not willing to commit themselves to the employment of a nurse practitioner may be willing to accept the FNP as a student. Through the preceptorship experience, the nursing student has the opportunity to demonstrate the role and educate the physician to the contributions which a nurse practitioner may make to his practice.

Before the student goes into a clinical setting, the faculty meets with prospective preceptors to discuss expectations. We explain that we would like students to have the opportunity to treat patients of all ages, male and female; they also need to assume some responsibility on a long term basis. In the ideal situation the student develops a caseload of patients with whom she or he will work during the entire preceptorship.

It is important for the student and preceptor to learn to share responsibility and develop mutually acceptable ways of sharing in the treatment of patients. In the beginning, some physicians prefer that FNPs observe, then gradually they accept the student's assumption of responsibilities for compiling a history, doing physical examinations, and planning care. Through this process, the preceptor learns to trust the FNP student.

One preceptor who was very effective allowed the student to choose patients as she desired. The FNP interviewed the patient and then made a physical assessment. Following that, the physician and student discussed the student's findings and assessment in the presence of the patient. Then the physician elicited additional information or confirmed findings as he deemed necessary. This positive approach to clinical teaching developed a great deal of trust in both the student and patients.

As trust develops, both participants become more open in the relationship. Students and preceptors then feel free to share both questions and knowledge. In some situations the physician acknowledges that he has learned to think of certain problems or approaches to care differently during the preceptorship, because of exchange of ideas with the FNP student.

Faculty supervise students in individual conferences in addition to frequent site visits. Through supervisory visits faculty observe the student functioning in a clinical setting, offer support, and maintain contact between the college and the preceptor. In addition, chart audits elicit valuable information about the level of student proficiency. Faculty review students' charts regularly as part of site visits during the preceptorship. Often the review is done by faculty and student together, and constitutes an important learning tool during which particular approaches to patient management can be reinforced, corrected, or improved. Chart audits are also part of the student evaluation process.

Students find the combination of classroom and clinical learning an intensive experience. Ideas and attitudes change rapidly as the student struggles to internalize these experiences.

PROCESS OF ROLE CHANGE FOR NURSE PRACTITIONERS

In the process of their education, FNP students undergo a role change. They develop different relationships with patients, with physicians, and with other nurses as they enact the nurse practitioner role. There is an added dimension to the self-concept, as the FNP student views the self in a different way as a result of new competencies, new scope of practice, and particularly having the others in the environment interact with the student differently. This role embodies a different approach to nursing than generally practiced by the registered nurse. The FNP is the one who must make the decisions about what care will be given, rather than carry out a plan of care which has been developed by the physician. It places the nurse much more centrally in the process of providing patient care and requires a different level of personal involvement.

There is a great deal of overlap of the FNP role into what has traditionally been thought of as medical practice, and this presents a challenge to students in integrating new knowledge and changed boundaries of practice. Nurses have long been taught that the practice of medicine and nursing are distinctly separate, that nursing has a separate body of knowledge and an area of unique function. A goodly amount of energy was spent in schools of nursing making distinctions between medicine and nursing, downgrading nursing's delegated medical functions, usually those functions connected with pathophysiology, and emphasizing nursing's unique independent functions such as counseling, support, and teaching. As FNP students, these registered nurses are required to embrace activities connected with disease management with great vigor, a startling and unsettling occurrence for those socialized into believing that this was really not a legitimate thing for nurses to do.

In addition to working through the medicine versus nursing dichotomy, FNP students must overcome their previous nursing socialization against decision making. The dictum that "nurses do not diagnose" is one of the more difficult barriers to overcome. Over the years, nursing education seems to have thoroughly inculcated this nondiagnosis into its products, although it runs contrary to everyone's common sense and daily observations. Nurses diagnose routinely in their practice in all settings, making a multitude of decisions about various aspects of care based upon their observations. These diagnostic decisions are more sophisticated when made by nurse practitioners, and require a broader body of knowledge and different diagnostic skills. The long semantic harange about what is a "nursing" versus a "medical" diagnosis has only served to reinforce the nurse's discomfort with physical treatment, as if nursing had nothing to do with the management of pathology. Thus, FNP students must overcome their reluctance to diagnose and use the proper names of diseases and conditions which they will treat, no small task for the well socialized nurse.

The FNP student can no longer take refuge in the common nursing tactic to avoid dealing with unpleasant or difficult situations by responding to a patient's question with "You'll have to talk to the doctor about that." By assuming responsibility for treating the illness or health need itself, as well as helping patient and family cope with the impact of illness, the nurse practitioner becomes the person for whom "the buck stops here." It is healthier for the nurse to deal honestly with all aspects of the patient's problem, rather than play the game of limited knowledge or authority. The patient can also benefit, as the nurse practitioner can present the facts from the standpoint of direct involvement in diagnosis and treatment, as well as utilize counseling skills to ease the impact and enhance coping mechanisms.

Decision-making expands for the nurse practitioner into other areas traditionally off-limits to nurses. Advising patients regarding specific procedures or practices to improve their illness was limited to relatively minor comfort measures, and these frequently had to be cleared with the physician first. The entire realm of medication was also prohibited for nurses, to the extent that a nurse could not even order aspirin without a written or verbal prescription by the physician. Nursing education includes pharmacology, and nurses have considerable knowledge about uses and actions of drugs. Nurses are expected to observe patients for adverse effects from medications, and evaluate their effectiveness. Certain judgments are required of nurses, including when not to administer a drug, sometimes variations of dosage, and time spans between repeat doses in certain instances. An artificial line has been drawn which permits a level of nursing decision-making, but limits nursing judgment in a way which is both inconsistent and inefficient in carrying out patient care. The FNP student is required to cross this artificial line and learn to prescribe drugs and other treatment modalities. It is a difficult thing for the FNP student to do, as it breaks with mores of both medical and nursing groups. Considerable anxiety surrounds this type of decision-making, particularly as the legal situation requires that a physician's signature be on all prescriptions.

The FNP Evaluation Study of Role Change

Because of the many questions still unanswered about FNP preparation, practice, and role change, an evaluation study has been intiated by the FNP project which is in addition to the five year longitudinal study of all Second Step students. Data about the educational process, levels of student competency, attitudes of students and personnel in the preceptorship, and the process of role change in students are included in the FNP study which is also assisted by Kellogg funds. While the study is presently still underway and all data have not been collected, we do have data to examine the process of student role change.

The role changes outlined above may be observed by the nursing supervisor or physician preceptor as he or she works with the student FNP over a period of several months. Documentation of this type of change, therefore, is frequently anecdotal, based upon observation. Another form of documentation and one which is easier to quantify but not necessarily more valid, is based upon the students' responses to tests and questionnaires, administered at various times within the training program.

Theoretically, as indicated in the above paragraphs, a nurse practitioner student may be expected to change in several dimensions as she practices her new role. Satisfactions expected from the profession will change as she or he undertakes new responsibilities and tasks. As these new experiences are internalized, she or he will undoubtedly indicate some awareness of personal growth. Finally, the image of nursing will be altered by new experiences and by the new way in which the practitioner is perceived by others.

Rather substantial changes have been documented through responses to a questionnaire administered upon entry to the program and at graduation. Responses to an item asking FNP students to indicate those professional experiences which they perceived as most satisfying or personally rewarding showed that the number of students finding great satisfaction through traditional work experiences was reduced over the period of the two years (Table 3). Being skillful in the keeping of records or the use of instruments or obtaining the approval of physicians became increasingly unimportant over this period. Satisfactions derived from the direct care of patients, however, increased. This very aptly reflects the student's increasing involvement with patient care and shift in focus from relationships with the physician to relationships with patients.

The student nurse practitioners also perceived they had changed through their educational experience. As shown by Table 4, growth was made in both the areas of intellectual and social attitudes and in personal attributes. The majority of students indicated they had grown in maturity, self-awareness, and a sense of identity, as well as in areas more closely related to academic experience, such as intellectual interests and social issues.

The image student nurse practitioners had of nursing also changed considerably during this period. As previously reported, the FNP students upon entry to the program at California State College at Sonoma had rather traditional views of nursing. Over two thirds of the practitioner students chose hard work, technical skill, authority, order, and routine as phrases describing their image of nursing (Table 5). While believing these were aspects of nursing as a profession, they were less willing to accept these values for themselves. Only a small minority of the students accepted close supervision, authority, and hard work as important for themselves. Within this category of traditional values, appreciable changes occurred over the two years from entry to graduation. Traditional values declined both in the image of nursing and in their importance to the nurses. Fewer nurses saw religious inspiration, technical skill, hard work, and close supervision as typical of nursing. They were also more willing to reject these values for themselves, particularly technical skill, emotional control, order, and routine. Clearly, their perception of nursing as a profession became less traditional.

The opposite trend was true for characteristics which are more appropriate to the contemporary view of nursing; upon entry the nurses chose these values as important to themselves but did not see them as typically true of nursing. At the time of graduation, while they embraced these values to a greater extent, they correspondingly perceived them as less descriptive of their image of nursing. Imagination and innovation are clearly not included in the picture most nurses have of nursing.

Nursing as an occupation became more important to the nurse practitioners. Although they were more willing to question the profession's ability to command respect, they felt it was more important to them at graduation that nursing was respected by the community.

123

Table 3. Changes in professional attitudes: Satisfaction derived from professional work experiences*

Professional experience	Number of students (in percentages) who perceive great satisfaction from professional experience	
	Entry (N = 18)	Graduation (N = 16)
Traditional nursing experience		
Being complimented by a doctor for a task you performed well	17	6
The feeling of being vitally needed and important to the patient	39	33
Performing your part in a tense surgical operation or emergency without a flaw or moment's hesitation or indecision	56	11
Mastering the technique of a difficult medical instrument or apparatus	22	11
Contemporary nursing experience		
Making accurate and perceptive observations on the relationship of family behavior to the patient's morale and progress	39	67
Instructing a patient and his family in self care and home care of his condition	50	56
Getting and implementing new ideas on more effective methods of patient care	28	50
Assisting a patient and family to make appropriate decisions about health care	39	67
Helping a noncommunicative patient to verbalize his feelings	39	67

*This table is based upon the responses of students in Class I and Class II to the following question in the Nursing Student Questionnaire: "Below are certain experiences which some nurses and nursing students find satisfying or personally rewarding. Please indicate how much personal satisfaction they give you." Possible responses: "Little, Moderate, Considerable, Great,"

124

Table 4. Changes in attitude toward self and others: Personal
changes from entry to graduation, as perceived by
students*

Attribute	Number of students (in percentages) who perceived increase in attribute from entry to graduation (N = 16)
Intellectual and social attitudes	
Intellectual interests in your field	94
Intellectual interests in general	81
Concern with social issues	50
Political liberalness	44
Personal attributes	
Maturity	69
Emotional stability	44
Firmness of sense of identity	81
Self-awareness, self-insight	100

*This table is based upon responses to the following item in the Graduation Survey: "Please
indicate whether you feel you've changed in the following attributes compared to when
you began college." Possible responses included: "Decreased, Changed very little,
Increased."

In attempting to reconstruct these responses into a picture of the
students' experience at Sonoma, it may be hypothesized that the
average FNP student enrolls in the program with fairly conventional
professional values. They have viewed nursing through the eyes of
the society in which they live. Therefore, they have perceived it as
an exacting profession requiring dedication, skill, and restraint. It
is very much confined within an hierarchy, bounded by rules and
persons in authority to enforce those rules.

Entering FNP students, however, are not at all sure they want to
accept these values for themselves. While they are willing to see
nursing as a profession requiring skill and restraint, they show signs
of questioning and rejecting the inflexible social position of their
profession. Order, authority and supervision are not accepted values.
Rather, they are looking to nursing as a profession requiring originality, imagination, and innovation. Possibly it is with this quest that
they return to college. Feeling somewhat frustrated with the position
they have occupied as nurses in hospitals or doctors offices, they are
willing to reject the image given to them by society and seek new ways
to express themselves within their profession.

In their two years at Sonoma, this quest becomes intensified. They
become even more sure of the creative values of nursing and increasingly reject the more traditional values offered them. As they grow
and change, however, they also begin to see the discrepancy between
their view of themselves as professionals and the public's view of

Table 5. Changes in the professional values of FNP students from entry to graduation*

Characteristic	Attribution of characteristics to image of nursing (nos. in percent)			Acceptance of characteristic as important to self (nos. in percent)		
	Entry	Graduation	Diff.	Entry	Graduation	Diff.
Stereotyped nursing ideals						
Dedicated service to humanity	78	73	− 5	50	67	+17
Moving ritual and ceremony	22	27	+ 5	0	0	0
Religious inspiration and calling	33	7	−26	17	13	− 4
Traditional views of nursing work						
High technical skill	83	53	−30	67	34	−33
Emotional control and restraint	78	80	+ 2	56	20	−36
Human drama and excitement	72	53	−19	22	27	+ 5
Clear-cut lines of authority	89	80	− 9	17	7	−10
Order and routine	89	87	− 2	44	13	−31
Hard work	94	53	−41	28	34	+ 6
Meticulousness	50	40	−10	34	13	−21
Close supervision and direction	72	40	−32	11	0	−11
Clearly defined work tasks, each person responsible for her job and her job alone	44	47	+ 3	22	0	−22

Contemporary views of nursing work

Demonstrating care and concern for others in an immediate and tangible way	83	80	+ 3	78	87	+ 9
Originality and creativity	34	13	-21	67	80	+13
Exercise of imagination and insight	56	20	-36	67	80	+13
Solid intellectual content	44	34	-10	56	67	+11
Frequent innovation in the solution of problems	78	27	-51	72	87	+15

Characteristics of nursing as an occupation

An occupation highly respected in the community	89	53	-36	39	60	+21
Job security	83	87	+ 4	61	60	+ 1

*Responses are based upon the classes of 1974 and 1975. (Entry, N=18, graduation, N=15)

them. Quite possibly they suffer some disillusionment as they begin to realize that most people will not see them as imaginative, original, or innovative, nor will they give them the respect they feel their profession deserves in the community.

The most painful changes within the educational experience may not be the reduction of traditional values, a process which apparently begins before entry to the baccalaureate program, but a disillusionment suffered as a consequence of a reassessment of public image accompanied by personal expansion and growth. They become more confident, capable, and sure of the value of themselves as a professional person; at the same time they recognize the public may not be willing to see within them the qualities they value so much.

The nurse practitioners, however, do not indicate in their conversations a feeling of defeat or resentment. In interviews with them they demonstrated feelings ranging from quiet satisfaction to exhilaration with their personal progress, and as a group were most optimistic and hopeful about their future. Obviously, their satisfactions with their own growth and the expansion of professional opportunities outweighed any disillusionment they may have experienced. Perhaps this is the best measurement of maturity and growth. They are quite realistic and able to acknowledge the difficulties in their profession, but are not overwhelmed by them. As they become more inner-directed and guided by an inner validation, they are less dependent upon the approval and direction of others.

RELATIONSHIPS WITH COLLEAGUES[15]

In the process of becoming a nurse practitioner, a significant role change occurs in which attitudes toward the self and the practice of the profession are altered. The greatest changes occur in the areas of increased authority, a more sophisticated level of decision making and judgment, and the assumption of real responsibility in the provision of health care. In any cluster or system of interfacing roles, when one changes there are reciprocal changes in others. One reason for the controversy created by the nurse practitioner movement among both medical and nursing circles lies in the profound implications of this new type of nursing practice for established professional boundaries and traditional scope of practice. All change causes a certain amount of stress, but change which challenges the basic tenets or shakes the foundations of any ideology inevitably poses a threat and engenders resistance. The nurse practitioner role threatens both medicine and nursing. Physicians are faced with relinquishing their monopolistic control over the delivery of health care, particularly in ambulatory practice, and having to share decision making authority with the nurse practitioner. Nurses are faced with the necessity to broaden their knowledge base and expand their responsibility in health care, stepping into the primary provider position and becoming accountable for managing the health need or illness rather than just counseling and advising about it. Understandably, many physicians and nurses resist these changes.

Relationships with Other Nursing Faculty

Other nursing faculty in the Department of Nursing probably experience a variety of feelings toward the FNP faculty. As this is not a homogenous group, it is difficult to generalize about attitudes, and perceptions described here are based upon scattered experiences involving many different individuals. The process of acceptance by non-practitioner faculty goes through several stages, beginning with the question of "What is a nurse practitioner?" When some understanding of the role is gained, the next response may vary from thinking that all nurses more or less do these things, to rejection of FNPs as nurses, condemning them for leaving the fold and migrating over to the practice of medicine. The "junior doctor" attitude is hard to overcome, because the nurse faculty must essentially change their definition of nursing to include instrumental and curative functions. This means questioning what one has learned and integrated through the long process of socialization into nursing.

The other attitude, though not immediately as troublesome, is equally dangerous. It has contributed to the "band-wagonism" now occurring as collegiate nursing departments scurry to incorporate physical assessment and call their products nurse practitioners. Faculty must address the issue of whether they believe nurse practitioner practice is essentially the same or radically different from traditional nursing. Or, are there many varieties of nurse practitioners, ranging from those who do well-baby examinations and counsel mothers on growth and development to those who assume primary responsibility for full management of common acute and chronic illnesses of all types of patients? If the nurse practitioner movement is to exert maximum impact in changing the health care delivery system and improving care available to people in this country, nursing should strive to encourage practice at the highest level. When practiced as described here, the nurse practitioner role is a marked change from the traditional nursing role. Simply adding some physical diagnosis to the nursing curriculum falls abysmally short of providing the extensive instruction in health maintenance and illness management with carefully supervised clinical and lengthy preceptorship necessary to prepare a fully competent high-level nurse practitioner.

Faculty may ultimately arrive at a level of acceptance which recognizes the differences inherent in the role but appreciates the integration of previous nursing knowledge and functions. Sometimes with this understanding comes the feeling that "it's all right for you, but it's certainly not for me." This is a real and legitimate position, for truly not all nurses wish to become involved in this type of practice. One can respect differences in philosophy and practice, understand the need for standards and reasonable controls, and can work cooperatively in the interest of improving health care. Different groups of nurses will offer different services to patients, and there is a need for all valid services.

Numerous other factors influence the relationship between the FNP faculty and other nursing faculty. On our campus, there is a lack of opportunity for contact due to the many off-campus obligations of all clinical faculty. Being present in a large group at faculty meetings twice a month does not really afford the opportunity to get to know someone well. FNP faculty miss many of the informal mechanisms of faculty interaction, because of their part-time status and because student supervision takes them off campus much of their two-and-a-half teaching days per week. When on campus, they are busy teaching the FNP course, holding course planning meetings, and counseling students. One FNP faculty who has been with the department the longest time, and underwent FNP preparation while a faculty member, notices some exclusion from her previous status with the other faculty. She is no longer automatically included in groups, but must make an effort to join them. While there is no sense of rejection, there is the feeling of not being a "regular" member, of now being somewhat in an out-group position.

Some pressure tends to be exerted upon FNP faculty to integrate their course better into prevailing curricular concepts. Some of these concepts do not "fit" comfortably, resulting in some stretching of intent in application. Ideas for curriculum revision have grown out of examining the place of the FNP course within the curriculum. The level of understanding a given faculty member has of the goals and processes of FNP preparation colors their notions about the curricular relationship of the FNP course. Closer integration has occurred with the development of the physical assessment course in the junior year and the incorporation of a beginning level of physical diagnosis into community health nursing courses. FNP faculty conducted a workshop for other faculty in which an introduction to physical assessment, including teaching the use of instruments for selected physiologic systems, was provided. This afforded other faculty the opportunity to increase their familiarity with FNP faculty and some aspects of nurse practitioner practice. Such increased understanding promotes more congenial relationships, as well as equips faculty to better assist community health students utilize a broader knowledge base in patient assessment.

Relationships with Physicians

The FNP faculty interact with physicians in two settings which include the teaching team at the college and the health care team at the clinic. The underlying dynamics of the problems are the same, however, whether the nurse and physician work together as teachers or clinicians. The FNP faculty often get a "double dose" of these problems, although only those associated with the educational setting will be discussed.

Physicians have a very difficult time learning to share. Partly this is a result of their education, which strongly conditions them that theirs is the sole and total responsibility, and partly it is a function of the dominant and independent personality type which goes into medicine. Doctors not only cannot share gracefully with nurses, but often also find it most difficult to share with other physicians. When they establish practices together, it tends to be two or more individual practices located in the same building, rather than a true team sharing patients. Thus, when the nurse practitioner enters the scene talking about being a "colleague" and working with MDs on a "team," most physicians have a built-in natural resistance to such an approach.

Besides the issue of sharing as a general principle, physicians not infrequently view nurse practitioners as heretical upstarts who are trying to cross well established boundaries of practice. Of course nurse practitioners are doing just that, and the character of physician response largely depends upon whether there is willingness to question traditions of practice and re-examine the standard allotment of tasks. Physicians have a long history of almost total control over the nature of health care delivery in the U.S., and are in general most reluctant to give up that control. The concern over competence and quality care is real and legitimate, but the concern over retention of power is unsupportable if one believes in democracy and principles of equality. That nurse practitioners, when properly prepared, can deliver an equal quality of care in most ambulatory and/or primary care settings has been well demonstrated. If, then, competency is removed as an issue, we are faced with the desire to retain power as the basis for physician opposition.

Sexist attitudes play a significant part in this particular power struggle. The fact that most physicians are male and most nurses are female strongly influences mores which in turn shape the broad behavioral spectrum of professional role enactment. Women have long been perceived as subservient to men, less intelligent, and less competent than men, and enacting a nurturant and supportive function so that men may carry on with the great things in life. When women step out of this sexist conception of role, and challenge the male definition of the world, the balance of power is upset. Thus the nurse practitioner who is a woman poses a double threat to the male physician, who must then deal with his identity as a physician and his identity as a man. Since the two are really inseparable and have been integrated in the physician's self-concept, a challenge to his conceptions of what the physician role should be also constitutes a challenge to his sense of masculinity. This is a very deep seated and profoundly troublesome challenge, and may shake the very foundations of male identity to the extent that the

131

physician must immediately close out any possibility of accepting the nurse practitioner. For some physicians, this unfortunately has been their method of coping with the nurse practitioner threat.

Among other physicians, one can find a continuum of comfort and acceptance of the nurse practitioner role. There are strong advocates who desire the broadest possible range of functions for FNPs, and indeed such brave souls instituted the nurse practitioner movement. There are many others who accept a certain level of shared responsibility and authority, but still view the MD as the "captain of the ship." While it is true that any team or group must have a leader, it is equally true that the leader need not be the same person in all circumstances. This concept will take some time before it is well integrated by physicians who are generally accepting of the nurse practitioner.

There are many small and some large problems in working day-to-day in a team relationship with physicians, if the FNP aspires to a truly collegial relationship. On the teaching team, effort must be expended to achieve equitable distribution of course work. Since the MD does not view teaching FNP students as his primary commitment and has a growing private practice, he may tend to minimize the amount of time put into teaching activities. This necessitates the FNPs setting quite specific expectations and spelling out responsibilities, with the implication that the MD could be doing more to enhance the learning experience. Trying not to fall into the old male-female doctor-nurse game is part of this problem as well as constituting a separate problem in itself. FNP faculty at times catch themselves "running and fetching" for the MD, whether it's getting instructional materials or a cup of coffee. In trying not to do these things for the MD, we had to ask whether we did not indeed do it for each other, and wherein was the difference. Perhaps part of the problem was in our perceptions, for FNP faculty do assist each other by making extra trips for forgotten materials. Once we were able to establish that the MD would also "run and fetch" for us, this problem dissipated.

Reminding the MD about class handouts, lecture topics, getting in exam questions, and locations of clinical experiences at times assumes a "nagging wife" character. The MD tended to be forgetful, or perhaps FNP teaching was a relatively low priority for him, and the FNP faculty had to contend with a certain amount of disorganization as a result. After some confrontation this situation improved, particularly when the FNPs simply let the MD face the consequences of forgetting to prepare with the students. The students did criticize the MD on several occasions, resulting in some changes in his behavior.

One residual of the doctor-nurse game which both faculty and students notice is the typical nursing avoidance of contradicting the doctor. At times during class the MD would make statements which were inaccurate or incomplete, or about topics in which FNP faculty were more knowledgeable. The fact that FNP faculty did not take issue more frequently with the MD is probably partly due to old mores that proscribe nursing contradiction of physicians. Although at times the points were small ones, lecture time was limited and the discussion would not be too fruitful, or the hassle simply seemed more than the issue was worth, FNP faculty recognize the need to be more assertive with their expertise. The students found it somewhat difficult to set limits on the MD, particularly in his style of teaching. They would listen politely while he went off on a tangent about some exotic disease which FNP's would hardly ever see much less treat, then verbalize later to the faculty about too much useless material in lecture. When faculty pointed out that students certainly interrupted them if lectures they presented strayed from the point, students had to face their role in the doctor-nurse game and accept responsibility for making their learning needs known to the MD. This they did, and as a result the MD's lectures improved and became more relevant.

The problem of salaries is a touchy one when FNP's and MD's are on a teaching team. With much more teaching experience, the FNP's full salary is about the same as the MD's half-time salary for teaching. This irksome situation grows out of the basic disparity between physician and nurse income, with its historic roots in the differential wage paid to women and service professions. While salary is certainly not the predominant motivation for most nurse practitioners, it is important both in the practical economic sense and as a measure of society's valuation of one's contributions. Nurse practitioners are making a substantial contribution to the quality and extensiveness of health services, and need to be properly reimbursed for this. Schools of nursing have notoriously underpaid faculty, again with a sexual differential, and must compete with higher-paying practice positions for the best qualified nurse practitioners.

The power struggle with medicine continues on a philosophical and in some cases very practical basis, although in individual situations cooperation seems much more the prevailing mode. The issue of who shall control and regulate nurse practitioner education and practice is far from resolved. Most nursing educators tend to believe that nurse practitioners should be prepared in baccalaureate or higher degree schools of nursing, primarily taught by nurse practitioners with physician input into curriculum and instruction. Physicians seem to generally accept collaborative practice, but desire regulations regarding physician supervision of nurse practitioners and prevention of independent practice. Some physicians and nurse practitioners would like to see nurse practitioners licensed separately from other nurses, probably under the Board of Medicine similarly to physicians' assistants, or under a joint board of nursing and medicine. Others prefer that nurse practitioners remain under the general nursing license, but that regulations be written to assure minimum standards for education and competency to practice. Still others visualize a merging and blending of the nurse practitioner role into nursing as a whole, without the need for clear distinctions, allowing the economics of jobs to define the scope of practice.

FACULTY PREPARATION AND JOINT APPOINTMENTS

Schools of nursing have historically not built in a practice component for faculty. Most teaching positions fill the faculty member's time with instructional activities, meetings, and student counseling, leaving little or no time for practice. Even with time available, however, the lack of a support structure for faculty practice discourages individual efforts. There are very few faculty positions today in which a practice component is integrated and fully supported within the expectations of the teaching role.

In nurse practitioner education, faculty practice is seen as an essentail component for effective instruction. Continuing involvement of those who instruct in the actual practice of their profession enriches the learning available to students in many ways. Such involvement should also be beneficial to the practice setting, as the newer developments and intellectual growth of the profession which often ferment in the educational system are brought directly into practice. The closer matching of educational ideals with the practical requirements of the real situation could also result from faculty involvement in practice.

Increased faculty practice might help improve a variety of problems in nursing. Nursing's alliance with schools of education rather than the sciences, although unavoidable in the early evolution of nursing preparation in the move from hospital to collegiate setting, did reduce nursing's involvement in the progress made in biologic and physical sciences. Nursing benefitted in the areas of learning theories and new approaches to curriculum development and teaching methodology, resulting in more innovative approaches to nursing curricula and instruction. But, physiology and pathophysiology received less emphasis as the psychosocial aspects of illness and health needs became the forte of collegiate nursing programs. The current trend is toward a more balanced approach as physical care is again seen as a legitimate part of nursing practice rather than a lower level of delegated medical function. Nurse practitioners certainly represent a balance between the physical and psychosocial, and involvement of faculty in practice may produce more research and writing about pathophysiologic problems in nursing.

The separation of nursing service and nursing education which resulted when nursing preparation moved from the hospital to the college was also an unfortunate, albeit unavoidable, event. It was necessary to free student nurses from service to the institution and develop a training process which focused on their learning needs, and it was necessary for nursing to break away from medical control of

134

education and outgrow the handmaiden role. In the process, however, nursing education lost its channel of influence upon the delivery of nursing services within the hospital and clinic setting. A long history of animosity between nursing service and education has served to keep the two separate, and little has been done to encourage a mechanism to reunite them. If nursing faculty become involved in practice on a regular and widespread basis, this gap would probably be bridged rapidly as common concerns would become more apparent. No doubt the care given to the patient would improve.

Advantages of Joint Appointments for Faculty

Practice permits continued development of clinical skills, both in the areas of physical assessment and clinical judgment. Using the instruments, hands, eyes, and ears to provide information which contributes to diagnosis is new to nurses. The usefulness of eliciting physical examination data and its direct application to the care provided by the FNP are of a different magnitude than before. This is a fine skill requiring deftness and great dexterity. Repeated opportunity to practice in the real situation is the only way to truly refine the skill of physical diagnosis. Watching other expert clinicians in action, then trying the techniques oneself with new awareness is essential to this learning. It cannot be obtained without continued opportunity to practice. Clinical judgment, the very core of quality care, also needs repeated practice to achieve levels of excellence. Judgment is such a complex ability, gleaned slowly through years of drawing subtle inferences and making intricate associations, that one must indeed have years of practice in order to become expert. Nursing educators have appropriately asked "how many beds must the student make in order to know how to make a bed," and questioned established lengths of time spent teaching various nursing activities. The level of cognitive processes involved in the skills of physical assessment and clinical judgment as practiced by the nurse practitioner so far exceed most ordinary nursing procedures, however, that no comparison may be made. In these areas experience truly is the best teacher, and faculty must continue their experience if they aspire to the status of expert in the field.

Continuing in practice gives the FNP faculty member authenticity as a teacher. Being involved oneself in the practice of a role being taught cannot but increase understanding and intimacy with the small details. Nursing educators are infamous for being theoreticians who are unable to perform in the practice setting, a reputation which has reduced their credibility with students and colleagues of all disciplines in practice. Although this situation has improved during the last decade, as internal values among nurses dictated that faculty should have experience before teaching and be expert clinicians before trying to impart clinical knowledge to students, faculty will lose expertise and fall behind current developments without a continued mechanism for practice. For nurse practitioner faculty, the need for authenticity cannot be overemphasized. Because the role is so new, those involved in teaching it must be closely allied with practice in order that congruent evolution may take place.

Faculty who practice also are provided with a growing pool of clinical examples which enrich their teaching. They are always encountering new cases which may better illustrate the content and provide more understanding of the problem. These are brought fresh to the classroom or conference, where students and faculty alike benefit from this shared learning. Faculty can keep in better touch with the problems in the practice setting and the development of the FNP role in practice. They can add their perspective and expertise to the solution of problems and directly influence role development. Having this close association between practice and education keeps the FNP curriculum closely related to actual practice, so that what students learn has more applicability to the real situation, with a constant compromise between idealism and pragmatism. This reduces the credibility gap in nursing education.

One final advantage for faculty involves personal satisfactions. Giving direct care to patients is a leading source of satisfaction in nursing and a major reason why people go into nursing. Teachers largely give up this source of satisfaction, for their role requires a secondary relationship with the patient as they facilitate the student's giving the direct care. When faculty have the opportunity to practice, they are once again able to use their personal skills directly, with the many rewards of "a job well done" available to them. This also reinforces their skill in practice, enhancing self-respect in a central area of professional nursing identity. Although also subject to the agonies of personal errors and inadequacies in practice, the rewards of direct patient care generally outweigh the drawbacks for those who identify practice competencies as an important part of their nursing role. Some people like the change of pace and variety which accompany joint appointments. The pace of daily routine differs greatly in educational and practice settings, and the physical locations communicate different atmospheres. This can be quite stimulating for some, but might be simply draining for others. A mental "shifting of gears" occurs when moving from one to another setting, particularly if involved in both on the same day. It certainly prevents getting into a rigid routine and breaks up habit patterns. Although an exciting process, it does require a considerable amount of mental energy.

The FNP faculty in a joint appointment sets an example for professional and public acceptance of the nurse practitioner role. The image of the educator is changed to one of greater authenticity, and qualifications for clinical teaching improve. There is also much opportunity for personal satisfaction.

Disadvantages of Joint Appointments for Faculty

There are some problems with joint appointments, however, and certain of these elude ready solution. Working out a sane schedule is one of the more chronic problems. Each employing institution must have a reasonably predictable schedule, which at times results in conflicting demands upon the FNP. There are traditions about scheduling classes, and traditions of which types of clinics will be held on which days. Students have other demands on their time which further complicate the situation, for FNP faculty and students must be available at the same time for classes and portions of the clinical experience. The more individuals who become involved, the more intricate the variables involved in scheduling. Practice schedules may fluctuate from month to month, while academic schedules remain set for the semester. The times FNP faculty have available for meetings and conferences change monthly, to the frustration of secretaries, other faculty, and students. Because practice schedules fluctuate, it is hard to plan with much surety for more than a month in advance. Compromises obviously have to be made between the two settings, such as putting aside one day for classes and conferences during which no clinics are scheduled for FNP faculty. Despite such efforts, at times FNP faculty simply cannot attend other faculty activities, because classes, student supervision, and practice conflict with these and must take precedence.

There is often a sense of not being totally involved in either place of work when one holds a joint appointment. Part time people are not there as much as full time, and cannot devote as much effort to the full range of activities in the institution. The FNP faculty must set priorities at each place of work, and learn to decline involvement or maintain peripheral involvement when necessary. This is difficult, particularly when one believes in the item or issue and would, under other circumstances, become more deeply involved. One feels somewhat left out of things, and often hears about events after they occur. The setting of limits on oneself and others is a requisite for those who would span two different settings in their work.

That 50 per cent plus 50 per cent adds up to more than 100 per cent is an occupational hazard of the half-and-half position. Both employers tend to expect somewhat more than their alloted half, and when the employee sets limits upon expectations which go beyond what is equitable, a sense of disapproval may be conveyed by the employer. FNP faculty who practices may have to periodically re-explain other obligations to employers, and learn to stand firm about what constitutes an equitable work load in each setting. Learning to live with comments such as "Oh, do you still work here?" and "I can't ever seem to find you" is a talent the person in a joint appointment must develop. These comments invariably come on a day when the FNP feels this business of working in two places will simply never get coordinated, and is indulging in a little self-pity about being so over-worked. Despite the temptation to think that no one will really understand the strains of a joint appointment, the FNP faculty must make special efforts to keep people informed about location and activities. It is probably true that one setting will receive more attention than the other, despite one's best efforts to balance this out fairly. This is a result of personal interests or the extent of responsibility perceived in each setting. Or, the actual ability of the FNP to influence the power structure and the rewards available in the setting may sway primary loyalty. Hopefully, the interests of the two settings will not be contradictory, thus presenting a serious conflict for the nurse practitioner.

At present, there is a scarcity of family nurse practitioners who also hold a master's degree and are prepared for teaching. Courses have been developed in some parts of the country to meet this need, but the number is still small. As part of the FNP project, two C.S.C.S. faculty members were sponsored for study to become nurse practitioners, thus creating a pool of prepared instructors. The FNP faculty have also conducted physical assessment workshops to acquaint other faculty members with the physical diagnosis process.

CONCLUSIONS

The experiment at Sonoma with the FNP preceptorship indicates that nurse practitioner preparation at the baccalaureate level within an R.N. degree program is feasible. Such a project may be integrated into the nursing curriculum, and offers students an additional career option as they expand their nursing practice. The institution of physical assessment and an intensive pathophysiology course in the junior year provides a critical foundation on which FNP preparation can build. The junior experience in community health nursing also contributes an essential ingredient toward FNP education and practice.

During the two semester FNP preceptorship, students undergo considerable stress and significant role change. However, the outcome seems to indicate satisfaction in terms of personal growth, confidence in the ability to function as an FNP on a beginning level, and a positive outlook for the future. Acceptance of graduates by physicians and health care institutions within the community appears to be quite good.

Ours is a changing world, with changing relationships between physicians and nurses, men and women. Hopefully the outcome will lead to positive growth for all, so that a person can find expression of the full level of ability without sexist or professional territorial constraints as well as the full expression of the human personality. If such an outcome is realized, health care in this country will also improve through increased availability of services and increased ability of the health care system to respond to individual needs, whether physical, pathophysiologic, psychological, or social.

REFERENCES

1. Lewis, C. E., and Resnick, B.A.: Nurse Clinics and Progressive Ambulatory Care. *New England Journal of Medicine* 277:1236, 1967.
2. Connelly, J. P., Stoeckle, J. D., Lepper, E. S., and Farrisey, R. M.: Physician and Nurse -- Their Interprofessional Work in Office and Hospital Ambulatory Settings. *New England Journal of Medicine* 275:765, 1966.
3. Ford, P. A., Seacat, M. S., and Silver, G. G.: Broadening Roles of Public Health Nurse and Physician in Pre-natal and Infant Supervision. *American Journal of Public Health* 56:1097, 1966.
4. Silver, H. K., Ford, L. D., and Stearly, S. C.: Program to Increase Health Care for Children: Pediatric Nurse Practitioner Program. *Pediatrics* 39:756, 1967.
5. Charney, E., and Kitzman, H.: The Child Health Nurse in Private Practice, a Controlled Trial. *New England Journal of Medicine* 285:1353, 1971.
6. Spitzer, W. C., et al.: The Burlington Randomized Trial of the Nurse Practitioner. *New England Journal of Medicine* 290:251, 1974.
7. National Commission for the Study of Nursing and Nursing Education: *An Abstract for Action.* McGraw-Hill Book Co., 1970, p. 89.
8. Extending the Scope of Nursing Practice, A Report of the Secretary's Committee to Study Extended Roles for Nurses. November 1971, U. S. Department of Health, Education and Welfare.
9. Standard of Care: Glossary of Terms. California Nurses' Association, March, 1974.
10. Joint Statement on Family Nurse Practitioners in Primary Care. California Joint Practice Commission, 1975.
11. Feldman, M.: Cluster Visits. *American Journal of Nursing* 74:1485, 1974.
12. White, Martha Sturm: Psychological Characteristics of the Nurse Practitioner. *Nursing Outlook* 23:160, 1975.
13. Davis, Fred, and Olesen, Virginia L.: Baccalaureate Students' Images of Nursing. *Nursing Research* 13:8, 1964.
14. *Some Pathological Conditions of the Eye, Ear and Throat, An Atlas.* Abbott Laboratories, Chicago, 1946.
15. Based in part on ideas of Dorothy Blake, R.N., M.S., FNP, member of teaching team in Family Nurse Practitioner Program, California State College, Sonoma, Department of Nursing.

BIBLIOGRAPHY

Anderson, E. M. Leonard, B. J., and Yates, J. A.: "Epigenesis of the Nurse Practitioner Role." *American Journal of Nursing* 74:1812, 1974.
Cleland, V.: "Sex Discrimination: Nursing's Most Pervasive Problem." *American Journal of Nursing* 71:1542, 1971.
Heide, W. S.: "Nursing and Women's Liberation — A Parallel." *American Journal of Nursing* 73:824, 1973.
Linn, L. S.: "Expectation vs Realization in the Nurse Practitioner Role." *Nursing Outlook* 75:166, 1975.
Lynaugh, J. E., and Bates, B.: "Physical Diagnosis: A Skill for All Nurses?" *American Journal of Nursing* 74:58, 1974.
Malkemes, L. D.: "Resocialization: A Model for Nurse Practitioner Preparation," *Nursing Outlook* 74:90, 1974.
Martin, L. M.: "I Like Being an FNP." *American Journal of Nursing* 75:826, 1975.

Mauksch, I. G., and Young, P. R.: "Nurse-Physician Interaction in a Family Medical Care Center." *Nursing Outlook* 74:113, 1974.
Pierik, M. M: "Joint Appointments: Collaboration for Better Patient Care." *Nursing Outlook* 73:576, 1973.
Roberts, J. I., and Group, T. M.: "The Women's Movement and Nursing." *Nursing Forum* 12:303, 1973.
Stein, L.: "The Doctor-Nurse Game." *Archives General Psychiatry* 16:699, 1967.
"The Nurse Practitioner Question." Round Table Discussion. *American Journal of Nursing* 74:2188, 1974.

CHAPTER 7

Liberating the Curriculum from Stereotypes of Ethnicity and Femininity

Renée Romanko-Keller, R.N., M.A., and Christine H. Beaty-Morton, R.N., M.S.

THE ISSUES

The 1970s have brought increased demands from consumers for full participation in decision making in the field of health care. They are dissatisfied with rising costs and the quality and adequacy of health care. They are disenchanted with decision making that does not involve their communities which are so acutely affected by the outcomes of those decisions. Black communities in the 1960s and 70s gave leadership to ethnic peoples of color in expressing their discontentment with health services within their communities and pointed out the lack of community participation in health planning. The federal government attempted to lend support to local communities by not funding programs which did not include the participation of community people. Consequently, there is a growing movement to include all communities in federally funded health planning. The Women's Movement has put tremendous energy toward emphasizing the need for better health care for women. The nationwide development of Women's Health Collectives and Clinics is one of the outcomes of this concern. More women are recognizing and understanding the need for their participation in the health care of their own bodies. The influence of women as health consumers is seen in recent Supreme Court rulings on abortion rights for women. Hence, the evolution of the power of the consumer to influence the direction of events has been touching the lives of many Americans in the health field as well as in other areas.

Margaret Mead observed that the current questioning of the status of women is part of a larger process of re-evaluation. She believes that there is a worldwide concern regarding the political and economic exploitation of the land, the sea, and the air, and the endangered populations that depend upon them. As decision making has reached higher levels, half the harvests of the world have been bought and sold in

141

political and financial deals which have ignored the fact that food is grown to be eaten.[1] There seems to be an international awakening to our growing interdependence and the need for a shared responsibility in protecting the welfare and health of the world as a community. Hence, the Women's Movement is symptomatic of a move for more participation in decisions which affect the lives of us all.

Nursing's struggle to be involved in the decision making processes of patient care has been a long and arduous one. Presently, the Women's Movement has given psychological support to nurses who have seen the need for fuller participation in issues of patient care, client advocacy, and health care delivery. The nursing strikes in the San Francisco Bay Area hospitals in the summer of 1974 were mainly concerned with issues of professional performance and demands for more decision making power as it related to nurses' responsibilities for the health care of clients. Such extensive responsibility and the lack of participation in decisions affecting that and one's work domain have continued to feed a slow burning fire of dissatisfaction among staff nurses in hospitals and health care agencies not only in San Francisco but around the country. This unequal yoke of powerlessness has begun to chafe!

The exclusion of most women and ethnic peoples of color from participation in the decision making processes of our national life persists as a living reality. Opportunities for participation have not kept pace with the rate of rising expectations among these groups. The problems within the field of health reflect this overall attitude of exclusion. Hence, nurses and consumers alike are directly affected by stereotyped attitudes which control their access to positions of power and their participation in the definition and solution of community, state, and national health problems.

The process of stereotyping does not allow for critical thinking or personal variation. Stereotype can be defined as a simplified and standardized conception or image invested with special meaning and held in common by members of a group. The use of the word is synonomous with words such as lifeless, stale, worn, and dull.

Nursing educators are in an unique position to create programs that will dramatically change the present situation. But this will only happen if there is a clear understanding among educators of the power of stereotyped thinking in maintaining the status quo. Our concepts of ethnicity and femininity are barriers to our own participation in the field of health, the profession of nursing, and our national life.

It is our premise that the two most fundamental problems facing all levels of nursing today are the perpetuation of unexamined practices of sex discrimination and the exclusion of ethnic peoples of color. These practices have kept nursing a predominantly white, female occupation that has continued to attract women largely from traditional and conservative families within the middle class. To be a nurse fit society's image of woman's work and was compatible with

142

social expectations of women, that is, to care for and to nurture others. Furthermore, nursing's close work relationship with medicine has paralleled the relationship of men and women in society at large. Nursing was woman's work; medicine was man's work. And until recent years, medicine has dictated the perimeters of the education, supervision, and direction of nursing's practice. Except for a few outstanding nursing leaders, leadership in nursing has been mostly ineffectual and limited in vision. It has been bound to the image of woman's role in society. Consequently, stereotyped thinking within the leadership of nursing has limited nursing's future and isolated nursing from the mainstream of intellectual thought.

This evolution within nursing has created a situation in which the participation of men and ethnic peoples of color has been limited. By and large, this has meant the exclusion of groups of people of the same race or nationality who have shared a common and distinctive culture and who have been nonwhite. Blacks, Mexican-Americans and native Americans are examples of such groups who have not participated in nursing's past and present in any great numbers. Certainly financial considerations have been and are very real factors in limiting educational opportunities of ethnic minorities. But provided that there are opportunities for financial assistance, what else discourages participation in the world of nursing? We propose that nursing's images of ethnic peoples of color have been significantly dictated by social attitudes that have given predominatly negative characteristics to those groups. A distinct ethnocentrism can be observed within nursing. This unarticulated attitude implies a belief in the inherent superiority of one's own group and a feeling of contempt for other groups and cultures. Hence, it can be hypothesized that the climate within nursing has been prohibitive.

Nursing's ability to deliver sensitive and effective health care to all people within society makes participation of men and ethnic peoples of color a necessity. The participation of both groups in the education, administration, and practice of nursing holds the potential of liberalizing the profession and enlarging our potential for solving the health needs of all communities entrusted to our care. It would appear that unexamined practices within nursing have created a situation in which few men and ethnic peoples of color are attracted to the occupation.

Nursing educators stand in an uncommon position for giving leadership in the elimination of sex role and ethnic stereotyping within the field. At present, the movement toward recruitment of faculty and students who represent society at large is a direction that promises to encourage change. Yet traditional nursing education continues to perpetuate stereotypes by the designs of their curriculums. By such designs practices of sexual discrimination and exclusion of ethnic peoples of color are encouraged. In looking at that assumption about what closes our awareness as educators, two issues from among many appear and reappear like twin phoenixes. First, the unexamined practice by nursing faculties in utilizing societal norms in developing curriculums holds considerable controversy. We believe that the definitions commonly accepted do not reflect the pluralism or diversity of our cultural heritage. Secondly, because nursing still remains primarily an occupation of white females, the design of curriculums reflects a female world view. Unfortunately, women have been socialized to accept subordinate roles, to be passive observers, and to aspire to a future that defines one's life in terms of parenting and becoming someone's wife. Hence, a sense of passivity and powerlessness seem an undercurrent in the mainstream of nursing. It is interesting to note that this same sense of powerlessness and passivity can be observed within ethnic groups of color in the United States. It is as if those oppressed by social stereotyping eventually internalize negative images of themselves and become what is expected of them. Certainly, intellectual thought in nursing since *Notes On Nursing* by Florence Nightengale has confused the work of nursing with ideas of femaleness. Being a woman's occupation in a male dominated culture has not placed nursing in a position of influence, power, or political clout.

Therefore, we wish to limit our discussion to powerlessness as an outgrowth of sexual discrimination and the teacher as cultural agent as a consequence of exclusion of ethnic peoples of color. These two issues will be the focus of this chapter in our analysis of an approach to liberalizing nursing curriculums from stereotyped thinking. We will propose a model adapted from the Peace Corps that holds possibilities for use in curriculum design for the teaching of pluralistic concepts and values. We will make inferences regarding the feasibility of its use in nursing with examples of its application within the Second Step curriculum. And finally, we will discuss Sonoma's approach to liberalization in dealing with these issues.

POWERLESSNESS

Turning now to the first issue, the problem of powerlessness and passivity which unconsciously binds the occupation of nursing, we wish to explore briefly the evolution of the phenomena and then to focus upon the role of education in effecting a change in this area specifically. This sense of powerlessness within nursing parallels the experience of women and ethnic groups of color in the United States. This parallel is not surprising if one views women as a minority group within a paternalistic society. It is our intention to explore the impotency, lack of assertiveness, and conformity that is generally seen in women in nursing and to draw a parallel with the experiences of others within the society who are also seen as less valuable members.

Pauline Bart[2] notices that a child's image of the future is pieced together from many sources, including historical evidence about what was possible in the past. History textbooks examined by Bart depicted women as passive, incapable of sustained organization and work, satisfied with their role in society, and well supplied with material blessings. They rarely fought for anything. Children's literature, when examined for sex role stereotyping, has revealed the overall impression that females are mainly in the background and essentially invisible and that girls will not be very important. Education, as it exists today, implies that nothing significant is likely to occur in the future with respect to the place of women in society. Its central message to young girls is that they should look forward to a life of submission, housework, and childbearing.[3]

Should a woman not get the message about her place and work, attempts are generally made to "cool" her interest in occupations seen as traditionally masculine. This inhibition of opportunity for intellectual development and independence of alternate life choices produces a fatalism and passivity within women.[4] Ironically, the process is one of assisting the women "to know her place" in society.[5] The paradox is that most women eventually buy the package and believe that it is the best of all possible bargains. Yet, there has been no conscious choice. Instead, women have clearly accepted social expectations with hardly an audible whimper.

Should a woman break from this mold, she is seen as exceptional and unusual by both men and women. She, in turn, becomes agressive toward other women because she, too, believes that she is exceptional and unusual. She does not welcome competition from other women in her field. This process is described by the authors of the article, "The Queen Bee Syndrome."

> The Queen Bee tries to be a superwoman, and is as eager to "win" in the traditional feminine role of wife and mother as in her career. The great majority of the married professionals do all or almost all of the housework and childcare, and tend to think it should be that way. When a career crisis might develop between her work and that of her husband's, she believes that the man's job has priority. Given a hypothetical situation in which husband and wife are each offered good jobs in different cities, half of the Queen Bees think that the wife should follow the husband — compared to 39% of the traditional women, 12% of the NOW members, and only 3% of the radical feminists. . . . The majority (of Queen Bees) believe that women can best overcome discrimination by "working individually to prove their abilities"![6]

Virginia Cleland[7] observes that women in a primarily female profession think they are not subjects of discrimination. Yet, she ponders, who really makes the important decisions for nurses and nursing? Generally, positions in nursing are available only with the approval of male systems in medicine, hospital administration, and higher education. Furthermore, she observes that autonomy in nursing is a sham! Because of nursing's utter isolation from all vestiges of power except within its own group, there is a parallel to the exploitation of Blacks in our culture. With women, as with Blacks, dominance is most complete when it is not even recognized. That is, there is an observable unconsciousness and unawareness within nursing regarding our own oppression and discrimination.

What Can Be Done to Redefine the "Good Life" for Women?

If behavior is a function of reinforcement while knowledge is a function of learning, it is conceivable that by the use of reinforcement, knowledge could be released into behavior.[8] With different patterns of reinforcement, women and men could develop more role freedom and hence more creativity, happiness, fulfillment, expansion, and personal growth. New social goals seem to be developing in which one needs a fusion of what have been "masculine" and "feminine" qualities.[9]

Ellen and Kenneth Keniston[10] believe that the following changes within our society can support a redefinition of life for women:

1. The development of social institutions to support and encourage those women who want or need to work.
2. A change in attitudes regarding working women by family and society to encourage women to work since most women will find themselves with nothing to do during the greater part of their adulthood.
3. Women's conceptions of their potentials might also be changed by alterations in the demands that men (their husbands and fathers) make upon them.
4. The greatest leverage for changing the image of women and their potential could be gained by providing more viable models of womanhood to girls in adolescence.

Role of Education

Studies reveal that most women will fully explore their intellectual potential only when they do not need to compete and least of all when they are competing with men. It is believed that a bright woman is in a double bind. It she succeeds, she is not living up to societal expectations about the female role. If she fails, she is not living up to her own standards of performance. Hence, a woman who is motivated to achieve is defying conventions of what "girls should do." Consequently, she pays a heavy price in anxiety.[11]

But for all women perhaps the most striking and harmful effect on the evolution of healthy, adult personalities are the effects of low status expectations on the development of self-esteem. Women

146

have traditionally accepted society's negative stereotypes. The outcome has been a belief that women are less intellectually capable, less important, less worthwhile, and less able to make decisions.[12] Is it possible to even think of such a person having any sense of personal power? It's the paradox that faces nursing, a separate but equal occupation for women.

One nursing educator[13] sees the following kind of personal qualities necessary for leadership within present day nursing: political and intellectual astuteness, good risk takers, fairly aggressive, active pursuers of issues, strong egos, and a positive sense of personal identity. She believes that future socialization practice within nursing must seek ways to provide equal male-female leadership opportunities rather than perpetuation of the past subordinate-superordinate pattern of relationship.

These are two approaches that we recommend for effecting a change in the education of nurses: (1) assertion training and (2) a bicultural model approach. Essentially assertion training is a method that can be used to overcome a sense of personal powerlessness. Behavior which enables a person to act in his own best interests, to stand up for himself without undue anxiety, to express his honest feelings comfortably, or to exercise his own rights without denying the rights of others is called assertive behavior. Assertion training attempts to assist the person in the development of a repertoire of assertive behavior so that he may choose appropriate and self-fulfilling responses in a variety of situations.[14]

Patrick C. Lee and Nancy B. Grooper[15] hypothesize that sex role can be viewed as a culture. They think that there are significant continuities between the sexes, as there are between any two cultures. Thus, while male and female cultures have many characteristics in common, they nevertheless present distinctive group identities, adaptive patterns, and world views. The bicultural model identifies cultural compatibilities and commonalities or how cultures coexist, accommodate, and blend. This underscores areas of constructive interaction which otherwise might go unrecognized and indicates the best points for further intercultural penetration. Hence, it is feasible that a bicultural model could be utilized to educate both men and women for more role flexibility.

Membership in a culture senstitizes one to perceive and interpret stimuli selectively and to practice selective responses. This process leads to a range of stimuli not necessarily represented in other cultures. Cultural differences are not so much structural as situational. A bicultural model gives us a third language for describing the interaction of sex role cultures. Focus is on acquired cross-cultural compatibilities, similarities, and consistencies.[16]

THE TEACHER AS CULTURAL AGENT

"Don't change beliefs. Transform the believer." Werner Erhard

Looking at the second issue of the controversy regarding societal norms utilized by nursing faculties in the development of the curriculum, we wish to look at the concept of the teacher as a cultural agent within his or her own culture, a culture of diverse heritages. It is known that nursing faculties usually tend to be female, white, Protestant, and middle or upper-middle class in background. This is a critical point. We create from our own world view. Robert Blauner notices a truism in the academic world.

The professor is oriented toward molding the student in his own image, and he is likely to feel that the only satisfactory training is the kind of education he himself received in graduate school.[17]

To further illustrate this point an example from an international experience may be useful in clarifying the concept of teacher as cultural agent. As a Peace Corps Volunteer teaching in a university school of nursing in Latin America, one of us experienced being a cultural agent. It took some time to understand and experience such a phenomenon. The intent of our work was to enculturate and to function within a world view different from our own. Because our skills and knowledges had root in another culture, the process of choosing to share and participate from that framework was a difficult and sensitive task. Although we were consciously aware of cross-cultural influences, attitudes, values, and views, our work was fought with unexpected cultural pitfalls. The following incident is an example of a cross-cultural confusion that occurred:

Cheating on examinations by the nursing students gave some concern to the faculty. The directions to the students were that each one was to write her own. Her score on the examination was used to evaluate her mastery of the subject by the faculty. Yet at each examination there was blatant cheating and considerable group collaboration on completion of the exam. Faculty efforts to control such cheating did not seem to be successful.

Cross-Cultural Analysis: The school had been set up by a group of American nurses who were members of the Sisters of Mercy of the Catholic Church. They were invited by the University and Ministry of Health to set up the nursing program since there were no nurses within the country with the necessary preparation at that time. Eventually, the Sisters of Mercy left and the leadership of the school was assumed by local nurses who had completed masters' level work in nursing. Consequently, the curriculum was gradually revised to reflect this change in leadership.

One of the American ideas left over was that group efforts on examinations were not permissable. Yet, the culture was totally group oriented. Consequently, ideas of individual performances and competition were especially strange and foreign to the students.

They derived their identity from their families and the network of social relationships of their families. Group collaboration and cooperation was encouraged.

The cheating persisted because both faculty and students understood how it was. The only confusion resided within my mind as an American working in the situation. When I grasped the situation, it opened up a whole new way of looking at evaluation of performance for me within that setting. It seemed strange that it took such a long time to understand such a basic and simple cultural difference.

From many such experiences it gradually became clear that the source of my world view, that of Canada and the United States, totally influenced and colored my education, socialization, self-image, and created a distinct perspective. It became evident that what I observed around me in my host country was dictated by those early experiences. Consequently, it was very hard to perceive and decode what was before me in that situation.

The inference that we are making is that teachers are also cultural agents within their own country. The educational system teaches from the constraints of the social and political system of which it is a powerful gatekeeper. It decides who enters, stays, and leaves. Hence, if the curriculum is going to reflect diversity then the faculty will need to be diverse. We believe that faculty behavior rather than content of the curriculum determines the general education of the students.[18]

Joseph Chilton Pearce in *The Crack in the Cosmic Egg*[19] analyses the formation and evolution of a world view. Essentially he makes the point that people adjust to each other and agree to what is objective reality. Language is an example of a cultural agreement or an agreed verbal framework for perception of the world. Language and culture cannot be separated. Because cultural agreements have their bases in the unconscious and are automatic, travelers in other lands have many stories to tell about their perceptions of strange and exotic customs that seems illogical, funny, and amusing. In other words, we tend to see only that which can be incorporated into our frame of reference and we reject anything that does not fit. Werner Erhard observes in the Erhard seminar training (EST) that we keep looking for a truth to fit our reality, but given our reality, the truth doesn't fit.

To be free from one's cultural or subculture is a painful and difficult path to walk. To make choices implies knowing of alternate ways. Yet, the inertia created by cultural customs influences and controls all of our lives. David Spitz notices the same phenomena of the impact of custom as a force in limiting our freedom of choice.

> . . . Everywhere custom is king, and everywhere men think themselves free even as they bend the knee to it. They mean to get along; they seek approval and success, they comply, therefore, with

149

customary ways and customary expectations. They do not so much submit as behave, for to submit is to yield one's inclination to custom, and they have no inclinations except for what is customary. And because they behave, and are comfortable in doing so, they are disquieted and irked by those who talk and act otherwise than they do.[20]

In conclusion we propose that there needs to be aggressive recruitment for sexual and ethnic diversity within nursing faculties. We believe that the interplay within such faculties holds the potential for the development of curriculums not bound to a single cultural perspective. We infer that there are many cultural perspectives within the American culture. Since nursing gives service to all communities, it is mandatory that the norms used in developing curriculums be as diverse as the communities that we serve.

THE PROBLEM OF ACCESS

Nancy Milo[21] discusses the problem of access to the health professions in her new book. She poignantly describes the social process of outcasting or rejecting that continues within the health professions for peoples from low income and rural settings, especially minorities and women. Even after admission to health programs, socialization pressures are felt keenly by ethnically diverse students. We are reminded of the experiences of a former student who for her duration of two years at California State College, Sonoma, remained angry and on the fringe of her peer group. Although she was a registered nurse, she exhibited the behavior of one who sees herself as an outcast within her own occupational group. She experienced difficulty in identifying with her classmates and the faculty. In a class assignment, she described her reactions to the term, "professional nurse." A few excerpts from this assignment are as follows:

One phrase that I vehemently react to is "professional nurse." Apparently, I have been reacting to it more so in the last two years, but I have been unable to express my outrage. It is so easy to know that I am angry, but not so easy to understand my anger. . . . Professional has been the most popular phrase around here or should I say propagandized phrase. . . . Most of my classmates seem to have soaked it in. . . . 'Professionalism in medicine is nothing more than the institutionalization of a male, upper class monopoly.' Professionalism in nursing follows suit. It also means that we must not confuse professionalism with expertise. . . . 'Expertise is something to work for and to share; professionalism is—by definition—elitist and exclusive, sexist, racist and classist'. . . . Now I can understand my anger and know why I do not refer to myself as a "professional" nurse. If anything, I vow to become an expert in women's health care and share my knowledge among my sisters so that we can all become experts. . . .[22]

Another student experienced release from her own unawareness of the oppression of sexual stereotyping in her life. Upon the urging of the writers, she shared her insights with the department chairperson and eventually the faculty in an open letter.[23] A few excerpts from this letter are included as follows:

. . . The experience at California State College, Sonoma, and the Second Step has facilitated growth and awareness for me that goes beyond the confines of this letter. Specifically, I learned:
(1) . . . my reason for entering nursing in my youth had been my need to take care of others (focus on others). By taking care of others, I didn't focus on myself, and take care of my needs. Not knowing my own need for being in nursing, I was resolved of any responsibility for myself and the assertion of my needs. I complained, whined, and played "Ain't it awful." I became a "drop out" for thirteen years. Learning this and accepting the past has made it possible for me to move on to other things such as:
  1.1 I have made a conscious choice to rechoose nursing.
  1.2 I have a better knowledge base of my professional needs and a stronger sense of self-assertion.
  1.3 I am more open to risk-taking with less concern of rejection.
  1.4 I have discovered that enjoying my work has intrinsic value.
  1.5 Responsibility for myself is my responsibility.
  1.6 I have a greater appreciation and understanding for the total process of being human.

Both students, through their educational experiences, became more aware of the roots of their own personal oppression within nursing. One viewed herself as outcast; the other viewed herself as not being able to choose. As Feire[24] says, concern for humanization leads at once to the recognition of dehumanization. He believes that the oppressed are the ones who ultimately will liberate themselves and those that oppress them. Within that context it is interesting to re-read the students' experience of liberation. We would like to acknowledge that these students have been instrumental in raising our levels of consciousness as their faculty.

TEACHING STUDENTS HOW TO LEARN IN CULTURALLY DIVERSE SITUATIONS: AN APPROACH

Because nursing is an applied field, application of knowledge in the practice of nursing becomes a critical skill for the success of the practitioner. Teaching students how to transfer information from lectures and textbooks into the experiences of their practice is one of the focuses of clinical teaching. The dilemma posed to the educator is how best to facilitate this process in the educational setting so that the student can transfer the process to other situations in the future.

The specific content that we are referring to in this paper is the knowledge of life-styles, attitudes, values, and cultural norms of women and ethnic groups of color in the United States. Are students given opportunities to learn the things that we want them to learn regarding themselves and cultural diversity within American life? A truism in nursing is that nursing care is for all people. Yet we maintain that nursing curriculums have not historically and do not presently provide content and experiences for students to raise their levels of awareness and sensitivity to their own values and the values of subcultural groups within our society.

There are some indications that this situation is beginning to shift with the inclusion of ethnic studies requirements within nursing curriculum and third world people on faculties of schools of nursing. Some examples of these changes are reflected in the following writings. Florence Martin Stroud and Teresa A. Bello in their chapter, "Community Nursing in Racially Oppressed Communities" of a recent publication[25] make a good point about how the application of the nursing process in minority communities can be oppressive. Also, Nancy Milo's experiences as a public health nurse in a Black urban setting are well documented by her writings. Although she is not Black, she has been able to function sensitively and effectively in a Black community. Her work is worth looking at carefully. Frances Storlie's book, *Nursing and the Social Conscience* is also a significant one. Her early years following the migrant circuit with her family gives her an unusual and sensitive point of view. And, finally, two psychiatrists who are Black, Dr. James P. Comer and Dr. Alvin F. Poussaint, have written a book on childrearing, *Black Child Care* (Simon & Schuster, 1975). They believe that Black parents need a different kind of child rearing advice than do White parents. The book includes problems common to all families; yet it does not ignore such urban realities as drug addiction, prostitution, and crime.

Given that there is an aggressive recruitment of men and ethnic groups of color within nursing as students and faculty, the problem of how to develop content and clinical experiences to promote multicultural learning continues to be a vexing one. How can we learn from each other? According to the perceptions of George Leonard,[26] humane, constructive change is multidimensional, involving the stuff of art, dream, and religion as well as hard thinking. He believes that the development of new perceptions by significant numbers of people within a culture may, almost unnoticed, turn that culture around. He further believes that some of the old assumptions that have shaped and limited our civilization are becoming visible and thus are being questioned. We believe that nursing is beginning to feel some of those social changes. Can we have a positive vision in nursing of what creates, maintains, and supports health and wellness for all people, not just a select few?

We believe that conscious inclusion of men and ethnic groups of color as students and faculty in the process of developing curricular content can assist greatly. An example of such collaboration is reflected in an article by Gertrude Hess and Florence Stroud.[27] They used seminars to surface racial tensions among students and faculty at the University of California in San Francisco. Such a process seems to have value in assisting faculty and students in raising their levels of consciousness regarding their own experiences.

Within the field of humanistic education, there recently has been more attention to the issue of the clarification of values. It is an attempt to assist students to be in touch with their own feelings and inner experiences and to choose for themselves. This focus has grown out of previous teaching approaches that have used moralizing, a laissex-faire approach, and role modeling as ways to teach values. Now the emphasis is upon the process of how to develop values. Implicit in this process is an effort to assist students in dealing with real values, such as helping them to become clearer about who they are, where they want to go, and how they are getting there. Students are actually studying themselves. They are the subject matter.[28]

The seven valuing processes according to Toffler[29] are:
1. Prizing and cherishing
2. Publicly affirming
3. Choosing
4. Choosing—after considering consequences
5. Choosing freely
6. Acting
7. Acting with a pattern, repetition, and consistency

Working through these processes with students holds potential for nursing educators. Might not this approach have some value in liberating the students and faculty from stereotyping?

Toffler[30] also discusses the problem of "overchoice" that faces western civilization. He recommends a cultural systems approach as a model for organizing significant areas of inquiry for students. He believes that all cultures are affected by seven different types of change or change factors: demographic, technological innovation, social innovation, cultural value shifts, ecological shifts, information-idea shifts, and cultural diffusion.

A general definition of systems includes four components: (1) elements, (2) relationships, (3) patterns, and (4) purpose.[31] This process is more difficult to apply in the social sciences than the natural sciences. Yet the systems approach has been of interest to nursing educators in

153

recent years and has been used commonly in the physiologic components of the curriculum. It seems to be a reasonable way to process a lot of data in a form that assists the students in the organization of significant information. Implicit in this approach is that the model can be applied widely. Its obvious limitation is that it is highly cognitive in orientation. It assists one in developing content. It does not deal with the issue of application.

There must be a focus of placing the responsibility for learning upon the student. By learning how to learn, a student has a higher probability of being able to transfer that process to future situations. It is noticed that this focus promotes self-reliance and an increased capability for solving problems. Some questions that need to be asked to support this are as follows:[32]

1. Could they learn the same materials on their own?
2. Could this series of lectures be replaced with reading assignments plus seminars?
3. Could students be assigned problems, the solving of which requires that they learn basic information on their own?

The Peace Corps has had to look at the problem of educating for application of learning across a barrier of culture and values. We believe that the cross-cultural learning model used by the Peace Corps has some value to nursing educators. A basic tenet of this model is the concept of working with another. Feelings of non-acceptance of the other must be resolved before there is a working with. Thus, on-going learning in the situation is a must for appropriately and sensitively giving service that is acceptable within that other cultural context. An example of the working through of this process is recorded by Moritz Thomsen in his own story as a Peace Corps volunteer in Ecuador, *Living Poor*.[33] Hence, we offer for your critical consideration our interpretation of the Peace Corps' cross-cultural training model and some examples of application of this model to nursing.

AN ALTERNATIVE MODEL*

The Peace Corps has had considerable experience in developing innovative approaches for training volunteers to work effectively in cross-cultural situations. The processes of learning how to enter another culture, to successfully work there, and then to re-enter your own culture once again are the bases of Peace Corps training. Intensive language training also is an essential component of Peace Corps training and to a lesser degree specific content (history, poli-

---

*The author, Renee Romanko-Keller, is a returned Peace Corps volunteer who trained at Camp Crozier, Arecibo, Puerto Rico, in 1969 in the last of the outward bound training camps. She also worked as a PC Trainer in Ponce, Puerto Rico in 1972.

tics, geography, etc.) are included. Most Peace Corps training now is done in-country.

It is my belief that the model for cross-cultural learning used by the Peace Corps is transferable to the teaching of faculty and students in nursing. There are parallels in the Peace Corps work experience to that of nursing which I have experienced in my practice and teaching. First, in both situations, one is expected to apply theoretical knowledge in ambiguous social situations and to take action often times under stress. Secondly, one is expected to have knowledge and skills required to carry out one's technical responsibilities. But the human aspects of one's work are equally as important as one's knowledge and skill. They are critical to one's success in the field. By human aspects, we mean functions such as establishing and maintaining trust, communicating, motivating, influencing, consulting, and advising.

When one works in another culture, all these interpersonal processes take place across differences of values, ways of perceiving and thinking, and cultural norms and expectations. Even if one has developed considerable communication skills in his or her own culture, there remains a great deal of learning that needs to be done before one can adapt his or her skill to operate cross-culturally. There is a direct relationship here to the problems of working in an urban ghetto if you are middle class or working in a rural setting if you are from an urban area. We believe much of nursing's failure in these areas comes from culture shock, and hence a high drop out rate from working in those areas. One could postulate that the experience of not knowing how to learn in those situations creates anxiety and depression (culture shock) within nurses.

Yet, it is not enough to understand how another culture differs from one's own. What is needed is an ability to feel one's way into intimate contact with those other values, attitudes, and feelings. The ability to work within the framework of the values of the other culture and not lose your own values is essential. One cannot protect himself or herself behind a wall of intellectual detachment. Personal involvement is necessary.

Roger Harrison[34] compared some generally accepted goals of university and cross-cultural education. It is useful to look at his work in clarifying the difference in focus needed for cross-cultural learning. It is as follows:

Some Major Goals of University Education

Some Divergent Goals of Overseas Education

Communication: To communicate fluently via the written word and, to a lesser extent, to speak well. To master the languages of

Communication: To understand and communicate directly and often nonverbally through movement, facial expression, person-

abstraction and generalization, e.g., mathematics and science. To understand readily the reasoning, the ideas, and the knowledge of the other.

Decision Making: To develop critical judgment: the ability to test assertions, assumptions, and opinions against the hard facts and the criteria of logic. To reduce susceptibility to specious argument and to be skeptical of intuition and emotion. To search for the best, most rational, most economical, and elegant solution.

Commitment: Commitment is to the truth. It requires an ability to stand back from on-going events in order to understand and analyze them and to maintain objectivity in the face of emotionally involving situations. Difficult situations are handled by explanations, theories, reports.

Ideals: The great principles and ideals of western society: social justice, economic progress, scientific truth. To value the sacrifice of present rewards and satisfactions for future advancement of these ideals and to find self-esteem and satisfaction from one's contribution toward distant social goals.

Problem Solving: A problem is solved when the true, correct, reasonable answer has been discovered and verified. Problem solving is a search for knowledge and truth. It is a largely rational

to-person actions. To listen with sensitivity to the hidden concerns, values, motives of the other. To be at home in the exchange of feelings, attitudes, desires, fears. To have a sympathetic, empathic understanding of the feelings of the other.

Decision Making: To develop ability to come to conclusions and take action on inadequate, unreliable, and conflicting information. To be able to trust feelings, attitudes, and beliefs as well as facts. To search for the possible course, the viable alternative, the durable though inelegant solution.

Commitment: Commitment is to people and to relationships. It requires an ability to become involved: to be able to give and inspire trust and confidence, to care and to take action in accordance with one's concern. Difficult situations are dealt with by staying with them, trying to take constructive action.

Ideals: Causes and objectives embedded in the here-and-now and embodied in the groups and persons in the immediate social environment. To find satisfaction, enjoyment, and self-esteem from the impact one has directly on the lives of others. To be able to empathize and work with others who live mostly in the present toward the limited, concrete goals which have meaning for them.

Problem Solving: A problem is solved when decisions are made and carried out which effectively apply people's energies to overcoming some barrier to a common goal. Problem-solving is a process, involving intelligence, creativity, insight, and a respect for facts.

social process involving communication, interpersonal influence, consensus, and commitment.

He further analyzed the meta-goals for university and cross-cultural training. By meta-goal is meant the approaches to learning, problem-solving and personal development which the learner acquires from being involved in a particular system of learning. Below are listed some meta-goals for university education contrasted with meta-goals appropriate for cross-cultural learning: [35]

Meta-Goals of Traditional College and University Classrooms

Appropriate Meta-Goals for Cross-Cultural Training

Source of Information: Information comes from experts and authoritative sources through the media of books, lectures, audio-visual presentations. "If you have a question, look it up."

Source of Information: Information sources must be developed by the learner from the social environment. Information-gathering methods include observation and questioning of associates, other learners, and chance acquaintances.

Learning Settings: Learning takes place in settings designated for the purpose, e.g., classrooms and libraries.

Learning Settings: The entire social environment is the setting for learning. Every human encounter provides relevant information.

Problem-Solving Approaches: Problems are defined and posed to the learner by experts and authorities. The correct problem-solving methods are specified, and the student's work is checked for application of the proper method and accuracy, or at least reasonableness of results. The emphasis is on solutions to known problems.

Problem-Solving Approaches: The learner is on his own to define problems, generate hypotheses, and collect information from the social environment. The emphasis is on discovering problems and developing problem-solving approaches on the spot.

Role of Emotions and Values: Problems are largely dealt with at an ideational level. Questions of reason and of fact are paramount. Feelings and values may be discussed, but are rarely acted upon.

Role of Emotions and Values: Problems are usually value- and emotion-laden. Facts are often less relevant than the perceptions and attitudes which people hold. Values and feelings have action consequences, and action must be taken.

Criteria of Successful Learning: Favorable evaluation by ex-

Criteria of Successful Learning: The establishment and main-

perts and authorities of the quality of the individual's intellectual productions, primarily written work.

tenance of effective and satisfying relationships with others in the work setting. This includes the ability to communicate with and influence the others. Often there are not criteria available other than the attitudes of the parties involved in the relationship.

To summarize the aims and goals of cross-cultural learning four main areas emerge as follows:[36]

1. The development of independence within the students so that they source their motivations, decisions, data collections, and definitions of problems (less support on authorities). In other words, the learners look to themselves as the originators of solutions and they gain confidence in their abilities to problem solve with limited and many times conflicting information.

2. The development of emotional resources within the learners so that they can deal constructively with the strong feelings aroused by cross-cultural conflict and confrontation.

3. The development of an ability to act from a position of conscious choice in situations of stress and uncertainty and to experience the consequences.

4. The development of an ability to use their own and others' feelings, attitudes, and values as information in the process of defining and solving human problems.

Essentially, the teacher is concerned with aiding the inductive learning processes of the students. An attempt is made to assist the learners in verbalizing what their feelings, perceptions, and experiences have been and in drawing out their own conclusions and generalizations from them. Teaching in this way demands a great deal of skill. It requires a sensitivity to interpersonal processes and an interest in the growth of the learner. It is a relatively private and unrecognized role, rewarded mostly by the relationships that develop between the students and the teacher.[37]

We have learned in the Peace Corp training programs that persons with practical experience do not necessarily become skillful teachers from that experience. The value of experienced persons is in their potential to conceptualize the cross-cultural learning experience in terms which can be applied to an experience-based learning situation. The key for effective teaching in these situations lies in the teacher's ability to use induction, to understand and develop a climate that facilitates learning, and to create situations where transfer of learning can be experienced by the learner. Unless students have received assistance in abstracting from the particular events, they will experience a great deal of difficulty in translating what they have learned.

This transfer of learning is essential in bridging theory to that which is concretely useful on the job.

We have found that problems at the level of feelings, motives, perceptions, and attitudes are quite similar regardless of cultural context. Therefore, getting a handle on one's own experiences in socially ambigious situations is a powerful tool in any cultural setting. Developing confidence in one's ability in such situations helps integrate the "head and guts" of one's experiences. So the need for expertise is less in the area of specific content about the culture, but rather more significantly in the area of developing skill in problem-solving processes. This includes particularly the development of strong feeling-thinking linkages.

Essentially, the cross-cultural training method used by the Peace Corp is the cultural immersion model. The student confronts and experiences that other culture in a variety of different ways. The trainers, in designing specific strategies, use the concepts of freedom and encounter in significant ways. Freedom is provided for the student to experience learning how to learn in another culture. Situations are also created for the student to encounter himself learning on an affective level. So personal involvement is encouraged and rewarded with attention to the aspects of self that are touched and changed in the process.

Overall principles used in designing strategies for training are as follows:[38]

1. *Problem solving:* No information is presented which is not relevant to the solution of some real problem which the learner is asked to solve in the here-and-now.

2. *Immediate data orientation:* Learners are required to develop information from the persons who are present with them in a given situation.

3. *Value orientation:* In the training situation, learners are asked to make choices among competing values which have consequences for their relationships with others.

4. *Experience-action orientation:* Understanding is not enough. Learners must experience the emotional impact of the phenomena with which they are dealing. They have to influence others to action as well as to act independently. Hence, training situations require discussion and analysis that lead to decision and action.

5. *Use of authority (trainers):* A delicate and unusual use of authority is called for. Students are rewarded by the trainers for engaging actively and wholeheartedly in the learning process. The negative use of authority is implemented as a "fencing in" to keep students in contact with the problem they are expected to solve. That is, the trainers realize that the students will only learn by remaining in the situation that is making them so uncomfortable.

6. *Use of expertise:* The trainers design situations to assist the students in being confronted with the processes and problems which they will need in order to function. They assist the students in reflecting about their experiences so that connections and generalizations can be

made about what they have learned regarding themselves, their own goals in a cross-cultural setting, their own culture, and the other culture.

Primary among important adaptive resources is the ability to take moderate emotional risks[39] in situations where one's sense of self-esteem is involved. The concept of moderate risk is characterized by a willingness to increase tension somewhat in order to obtain information about the difficulty. The important thing is not whether these attempts are successful in resolving the problem, but rather in giving more information without the risk of damaging the relationship much more. It requires more emotional ability to withstand tension over a period of time than that required for low or high risk positions.

SOME EXAMPLES OF APPLYING THIS MODEL TO A TEACHING-LEARNING SITUATION IN NURSING

For two years, one writer has had the responsibility for a clinical section of ten students in Community Health Nursing, a two semester course in the junior year of the Second Step curriculum. Within the framework of the course and the constraints of the clinical objectives, a number of teaching strategies were employed to assist the students in immersing themselves in the community and then reflecting upon and analyzing what was learned. There was an explicit expectation to be creative, to experiment, to involve themselves, and to eventually choose interventions based upon the students' own diagnoses of the situation.

Initially, in assisting the students to enter the community, I gave them a series of mini-immersion exercises so that they could personally experience the community in various ways. The exercises began with community observation, followed by group discussions, and moved to participant-observation in various health care facilities within the community. Then a client caseload was gradually selected by each student. To begin the process of caseload selection, each student was given the assignment of selecting a well family from the community. The intent of the assignment was to provide "space" for the students to focus learning upon health and wellness. Again, it was a way of involving the students in choosing and discovering what they needed to learn about health in order to do health promotion with clients. It also exposed the students to the process of case finding.

The well family selected was followed for one year. Clinical seminars focused periodically upon the students' learning of what created wellness within their own experiences as well as that of the families. The parallel of discovering wellness in themselves and the families was made explicit. In addition, the students were asked to creatively record their learning. One of the students at the end of the year

160

wrote a poem reflecting some of the process of her learning. Notice
the personal involvement that is revealed in such a tender way as the
student looks back at her own family experiences.

Well Family

How we see ourselves, more oft than not,
Differs greatly from others,
I wonder how you see yourselves. . .
    as individuals
    as a WHOLE.
Do you see the WHOLE I see. . .
and envy. . .with distant longings.
    Longings based in my own deprivation. . .experienced
    In needs unmet. . .unattended. . .
Yet, n'er expressed. . .thus, I allowed their existence to flow
    ignoring MY responsibility. . .
    in alleviating my pain.

And so,
I chose you on purpose. . .
    to get as close as I could. . .
    to your closeness. . .and experience it for myself.
    To live in YOUR world for a little while. . .
      with painful reflection on my past. . .
And what is this WORLD. . .this WHOLE. . .I experience in you?
    It is not stagnant. . .but ever changing. . .
    Enmeshed so acutely in your individualities. . .
    Mustn't I have that backwards?
    Does not your WHOLE stem from the parts of
    which it is composed?
    Or are the parts, rather, a result of that whole?
    The complexity is too great. . .
      I can't distinguish. . .which came first. . .
      And it matters not. . .in how I SEE you.
What, then, is this WHOLE I experience?
What is it's meaning. . .to me. . .
    What are it's teachings. . .it's revelations. . .
FAMILY. . .HEALTH. . ."WELLNESS". . .combined[40]

In the development of the general caseload of each student, the writer
encouraged them to select a family that was different from their own
life style. Some of the students' choices were as follows: a single
parent family; a migrant, multi-problem family; an elderly man living
alone; a Mexican-American family; a young couple with their first

child; and a young, homosexual divorcee with a school age child. Many discussions regarding clarification of values came up throughout the year. The students experienced their own values in conflict often times with those of their clients. We noticed a definite movement within the students toward nonjudgment as their own values were made conscious.

The use of the group in clinical seminar to expose students to the power of students helping students was another adaptation from cross-cultural learning. The climate that was created within the group was that of a "positive peer culture."[41] The aim was to assist the students in developing peer support, a critical relationship, also, needed in nursing practice. In other words, the idea was to develop each student's ability to use his or her own and others' feelings, attitudes, and values as information in the process of defining and solving problems. Students opening up to the personal benefits of peer support is an exciting process to observe! We believe such learning has a high probability of being transferred to future work situations.

Another assignment which lent itself to problem solving within the community was the community analysis assignment. Because of the nature of the assignment, students were required to become involved with the community that they were studying. Since it was a group assignment, it also required considerable cooperation and collaboration. Both years the writer experienced the students wanting to make the assignment work for them in ways that the faculty had not foreseen. So she encouraged them to attempt to define what it was that they wanted. The problem solving that they participated in as a group reflected social processes often seen in cross-cultural problem solving, that is, solution of a problem can be reached when people's energies are applied to overcoming some mutually decided upon barrier to a common goal. This process is partly reflected in the following example from a group of students who attempted to adapt and broaden a component of the community analysis assignment to enhance the direction of their own learning. They submitted the following proposal:[42]

We, the students of the Sebastopol Community Health Practicum group, in order to provide a more comprehensive community health experience, should like to present to the nursing faculty, a proposal for a student designed, student initiated, community involved pilot clinic that incorporates both medical screening and individual and group counseling as the need within the community is perceived.

Objectives

1. The provision of the opportunity for students to explore alternative methods of initiating health care delivery on all levels of

162

prevention within the community is determined by the changing needs of the community.
2. The encouragement of community participation in all facets of planning, implementation, funding and evaluation of this clinic.
3. An increase in student awareness of health care delivery and maintenance problems within the dynamic community.
4. The provision of a comprehensive, biostatistical assessment of health status and delivery problems of the community through a consumer survey.
5. A provision for follow-up care by referral as deemed necessary as a result of screening.
6. This clinic work will be in conjunction with a caseload of three families.
7. The exploration of ways for the dissemination of information within the community.
8. The possibility of expanding the initial pilot program beyond May 1975.
9. An increasing awareness of values, feelings, and attitudes of self and others.

The opportunities for learning provided to this group of students for actively experiencing themselves trying to create change was of no small consequence. They wrote an after thought to their final group paper as follows:

We, the students presently in the Sebastopol Community Health Group, wholeheartedly endorse this type of learning experience for the next group of students who will obtain their community health experience in the Sebastopol area. We feel that the processes experienced provided useful and enlightening insights into the community of Sebastopol and also into the dynamics of the research process.

In essence, teaching students how to learn or survive in socially ambiguous situations where action under stress is required is a key concept in cross-cultural learning. Thus, valuing and trusting one's own experiences and abilities are critical for the learner. Developing "emotional muscle" so that one can tolerate tension over a period of time in taking moderate emotional risks is another critical, adaptive behavior. And finally, to find satisfaction, enjoyment, and self-esteem from the impact one has directly on the lives of others is important. Hence, mini-steps can be taken into the real world in preparation for the eventual role of practitioner. Such education is a form of role rehearsal for future situations of complexity and ambiguity. The Peace Corps has learned that guided immersion exercises greatly assist the process of transfer of learning to other situations. From my experience as a volunteer and trainer, I have found it possible to adapt cross-cultural methods to teaching community health nursing within the Second Step curriculum.

SONOMA'S APPROACH TO LIBERALIZATION

One of the intents of the Second Step curriculum is to promote cultural and sexual diversity within nursing. Attention has been given to the recruitment of an ethnically diverse faculty and student body. The philosophy developed by the faculty as a basis of the curriculum's design attempted to make clear our beliefs. In part, it is as follows:

> We believe society is characterized by a variety of cultures and subcultures, each with its own value system. . . . We believe professional nursing is primarily concerned with the maintenance of humane, individualistic concern for people and their problems. . . . Professional nursing attends to the health needs of man within the framework of man's goals, motivations, and value systems. . . . We believe there are many different approaches to the same goal and that students may have traveled different routes, distances, and directions.[43]

The faculty also believes that the teaching-learning process is a dual interaction and reaction in which the teacher serves as a facilitator and the individual student and/or student group as active and contributing participants in the process. It is crucial that there are identification and capitalization upon the rich and varied experiences and backgrounds that the students bring to the program. In this way, students learn from their peers as well as from their teachers, and the faculty, in turn, gain new insights and knowledge from their students.[44]

Intention is important. The formulating of a philosophy assists the faculty in reaching consensus and making overt the major thrusts that the curriculum will potentially make. It also reflects the level of social consciousness of the faculty regarding contemporary issues. According to Werner Erhard, "Intention is the essence of communication. . . if you keep saying it the way it really is, eventually, your word is law in the universe."[45]

In an open curriculum the intent is to recognize and capitalize upon the diversity found within the students. Admission requirements are such that the students are not penalized by grade point average, age, sex, or pattern of previous education. Hence, the design of an open curriculum can foster the inclusion of ethnic groups of color and can provide opportunity for more men to study nursing. This has been a deliberate attempt of the Second Step program at Sonoma State College.

164

Yet, the difficult question of how to individualize the curriculum to meet the diverse needs of all students continues to challenge the faculty's ingenuity, creativeness, and resources. What kinds of faculty development are needed to assist in the creation of materials that reflect cultural and sexual diversity? There is an awareness of the effect upon all students when culturally diverse points of view are absent from the classroom and clinical experiences, yet how to incorporate teaching models that reflect varying cultural patterns is not clear.

In an effort to assist the faculty in the development of materials for teaching culturally diverse values, attitudes, and knowledges, the department in February 1975 joined the WICHEN (Western Interstate Commission for Higher Education in Nursing) project, Models for Introducing Cultural Diversity Within Nursing Curricula.[46] The department was chosen as one of the demonstration schools for this project.

In further recognition of the need for nurses to have a knowledge base of the influence of culture upon health practices, all students in the Second Step are required to take four units in ethnic studies. They may choose from the following courses: Health and Culture; The Black Family; The Mexican-American Family; Cultural Conflicts; Seminar: Ethnic Interactions; Black Cultures in the Americas; Asian-American Education and Child-Rearing Practices; Identity and the Asian Americans; Native Californian Cultures; and Native American Cultures of the American Southwest. Knowledges gained from exposure to such courses can be applied if the student so chooses in clinical work in Community Health Nursing in the junior year or in the Senior Preceptorship.

Becoming Liberated

To liberate one must make conscious that which is not obvious. One is liberated when one is consciously aware and can make choices for participation from a position of responsibility. The extent that one loses his ability to make choices by choosing to be subjected to the choices of others is the extent of his oppression.[47] To critically confront one's own problems and to be responsible for one's own recuperation is the essence of being liberated or enlightened. Naive consciousness considers itself superior to facts, in control of facts, and thus free to understand as it pleases.[48]

It is our premise that there is a great deal of unconsciousness within the ranks of nursing regarding sex discrimination and the exclusion of ethnic groups of color from nursing. It is our intention to assist in raising the level of consciousness of nurses regarding their oppression and their participation in oppression. We believe that the gap between awareness and experience can be bridged. It is a process

165

of valuing one's experiences and coming responsibly from the position of one's experiences. That is being liberated and enlightened.

Being Alienated from One's Experiences

There is a subtle seduction in higher education. It is the unconscious internalization of the importance of the "expert's" opinion and the devaluation of one's own personal experiences. This overconfidence in sources other than one's self is a disturbing and frightening process. It leaves the student and practitioner afloat in uncertainty and anxiety when an expert is not readily available to give an opinion. There is a sense of powerlessness when one cannot trust one's own experiences as being valid.

The power of communicating from one's own experiences is not clearly understood. If one falls into the position of listening and reacting to all the various opinions of what to do, and does not observe what is working in his own experiences, he is an "ass." If a teacher realizes that what a student needs to know is in his experiences, the relationship between the two takes a curious turn. The process of dialogue becomes important. Both become more in tune with their own experiences. A valuing of each other and of their own experiences is a significant outcome of this process.

Dialogue according to Paulo Freire infers a horizontal relationship between two persons. A sense of empathy is developed when you are engaged in a joint search. On the other hand, a vertical relationship between two people impedes communication. A climate of distance and distrust can develop. Usually one issues communiques; the other receives communiques.[49]

The essence of dialoguing implies mutual participation. Success in moving into an equal, sharing relationship provides opportunity for the learner to experience himself and to grasp the power of his own experiences. A sense of control over one's self is an outgrowth of this process. Valuing one's experiences catches on. One becomes more assertive and alive.

SUMMARY

Our work as a faculty has just begun in the long journey of exploring ways of liberating ourselves and our students from the deadness of stereotyped thinking. Our exposure to the challenges and complexities of a diverse student body has opened up doors to our own learning and continues to act as a gadfly to our growing awareness. We value the full participation of our students in this arduous walk into the frontiers of social change.

REFERENCES

1. Mead, Margaret: Needed: Full Partnership for Women. *Saturday Review* June 14, 1975, pp. 26-27.
2. Bart, Pauline: Why Women See the Future Differently From Men, in Toffler, A. (ed.): *Learning for Tomorrow.* New York, Random House, 1974, p. 38.
3. *Ibid.*, p. 37.
4. *Ibid.*, p. 42.
5. Bem, Sandra L., and Bem, Daryl J.: Training the Woman to Know Her Place. The Power of a Nonconscious Ideology, in Garskof, Michele H. (ed.): *Roles Woman Play: Readings Toward Women's Liberation.* Brooks and Cole Publishing Co., Belmont, Calif., 1971.
6. Staines, Graham, Tavris, Carol, and Jayaratne, Toby Epstein: The Queen Bee Syndrome. *Psychology Today* Jan. 1974, p. 58.
7. Cleland, Virginia: Sex Discrimination: Nursing's Most Pervasive Problem. *American Journal of Nursing* 71:1542, 1971.
8. Lee, Patrick C., and Gropper, Nancy B.: Sex-Role Culture and Educational Practice. *Harvard Educational Review* 44:396, 1974.
9. Bardwick, J.M.: *Psychology of Women: A Study of Bio-Cultural Conflicts.* Harper & Row, New York, 1971, p. 218.
10. Keniston, Ellen, and Keniston, Kenneth: American Anachronism: The Image of Women and Work. *American Scholar* 33:372, 1964.
11. Horner, Natina S.: A Bright Women Is Caught in a Double Bind. *Psychology Today* 3:38, 1969.
12. Mandle, Joan D.: Women's Liberation: Humanizing Rather than Polarizing. *The Annals of the American Academy of Political and Social Sciences* 397:121, 1971.
13. Leininger, Madeleine: The Leadership Crisis in Nursing: A Critical Problem and Challenge. *Journal of Nursing Administration* March—April 1974, p. 29.
14. Alberti, Robert E., and Emmons, Michael L.: *Your Perfect Right (A Guide to Assertive Behavior).* Impact, San Luis Obispo, 1974, p. 2.
15. Lee and Gropper, op. cit., pp. 369-370, 376.
16. *Ibid.*, pp. 386, 396.
17. Blauner, Robert: *Racial Oppression in America.* Harper & Row, New York, 1972, p. 261.
18. Burnett, Collins W.: The Myth of Change in Higher Education. *Intellect* 102:424, 1974.
19. Pearce, Joseph Chilton: *The Crack in the Cosmic Egg.* Simon & Schuster, Inc., New York, 1973, pp. 49-62.
20. Spjtz, David: Politics, Patriotism and the Teacher, in *Patterns of Power,* 2 ed. Pitman Publishing Co., New York, 1974, p. 417.
21. Milo, Nancy: *The Care of Health in Communities—Access for Outcasts.* Macmillan Publishing Co., New York, 1975, p. 154.
22. Brennan, Lori: REACTION Paper No. 3, N422B, Department of Nursing, CSCS, Spring 1975, unpublished document.
23. Chipps, Ernestine: Letter to faculty members. San Rafael, California, May 1975 (unpublished).
24. Freire, Paulo: *Pedagogy of the Oppressed.* Herder Co., New York, 1971, pp. 27-28.
25. Fleshman, Ruth, and Archer, Sarah E.: *Community Health Nursing—Patterns & Practice.* Wadsworth Publishing, Inc., Belmont, Calif., 1975, pp. 294-305.
26. Leonard, George B.: How We Will Change. *Intellectual Digest* June 1974, p. 15.
27. Hess, Gertrude, and Stroud, Florence: Racial Tension—Barriers to Delivery of Nursing Care. *Journal of Nursing Administration* May/June 1972, pp. 47-49.

28. Toffler, Alvin (ed.): *Learning for Tomorrow*. Vintage Books, New York, 1974, pp. 266-270.
29. *Ibid.*, pp. 263-266.
30. *Ibid.*, pp. 109-117.
31. *Ibid.*, p. 110.
32. Bryant, John: *Health and the Developing World*. Cornell University Press, Ithaca, N.Y., 1969, pp. 204-205.
33. Thomsen, Moritz: *Living Poor (A Peace Corps Chronicle)*. University of Washington, Seattle, 1969.
34. Harrison, Roger: *The Design of Cross-Cultural Training: With Examples From the Peace Corps*. The National Training Laboratories, Washington, D.C., 1966, pp. 5-6.
35. *Ibid.*, pp. 7-8.
36. *Ibid.*, p. 13.
37. *Ibid.*, p. 18.
38. *Ibid.*, pp. 13-16.
39. *Ibid.*, p. 11.
40. Renfrew, Cynthia: Class Assignment for N311B, Department of Nursing, CSCS, Spring 1975 (unpublished).
41. Vorrath, Harry H., and Brendtro, Larry K.: *Positive Peer Culture*. Aldine Publishing Company, Chicago, 1974.
42. N311B, Sebastopol Group Project submitted to the Community Health Nursing Faculty, Department of Nursing, CSCS, Spring 1975 (unpublished). (Students involved were as follows: Hannah Pressler, Mary Hineline, Susan Cranmore, William Stephens, Dorothea Vigil, Cynthia Renfrew, Rufina Wall, Carol Hammari, Harriet Ingham, and Barbara Tirpak).
43. *The Second Step: A Self Evaluation Study*. Rohnert Park, Calif., 1974, pp. 39-40.
44. *Ibid.*
45. Erhard, Werner: *If God Had Meant Man to Fly He Would Have Given Him Wings*. Erhard Seminar Training, San Francisco, 1973.
46. WICHEN: "Models for Introducing Cultural Diversity in Nursing Curricula." Marie Branch, Project Director, Boulder, Colorado, 1975-77.
47. Freire, Paulo: *Education for Critical Consciousness*. The Seabury Press, New York, 1973, p. 4.
48. *Ibid.*, p. 44.
49. *Ibid.*, pp. 45-46.

BIBLIOGRAPHY

Annas, George J., and Healy, Joseph: The Patient Rights Advocate. *Journal of Nursing Administration* May/June 1974, pp. 25-31.
Bardwick, Judith M., et al.: *Feminine Personality and Conflict*. Brooks-Cole Publishing Company, Belmont, Calif., 1970.
Benoliel, Jeanne Quint: Scholarship—A Woman's Perspective. *Image* 7:22, 1975.
Bergquist, William H., and Phillips, Steven R.: Components of An Effective Faculty Development Program. *Journal of Higher Education* 46:177, 1975.
Billingsley, Andrew: *Black Families in White America*. Prentice-Hall, Inc. Englewood Cliffs, N.J., 1968.
Cofer, Audre: Autobiography of a Black Nurse. *American Journal of Nursing* 74:1836, 1974.
Cott, Nancy F. (ed.): *Root of Bitterness (Documents of the Social History of American Women)*. E. P. Dutton & Co., Inc., New York, 1972.
Cowan, Paul: *The Making of An Un-American (A Dialogue with Experience)*. The Viking Press, Inc., New York, 1970.
Ehrenreich, Barbara, and Ehrenreich, John: *The American Health Empire: Power, Profits, and Politics*. Random House, New York, 1970.

Ehrenreich, Barbara, and English, Dierdre: *Complaints and Disorders, The Sexual Politics of Sickness.* The Feminist Press, Old Westbury, N.Y., 1973.

Friedan, Betty, and de Beauvoir, Simone: Sex, Society and the Female Dilemma. *Saturday Review* June 14, 1975, pp. 14-20, 56.

Garskof, Michele H. (ed.): *Roles Women Play: Readings Toward Women's Liberation.* Brooks-Cole Publishing Co., Belmont, Calif., 1971.

Gomez, Rudolph (ed.), et al.: *The Social Reality of Ethnic America.* D. C. Heath and Company, Lexington, Mass., 1974.

Hart, Edward, and Sechrist, William (eds.): *Dynamics of Wellness.* Wadsworth Publishing Co., Inc., Belmont, Calif., 1970.

Jacobs, Alfred, and Spradlin, Wilford W. (eds.): *The Group As Agent of Change.* West Virginia University Press, Morgantown, 1974.

Keller, Suzanne: Does the Family Have a Future? *Journal of Comparative Family Studies* Spring 1971.

Kushner, Trucia D.: The Nursing Profession—Condition: Critical. *Ms* 11:72, 1973.

Leininger, Madeleine: *Nursing and Anthropology: Two Worlds to Blend.* John Wiley and Sons, Inc., New York, 1970.

Menges, Robert I.: Cognitive Bias and College Admission. *Integrateducation* 12:30, 1974.

Moffat, Mary Jane, and Painter, Charlotte (eds.): *Revelations: Diaries of Women.* Random House, New York, 1974.

Morgan, Robin (ed.): *Sisterhood is Powerful.* Random House, New York, 1970.

Newman, Katharine D. (ed.): *Ethnic America Short Stories.* Pocket Books, New York, 1975.

Norman, John C.: *Medicine in the Ghetto.* Appleton-Century-Crofts, New York, 1969.

Otero, Lorraine M.: The Mechanics of Exclusion: The Lack of Spanish Speaking Nurses on Hospital Staffs in Sonoma County, California. A thesis submitted to California State College, Sonoma in partial fulfillment of the requirements for the Master of Arts in Political Science, California State College, Sonoma, 1974, Rohert Park, Calif. (unpublished).

Peplau, Hildegarde, and Sado, Robert: A Debate: Is Health Care a Right? *IMAGE* 7:4, 1974.

Phelps, Stanlee, and Austin, Nancy: *The Assertive Woman.* IMPACT Fredericksburg, Va., 1975.

Postman, Neil, and Weingartner, Charles: *The Soft Revolution.* Del Publishing Company, New York, 1971.

Shoben, E. J., Jr.: Academic Standards: A Problem in Values, in Vermilye, D. W. (ed.): *The Future in Making.* Jossey-Bass, San Francisco, 1973, pp. 160-173.

Sarason, Seymour B.: *The Creation of Settings and the Future Societies.* Jossey-Bass, San Francisco, 1972.

Seligson, Marcia: EST—The New Life—Changing Philosophy That Makes You the Boss. *Cosmopolitan* June, 1975, pp. 165-167, 172-173, 204-205.

Staples, Robert: Sex and Racism. *SIECUS Report* 3:1, 1975.

Stringfellow, William: *My People Is the Enemy.* Holt, Rinehart and Winston, New York, 1964.

Textor, Robert B. (ed.): *Cultural Frontiers of the Peace Corps.* The M.I.T. Press, Cambridge, Mass., 1966.

Toffler, Alvin (ed.): *Learning For Tomorrow; The Role of the Future in Education.* Random House, New York, 1974.

Weitzman, Lenore J.: Sex-Role Socialization in Picture Books for Preschool Children. *American Journal of Sociology* 77:1125, 1972.

White, Earnestine Huffman: Health and the Black Person: An Annotated Bibliography. *American Journal of Nursing* 74:1839, 1974.

CHAPTER 8

Faculty Group and Interpersonal Processes

Sue A. Thomas, R.N., M.S., and Janice Hitchcock, R.N., M.S.

The purpose of this chaper is to describe and interpret faculty behavior and interaction in the light of group dynamics. The evolutionary development of the faculty will be explored and individual behavior explained in terms of the group process. Particular emphasis will be placed on the significance of the on-going support group that began at the end of the first year. It is our hope that a picture of our dynamics may be helpful to other faculties as they explore their own interpersonal worlds.

THE FIRST YEAR

Group dynamics has influenced our behavior as a faculty since we first met three years ago in 1972, although the knowledge that we needed to consider the impact of the group process on faculty development didn't come until later. Seven of us met for the first time one month before the first students arrived and began then to work together as a group. None had close associations with the others, although several had been previously acquainted. We all had master's degrees but our clinical backgrounds were quite varied. One had extensive experience in medical-surgical nursing, both clinically and academically. She and two others also brought with them administrative expertise. Of these other two, one had been a director of psychiatric nursing in a county agency. The other had taught public health nursing and had been a staff nurse and supervisor in a public health department. A fourth member also had a master's degree in community health nursing but was new to professional nursing practice. The remaining three faculty had both teaching and clinical experience in, respectively, maternal-child health, nurse-midwifery, and community mental health nursing. All the faculty has a strong interest in the community and in working with the total needs of the

170

family. Our varying clinical backgrounds meant that we brought a variety of perspectives and levels of teaching skills to the program.

Preplanning

Initially, we were faced with the overwhelming job of developing a curriculum to be ready in one month, with freedom to develop the curriculum in our own way. From time to time the chairperson would suggest approaches that were of particular interest to her but the final decision was left to our judgment. As happens in any newly formed group, we tested each other as we explored our frames of reference and views on education while developing course objectives, content, teaching tools, and evaluation criteria.

Although we had a task to accomplish, one can see in retrospect that we were still moving through group process. Yalom[1] points out that every group must work through three stages of development. The first stage has to do with orientation, hesitant participation, and search for meaning. "Goblet issues" are common during this stage, that is, sizing up one another through discussion on nonemotionally laden topics. The term comes from the activity at a cocktail party whereby each participant sizes up the others by looking through a cocktail "goblet." For us, planning curriculum served as our goblet issue. During the second stage, issues regarding dominence, control, and power come to light. Hostility to the leader also emerges as one realizes he won't be chosen as the favored one and that the leader is not perfect. Although these issues emerged from time to time, usually in the form of jokes about how we were changing the ideas of of the chairperson, we were too busy with the immediate task to deal with them until much later. In the third stage, members have concerns about intimacy and closeness. As both negative and positive affect is more directly addressed, the group grows more cohesive and matures to the point that all affect can be expressed. We continued to grapple with this stage of development, however, and the establishment of our support group at the end of the first year (to be discussed in more detail later) was our first formal recognition of a need to deal with the deeper feeling levels of our relationships with one another.

Our interaction can also be interpreted in the light of Schutz's concepts.[2] He describes the three major concerns of groups as having to do with inclusion, control, and affection needs. The members must first decide how much contact they want with one another in terms of social and work relationships. Control issues deal with decisions regarding competition vs. cooperation, how much power is any member allowed, and what are the dominant-submissive relationships within the group. Affection needs relate to emotional closeness rather than the physical closeness implied in inclusion needs; issues of self-disclosure must be decided.

Although our mode of operation, by necessity, was for all to be included in all decisions, it was also a personal need of each member. We were all equally new and inexperieneed in developing this new approach to baccalaureate education and we wanted to be a part of every decision. Later, as we were forced to subgroup for efficiency's sake, we became acutely aware of how difficult it was for us not to participate in every activity. Our need to be a part of decision making could be interpreted as a need to control. Actually, we were quite open to the ideas of others and generally very able to compromise. It was the wish to be involved in the process of decision making that seemed to be paramount. Our group was too small to divide into task forces so that all major decisions were made in faculty meetings. We met weekly and discussed all issues. Since time didn't allow us to indulge in major disagreements and since we did not feel any strong hostility to one another at that point, decisions were equivalent to consensus. Most of us were quite verbal about our ideas and able to present them for discussion. We also could disagree with one another but with respect for the idea presented and the person who presented it. Values and commitments were not at first closely challenged, nor was negative feedback expressed. We looked to the authority figure, the department chairperson, for direction and had few questions regarding her curriculum outline. We closely resembled the dependency phase of group development in which the leader is expected to provide for our needs. All of us were aware that as we proceeded into the first semester, conflicts would arise and we would have to deal with them.

While we were still working through the first stage of early group development, we were at the same time beginning to move into the second. The leaders among the group had started to emerge. They tended to be members who had the most experience. Two were formal leaders in that one coordinated the main course in community health and the other assisted the chairman with administrative duties. Several members took on leadership roles in different situations although not formally identified as leader. For example, one functioned as coordinator of a course although another had been originally appointed to this role. While this situation had the potential for conflict, none emerged because the designated coordinator had developed interests in other areas and was very glad to abdicate. Since she was perceived by other faculty to make a valuable contribution, this change did not make a difference in her relationship with other members.

First Semester

As we moved into the fall semester, each of us had some separate course commitments, but we all were involved with the community health nursing course. We continued to meet together weekly to work on course-related tasks. By this time, certain coalitions, antagonists, and roles were developing. One faculty member seemed to consistently leave herself out, usually with no explanation to us, by going her separate way at lunch time, coming late or leaving early, and seldom initiating an opinion in planning meetings. Our decision making was based on the input from all and each was expected to contribute according to his own knowledge base. In retrospect, it is clear that she was violating one of the group rules: everyone contributes to discussion without waiting to be asked. The rest of us seemed to accept this rule. Her isolating behavior broke another rule: we all stick together. While some faculty seemed to spend more time with certain other faculty rather than with all the members equally, these contacts were loose and shifting and always open to including another person, and interestingly, pairing had little to do with clinical orientation.

Roles are patterns of behavior that people take[3] and are usually defined in terms of that behavior. They may be disruptive or facilitative, i.e., they can restrict the group or help it to grow.[4] Several roles began to particularly stand out; most of them facilitative. Three faculty seemed to take the role of coordinator, each in different areas and related to their job commitment. One, who liked administrative detail, took over some of the responsibilities that the chairperson had been carrying, particularly the admission process. The other two members, one assigned as community health coordinator and the other who took over as coordinator of another course, have been previously discussed. These three also accepted the role of information giver. One was very helpful in exploring the intricacies of admission procedure and how to deal with the college bureaucracy in general. The others immediately began to help us explore possible approaches to teaching the courses for which they were responsible.

As our group rules imply, most of us accepted the role of initiator in one way or another. All had expertise in different areas and freely shared their knowledge and ideas. One member, new to teaching, tended to be quieter, more of an information-acceptor and follower. No one person stood out as a leader at all times, this role shifted according to the task and, consequently, so did the role of follower. One member in particular frequently took the role of evaluator. She was more involved with administration and this emphasis placed her in a good position to raise questions about the feasibility of our ideas and make helpful alternative suggestions. No one specifically took the role of harmonizer but whenever it seemed that someone was getting the brunt of a controversy, there was always someone to come to the rescue and help to settle the issue. Although no one clearly blocked interaction, one member did tend to avoid directly stating how she felt. We all avoided underlying conflicts for the time being in order to accomplish our task.

173

It wasn't until the second month of classes that the group had its first crisis. Due to an administrative oversight, and through no fault of her own, the quiet member learned that the Board of Nurse Education and Nurse Registration declared she could not teach because she lacked sufficient clinical experience. When the faculty rallied around to support her in this difficulty, she was unable to express herself and denied that she was experiencing undue stress. From this situation another group rule emerged. One should be able to recognize and express one's own feelings. She further deviated from accepted behavior, in the eyes of the rest of the faculty, because she chose to challenge the decision, rather than seek clinical experience. The school offered her a year's leave of absence to gain professional work experience. She chose her other alternative which was to prove to the BNENR that her volunteer and student experience was equivalent to work experience as an R.N. We felt that there was much she needed to learn through work, that her prenursing experience was not equivalent, and that she had difficulty acknowledging her limitations.

We were strongly in favor of her choosing a course that would allow her to improve her abilities. When she did not accept that option, a clear hiatus between her and the rest of the faculty was established. Because she was from a minority group, she and others on campus were quick to imply that our conflict stemmed from racism, and this issue became a red herring. That is, a false motive, racism, was attributed to our response to her problem and because racism is such an emotionally charged issue, energy was directed to exploration of that aspect while the real issue of professional performance was submerged.

In response to the questions being raised about our possible racism, we spent much time examining our own motives and questioning our attitudes. Every time, however, we came to the same conclusion: it was not her ethnic background but attitudes and behaviors separate from that to which we were responding. Issues that surfaced during this crisis continued through the second semester into the second year.

Second Semester

While we were still dealing with this situation, the second semester began and with it came two new faculty members. One joined the community health team and the other was hired to develop a new facet of the curriculum for the senior year. These work assignments as well as the individual personalities of the two people played an important part in how they were incorporated into the faculty group. The member who was a part of the community health group was forced to relate to all the faculty since at that time everyone taught a component of this course. She was an individual who enjoyed

174

being with people and was willing to share herself with others. She could acknowledge her need for support and inclusion and was also supportive of others. In other words, she adhered to our rules.

On the other hand, the second new faculty member preferred to work independently and her responsibilities put her in a position to do so. When members approached her to develop a relationship, the focus was kept on a task. Contact was additionally difficult because she was housed separately from the rest of us. She made a few attempts to develop informal personal relationships with faculty. This attitude, while valid in itself, conflicted with our rules. As the semester continued, there was also a beginning concern that her work production was not adequate or appropriate to the program objectives.

With the addition of these members, roles became further delineated. The member who joined the community health team became the harmonizer. That is, she could tolerate conflict when necessary but was pained by it and made every attempt to diffuse it. The attitude of the second new member was similar to that of our quiet member so that we now had two avoiders. The two with strong psychiatric background seemed most able to confront, although their styles were different. The mediator remained the same and was the member most removed from the community health team subgroup. One remained primarily an observer, although giving definite input in decision making. The community health coordinator and another member tried to be a harmonizer, by facilitating problem solving. When indicated, however, they were able to confront issues directly.

As the conflicts emerged, the faculty began to be aware of the need to consider ways to deal with these interpersonal concerns in a space and time separate from the curricula tasks. We began to realize we were using much of our energy to deal with these problems but the reality demands of the program prevented us from working through any of them. We all agreed that we would only begin this working through process if we set time aside for that purpose, and that we must take this time because these issues were interfering with our work. We all believed in the value of the group problem solving method and could support the validity of establishing a regularly scheduled time to meet to discuss our interpersonal concerns. By this time, we had one set of relationships (with our quiet member) which was rapidly deteriorating and had hired a new faculty member midsemester who was having trouble relating to the group and we to her. A third issue was also eminent; we were about to double faculty to begin our second year thereby incorporating seven strangers into what had become, in effect, a closed group.

Parloff[3] states that the major aims of small groups can fall into three categories: (1) enhancing organizational efficiency through experiencing and recognizing group forces, (2) enhancing interpersonal skills, for example, increasing skills in communication, independence, flexibility, increased self-awareness, and sensitivity to other's feelings, and (3) enhancing the sense of well-being, i.e., providing an intense emotional experience.

Our rationale for the group speaks primarily to the first two categories. Although we wanted to enhance our sense of well-being, whether or not the experience would be an intensely emotional one was left up to the individual. Lack of agreement about optimal group intensity has led from time to time to some misunderstandings about the purpose of the group.

Rationale for organizing a group was never formally delineated but seemed to consist of the following:

1. Provide a supportive forum to discuss our interpersonal concerns with one another as we experienced them in our day-to-day work.

2. Reduce our isolation from one another. This was a primary preventive measure in that we could foresee that the tasks of the coming year (accreditation and development of a senior year) would necessitate the development of many subgroups with little opportunity to function as a committee of the whole.

3. Increase our sensitivity to the needs of others.

4. Increase our sensitivity to our own behavior and its impact on others.

Our motivation to learn and our dissatisfaction with our interpersonal situation is described by Miles when he points out that for an individual to change and learn, he must first believe in the value of the group work and be at least somewhat dissatisfied with his own "attitudes, understandings and behaviors as a participant in working groups."[5]

Marram further describes our position in her discussion of growth and self-actualization groups. She states that the groups are related to the education and self-enhancement of individuals in the group setting. The emphasis is on conscious, here and now behavior, and the realization of new facets of one's behavior and feelings. Participants are healthy individuals who want to improve their working relationships and "who benefit from cognitive changes provided by the group experience."[6]

The process of getting the group going turned out to be fairly simple. Toward the end of the first semester, we met for the first time at the home of the chairperson. We planned an all-day meeting with pot-luck luncheon. Our facilitator was a faculty member in another department on campus. He was known to the chairperson as someone who had done a number of workshops for nurses on creating a climate for working. She had attended one of these and was impressed with his ability to relate to nurses yet maintain an objective and inquiring point of view.

On the face of this, one might question the propriety of including the "authority figure" in the faculty group process, much less utilizing a facilitator recommended by her and meeting at her home. In fact, it seemed like a very natural way to proceed. From the

176

beginning, we had worked closely with her. She was the one who had laid the groundwork for the program and had been instrumental in our hiring. She had never presumed to take over our curriculum planning, although many times she watched her ideas modified beyond recognition. We were not knowledgeable about the campus and she had an appropriate facilitator to recommend. No one questioned her involvement; she had recognized our need, supported this use of our time, and we considered her to be a member of the group. We acknowledged the authority issue as one with which we had to deal and considered it to be further "grist for the mill."

The initial meeting was very intense. It was the first time that feelings and opinions had been expressed for all the group to explore. The issues that were raised had been previously discussed in small groups but only occasionally had they been expressed so directly to the persons involved. The two "avoiders" bore the brunt of the feelings because most of the issues related to them.

These members fit the description of what Yalom[7] describes as deviant or peripheral. Deviancy within the group occurs when a member participates in group tasks in a way that impedes group movement to complete the task. The individual lacks psychological mindedness, is less introspective, less inquisitive, and is more likely to use defense mechanisms that are self-deceptive. This role was particularly stressful because of the group's high priority on coordination and cooperation. Peripheral members seem unable to perceive how others view them. Communication to the deviant member is great initially and drops off sharply as the deviant behavior remains the same and the group rejects him. In the studies of deviant members described by Yalom, the members were unable to meet the requisite skills for group membership: "the ability to face one's deficiencies, even to the point of undue self-criticism" and to have "a degree of sensitivity to the feelings of others."[8]

In retrospect, it is clear that we perceived these members in the way just described and responded accordingly. At that point in time we were much more hopeful that our difficulties could be resolved than we were to be during the second year, at least with regard to the newer member of the two.

A good deal was discussed in regard to the member who had been removed from teaching. Her dilemma had had such an impact on the community health team that we decided this history needed to be shared with the new faculty arriving in the fall before it could completely be laid to rest. In regard to the other isolated faculty member, we began to see how our philosophies of interpersonal relationships were discrepant. There was a sense of hope that further discussion in the fall would also lead to a resolution of our difficulties with her. At the same time, we left with a feeling of frustration that we had not come to an understanding.

The issue of incorporating new members was discussed to some extent. We found that much of our work with this issue centered around termination of our present group experience and recognition that the next year, while exciting to contemplate, would be very different. Our closed group would on the one hand become bigger and, on the other, be broken into many subgroups.

We determined that in order to weather the interpersonal complexity of all these changes, we needed to establish permanent monthly meetings of at least three hours in duration. The authority issue surfaced briefly at this point in that several members preferred it to be a classroom on campus. The remaining members recognized a need to get away from our work environment and eagerly accepted the offer of one faculty who lived near the campus to meet in her home. Her home continues to be our meeting place every third Monday morning, 8:30-12:00 noon.

We left the meeting feeling that an important decision had been made that would have a significant effect on us all in the year to come. Some members were more enthusiastic about the future value of the group than others, but it was a group decision made with thought and commitment.

The end of the second semester brought us further into the second stage of group development. We recognized the need to establish committees and divide up the tasks that were mounting as accreditation grew nearer. There would be new members coming in the fall to help us carry the load. Ambivalence ran high as we looked forward to their arrival, yet worried that they would bring a point of view that would "interfere" with out progress. However, we moved on to establish a Committee on Committees which met during the summer to identify standing committees. No longer would group consensus be so easy to achieve. We discussed our feelings that with the new organization we couldn't control all the issues as much as before although we'd still have a say in the final decisions. We were ready to move into the changes and challenges of the second year.

THE SECOND YEAR

During the second year of the program, a number of events occurred which effected changes in the structure of the group, in the feelings, attitudes, and behaviors of the various group members, and consequently in group functioning. This discussion will focus on those events that produced the changes and subsequent processes that evolved in relationship to them. The events that occurred were: (1) increase in faculty size; (2) structural changes in clinical assignments; (3) crystallization of the conflict with the faculty member who had been hired at mid-semester of the first year; (4) repercussion of the conflict on new faculty members; (5) energy expenditure in the movement toward accreditation; and (6) addition of a new faculty member the second semester of the second year.

As was anticipated at the end of the first year, when the following year began to unfold, members of the first year faculty began to experience changes in their previously established communication systems. These systems changed not only because of increased faculty size but due to other structural changes as well. During the first year all faculty had community health clinical assignments on the same week days. The second year this did not occur. Faculty who were teaching the community health course were assigned to different days during the week. Since the majority of the faculty were involved in this course, this change created a force that added stress to the complexity of the situation. Many of the previous modes of communication no longer existed, particularly those that had functioned on an informal basis. New channels had to be developed. No longer could every faculty member be involved in all faculty decision making. Committees were developed to deal with organizational issues, with the result that subgroups were formed as had been anticipated. The majority of the first year faculty experienced the change in the small group structure and the necessitated organizational changes with a concomitant sense of decreased communication, a sense of isolation, and a loss of the closeness shared the first year. Reactions to these changes were quite openly expressed within the group context. The members were able to accept the new faculty more easily than might have been the case if the acknowledgment of these feelings had not been sanctioned.

Part of the initial adaptation phase to the doubling of faculty size dealt with issues surrounding "sibling rivalry." A period of time occurred which could be compared to this phenomenon in sibling relationships. Some of the first year faculty perceived themselves to be in the ordinal position of the first born, and the new members were viewed as newcomers to the scene. A number of months elapsed before faculty were able to look at themselves as a whole and not divided into "old and new" faculty, although periodically the difference continues to surface.

The first group session, as had been planned at the end of the first year, was held the third week of the beginning month of instruction. As had previously been decided, the group's history was shared with the new faculty coupled with a clarification of the rationale for the group meetings. There was a variety of reactions from the new members of the group, ranging from acceptance of the idea to an expression of doubt about the value for it. All of the seven new faculty members agreed, however, to participate in the sessions.

As the second year evolved, it soon became apparent that the greatest expenditure of faculty energy was directed to the movement toward accreditation. This major force, plus the increase in faculty size and structural changes in the group, all contributed to high stress levels. One faculty member consistently functioned as a facilitator to encourage expression of feelings regarding the internal reactions to the process. Through expression of her feelings about what she was experiencing, others were able to express theirs also—negative as well as positive. Due to this ability to verbally acknowledge the stress levels inherent in the complexity of the situation, many of the faculty were able to deal with the anxiety more effectively.

During the regular academic work week most of the energy was focused on accomplishing tasks. Little time was available to deal with interactional issues. Thus, the built-in mechanism of group meetings became even more vital, in the eyes of many of the faculty, in order to deal with the interpersonal concerns. Issues that might have remained at a covert level and further eroded faculty functioning surfaced in the meetings that were set aside to deal with these concerns.

At the beginning of the second year, one of the events that emerged and crystallized as a carry over from the first year dealt with the faculty member who had been hired to develop a facet of the senior year. Although she had been able to work independently at first, faculty input into the process became imperative as we moved into the second year. Attempts to increase communication created some difficulty, because her preferred mode of operating was one of independence rather than interdependence.

Early in the semester, feelings surfaced in the group meetings surrounding the above issue. Negative feelings were expressed with the issue confronted directly in the group. Several of the new members of the faculty indicated discomfort with the expression of negative feelings and indicated that they perceived the behavior to be one of scapegoating. In the beginning sessions where conflict became an overt issue, they moved into buffering positions with the faculty member who was being confronted. Pairing occurred with support being provided by one new member particularly. Some of the other members of the faculty experienced varying degrees of discomfort during these intense sessions. During this time, the facilitator of the group, the same man who had been selected the previous year, functioned primarily as a safety valve for faculty during the intensity of these sessions. The facilitator helped to clarify the issues and provide feedback as to what he observed in the group interaction.

A number of group sessions revolved around the attempt to come to grips with the interpersonal conflict that had been identified. The issue peaked in intensity at the end of the calendar year. Basically, due to different beliefs about interpersonal functioning, the "deviant" faculty member chose not to return to the group. A number of individual attempts were made to initiate a relationship with this faculty member, however, the issue was dropped by the group. The issue was dropped because of the energy that was required to move through the accreditation process and because the faculty member

180

essentially withdrew from the group. Due primarily to accreditation and the fatigue levels associated with this process, the inclination to deal with the isolated faculty member shifted from the group context to an individual basis. The conflict that had been generated was unsuccessfully resolved. The faculty member's difficulty in meeting the program objectives led to her subsequent resignation from the faculty at the end of the academic year.

Following her departure from the group, feelings of guilt were expressed by some of the faculty members as we reviewed what had happened. A number of the members thought that other approaches might have been taken to deal with the conflict, that "something more might have been done," and that failure had occurred in the attempt to resolve basic interactional differences. The facilitator of the group was particularly helpful at this point in the situation. He helped the group to deal with their feelings, to realize that various members had attempted to deal with the problem in an overt way, and to encourage the group to move on to other issues.

One spin-off from these intense confrontative sessions was the ability to deal with individual interpersonal issues on a one to one basis. There were a number of minor conflicts that emerged which were not explored during group sessions because of limited time. As these conflicts became apparent during the group meetings, the individuals involved worked them out on their own at a later date. One member in particular asked that we talk with her outside the group one at a time if we had issues to take up with her. She though we were scapegoating the "deviant" member and expected that she would be next.

Much of the preceding behavior can be explained in terms of theory regarding advanced groups.[9] Subgrouping may occur and is usually disruptive. Such pairing develops when two or more members believe they can derive more gratification from each other than from the group. Coalitions between certain members may also develop. These behaviors occurred between old and new members. They would sometimes agree with one another regardless of the issue and avoid confrontation among themselves while in the group. At times, some members were in conflict between loyalty to the group or to particular individuals.

A positive activity of advanced groups is the extra group social meetings of dyads or cliques. Such meetings began to develop during the first year. They frequently took place now as the old and new members got to know each other. As is also true of groups taking in new members, the new members did not disrupt our progress and, in fact, moved through the early stages of group to become a part of the whole much more rapidly than expected.

After the previous events were over, the group priorities shifted and accreditation issues took the lead. As the faculty worked together to complete the report, beginning signs of cohesiveness were once again

181

observed. This specific goal was the major driving force which drew faculty together as a unit. After the accreditation process was completed and accreditation received, the faculty experienced a period of elation and, as would be anticipated, a subsequent let down following the event. Throughout this experience, the group moved further along in its process as faculty as a whole experienced a sense of closeness and cohesiveness. One faculty member acknowledged that we would soon need to be thinking about our next goal, which further supports the evidence that as one goal is met, human beings begin to look for another. Interestingly, the idea to publish the findings of our program, its processes as well as content, emerged toward the end of this second year.

Another event occurred during this year which again changed the configuration of the group. A new member was hired mid-semester of the spring term to help develop a facet of the senior year. She was open, supportive, and initiated contacts with the faculty. She, in essence, met the group rules and was easily accepted in the faculty group. She believed in cooperation and coordination and since her actions supported these beliefs she once again met another of the group rules.

The end of the second year brought about the need to review the group's functioning and to consider faculty views as to the need for continued monthly meetings to deal with process issues. General group consensus indicated the need for the meetings to continue in the third year of program operation, with the same facilitator being selected to remain within the group. A number of the members viewed the meetings more enthusiastically than others, however, for the most part the group decision was one of continued commitment.

THE THIRD YEAR

The third year emerged with fewer urgent issues to deal with than had been identified during the second year of the program. Several new members were added to the faculty, one full time and three part time. The increase in faculty size did not constitute a major event this third year due primarily to the established systems of communication. Prior to the hiring of these faculty, they were questioned as to their beliefs about the monthly group meetings and whether they saw themselves participating in such an organizational process. A part of the decision to hire faculty was based on the applicant's responses to these questions. This component of the hiring process indicated once again that the group valued dealing with interpersonal issues on an overt level. The explicit group value further crystallized faculty's beliefs in the significance of dealing with process issues as an important concomitant to effective group functioning.

182

Several mechanism were developed to deal with faculty hiring. During the first year all of the faculty were involved in interviewing new applicants. This involvement was one additional example of the attempt to meet the inclusion and control needs of individual members in group functioning. As we moved into the second year it was readily apparent that this system was not efficient, therefore several changes took place. Teams consisting of course members were organized to interview each applicant. Other faculty members were encouraged to attend the interview sessions, or if that was not possible, to meet the applicant informally. Perceptions of the applicant were shared among faculty members. The decision to recommend for hiring was essentially the responsibility of the course interview team, however, input from others was considered in making the final decision.

The system that we used during the second year for hiring purposes proved to be successful. With this in mind, we continued with the same type of organization in the third year. It might be interpreted that because of our faculty's commitment to teamwork, the significance of selecting faculty who could function effectively within the group context became an increasingly important issue in hiring new faculty.

The third year of the faculty functioning might best be described as a resting phase. Due to the high level of energy expended during the first two years of program development, the third year emerged as an essentially quiescent one. No major interpersonal issues or conflicts surfaced in the group meetings the third year. Faculty needed to experience the resting phase with some inputs to balance the outputs of the previous two years. A number of the group meetings revolved around providing support to faculty members who were experiencing issues dealing with student-faculty concerns, while others were spent focusing on getting to know each other as individuals.

The subgroupings that had been forged the second year were operational because of the necessitated organizational structure. Some of the communication systems that had been devised in the second year required some change during the third year. The first day of the week was devoted to committee meetings, faculty meetings, and team meetings. This constituted a change from the second year. During the second year no such plan had been organized, other than for general faculty meetings, with faculty attempting to function within various faculty committees on different days during the week. This schedule usually resulted in conflict because of difference in teaching assignments. It became apparent during the second year that this component of the organizational structure needed to be changed because of its ineffectiveness. The resultant change in the third year provided increased efficiency in time expenditure.

As the year drew to a close, three members announced they would not be returning the following year. One was the faculty member hired to teach community health during the second semester of the first year, the second was the member hired at midsemester the spring term of the second year, and the third had been hired to teach part time the third year. The forthcoming departure of these three faculty brought about the need to deal with termination issues in the group context. Several group sessions were utilized to focus on termination, where feelings were openly discussed, feelings ranging from loss to anger. These various feelings were explored with the resultant effect that the termination process was dealt with effectively. One of the departing faculty members expressed that she sensed some members were angry about her leaving, however, the issue had not surfaced during individual interactions. When this concern was explored in the group, it came to be seen as a normal part of the process of separation from a valued member.

A remaining issue has yet to be dealt with in the group. This is the question of "authority." During the second and third year the chairperson has remained an active participant in the group meetings. Her membership has not been openly explored or questioned. She has been supportive of the group since its inception and has valued its continuation as a useful vehicle to deal with process for herself as well as for the faculty. Perhaps because of her support and personal interest, the issue has not surfaced in any significant way.

At the last group session of the year, faculty commitment to on-going group meetings was again discussed. The mechanism received continued endorsement for the fourth year of program operation. This endorsement seems to further indicate that one central theme has persisted since the inception of our program. The theme is the belief that group functioning and morale are effected by the ability of the group to deal with interactional issues in an overt way rather than in covert mechanisms, that mechanisms need to be built in to deal with these issues at the primary or secondary stages of prevention rather than wait until the tertiary stage to intervene.

As this chapter draws to a close, we would pose a number of suggestions for other faculties, particularly those who may be newly formed groups. It is hoped that what we have learned might be helpful to others in exploring their own worlds. We would stress the importance of:

1. Developing an awareness of the implications of the interpersonal processes and dynamics specific to your group.

2. Devising a vehicle to deal with group process issues early, rather than coping with them in covert ways at later points in time.

3. Choosing a facilitator with whom you can work comfortably. Our choice was a man whose leadership behavior most closely resembled a laissez-faire model.[10] He gave the group complete freedom for decision making. While he made no attempt to regulate the

course of events, he would provide feedback when asked and sometimes would interject an observation or make a clarifying statement that was helpful. It was important that he come from outside our department system, yet have some understanding of nursing. He could maintain an objective viewpoint but with a comprehension of our problems and concerns.

Whether or not sex is a factor is difficult to say since we have no other experience for comparison, but it has been pleasant to have a man among a group of women. For us, the nondirective approach has been effective because we are quite self-directed in our discussions. However, we need to know that the leader is there to buffer our interactions should we need help.

4. Including the authority figure in group oriented meetings. Since the authority figure plays a role in the dynamics of any group and is a significant member of the group, we have found that by including the authority figure we not only have gained a clearer understanding of her interpersonal world but that she has developed a perspective of ours as well.

5. Anticipating proposed changed in faculty size, organizational components, and geographical settings, such as physical location and space factors, with a projection of the possible implications in relation to faculty behavior. This anticipation of periods of increased stress due to change, with the concomitant acknowledgement of this verbally, undoubtedly helped us to cope more effectively with the number of changes we experienced as a growing faculty.

6. Identifying your group rules and values relating to interpersonal dynamics with the subsequent acknowledgement of these in interviewing faculty applicants. We have found that consideration of interpersonal rules as well as professional perspectives is significant, primarily because this world of faculty interaction plays a major role in morale factors and effectiveness of group functioning.

From our curriculum, one can see that we believe in the validity and usefulness of the group process to effect positive change. Our commitment to our own group process and our recognition of faculty behavior as a manifestation of that process in action is a reflection of one way in which we work toward making our own behavior more congruent with our approach to teaching. Communication is vital to a healthy functioning group. We think we have found a way to deal with our "interpersonal underworld."[11]

REFERENCES

1. Yalom, Irvin: *The Theory and Practice of Group Psychotherapy.* Basic Books, Inc., New York, 1970, Chap. 10.
2. Schutz, William: *The Interpersonal Underworld.* Science and Behavior Books, Inc., Palo Alto, California, 1970.

3. Parloff, Morris: Group Therapy and the Small Group Field: An Encounter, in Sager, C., and Kaplan, Helen: *Progress in Group and Family Therapy.* Brunner/Mazel, New York, 1972, p. 174.
4. Kaplan, H., and Sadock, B. (eds.): *New Models for Group Therapy.* Jason Aronson, Inc., New York, 1972.
5. Miles, Matthew: The Training Group, in Dennis, Warren, Benre, Kenneth, and Chin, Robert: *The Planning of Change.* Holt, Rinehart and Winston, New York, 1966, p. 719.
6. Marram, Gwen: *The Group Approach in Nursing Practice.* The C. V. Mosby Co., St. Louis, 1973, p. 56.
7. Yalom, *op. cit.* pp. 163-164.
8. *Ibid.*, p. 164.
9. *Ibid.*, Chap. 11.
10. Cartwright, D., and Zander, A.: *Group Dynamics, Research and Theory.* Harper & Row, New York, 1968, p. 319.
11. Schutz, *op. cit.*

CHAPTER 9

The Sonoma Experience: A Student's View

Harriet Lionberger, R.N., B.S.

The purpose of this chapter is to present the student's view of the Second Step experience. That experience is examined from several perspectives—all related to the program as a learning, growing process. Since there are as many student views as there are students, I attempt here to bring together some of the common threads, identify and elaborate upon the more outstanding characteristics of student participation, and compare some differences of opinion. Two aspects of the program form the continuing background for these remarks, and are basic to the experience. First, all students in the program are registered nurses. Second, the emphasis is on self-directed study culminating in a contractual senior preceptorship which provides individual focus on an area of interest for each student.

Being one of the first students in the Second Step Program at C.S.C.S. is obviously an opportunity already lost in oblivion, as far as prospective students are concerned. Yet, it may be well to bear in mind that it is the perspective from which I write. My classmates and I lay claim to an experience seldom available, or at least seldom recognized: the experience of helping to mold the academic future for the growing number of R.N.s returning to school for higher degrees. If a sense of self-satisfaction occasionally intrudes between these lines, give it its due. It is one measure of the degree to which Second Step students participate in the evolution of their educational futures. But that is getting ahead of my story.

First, a word about the problem of separating the *experience* from California State College at Sonoma. The experience of Sonoma's Second Step has a powerful impact on students. The impact of the program would be similarly powerful in any other academic setting, however, it would be different. Transfer to the Second Step from Sonoma to Any College, USA, would demand certain changes in emphasis, some re-evaluation of evolving policies. The effect would be change. But that's okay. The result (if the program of Any College really *is* the caliber of Sonoma's) would be a program congruent with the nature of its parent institution. Now, I know nothing about the nature of Any College, USA. I do know something about Sonoma State. Indeed, something about Sonoma State has become a part of me, and surely pervades this paper. So, for the best results, if you're fantasizing the Second Step in the milieu of Any College, remember to adjust your perspective according to your own reality.

THE PHENOMENON OF AN R.N. RETURNING TO SCHOOL

Students arriving at the Second Step bring with them work experiences ranging from none, to staff nurse, to administrative positions. Some have been free to grow and to influence the direction of health care. Others are reacting to pressures to practice at less than a professional level. Virtually all have confronted rigid, established health care delivery systems, and felt the frustration of road blocks to their personal satisfaction in nursing. A variety of factors impel them into a baccalaureate program. Some, the fortunate ones, find and take the Second Step.

The question at hand, then, is "What brings students to the Second Step?" Close on its heels, "What happens when they arrive?" and "After the Second Step, what then?" In short, what is the Sonoma Experience?

In order to answer these questions, let us meet three prospective students. They are composite figures and are drawn from the experiences of Second Step students as I perceived them and who will illustrate this saga of the Sonoma experience. After we're acquainted, we can gossip about them a bit.

Jane has two basic reasons for returning to school. They are Tommy, age five, and Joanne, age seven. Now that her husband has left her, and she and the children are on their own, Jane's previously ignored urge to develop her career has emerged as a necessity. It doesn't matter that there is too little money, or that she will have too little time with the children. The future looms, menacing. The past offers no answers. The present discourages optimism. And yet, Jane has an idea that with a bachelor's degree, she could broaden her horizons. And she's heard that the new program at Sonoma State even has some kind of provision for allowing her to develop the new ideas that never got off the ground at the hospital where she has worked part time for the past four years. She is certain that, given the opportunity to develop those ideas, she can offer some patients an improved level of nursing care.

There has been no particular social calamity in Phil's life. Indeed, a depressing sameness prevails. He and his wife both work. His job offers little prospect for advancement. His work is similar to that for which other employees receive more pay, but he is not qualified for an upward change in job classification because of educational deficiencies. The obvious answer is to return to school for a bachelor's degree, even though the whole idea seems to be an exercise in redundancy. Obviously, he already knows all that is necessary for the competent execution of his job, or he wouldn't have been given the responsibility that is already his. Fortunately, Sonoma State is in commuting distance from home, so it is possible to get the degree with a minimum of upheaval in the job or home situation.

Social and employment factors have little apparent pertinence to Margie's decision to apply for admission to Sonoma's Department of Nursing. Her application was submitted before her graduation from an associate degree program. Sooner or later she is going to want to get a bachelor's degree, so, why not now when money is available to cover her fees and expenses. Anyway, Margie isn't so sure she really feels like a nurse, yet. Maybe with a bachelor's degree . . . and while she works on that, there will be time to explore new relationships before tying down to a long term job that might limit her horizons.

I suspect that Jane, Phila, and Margie aren't very different from R.N. applicants to other schools. Except for Jane, whose decision is influenced by what she has heard about the Second Step program, their motivations at least loosely fit those of R.N.s returning to Any College for a bachelor's degree. They are in flight from some intolerable situation, in a fight for improved academic or professional standing, or in the plight of pursuing satisfaction of some poorly defined expectation of one's self as a nurse. But because the motivations can be generalized for a broad population, the particular effect of the Second Step should stand out a bit, against the background of traditional programs, as a setting in which an R.N. may qualify for a bachelor's degree.

WHEN STUDENTS ARRIVE AT THE SECOND STEP

The unique effect of the Second Step is apparent to its students from the outset. Preliminary interviews with the program chairman or other faculty member delineate the difference for some of them.

For Jane, the interview is a moment of confrontation. She is expected to identify some of her ideas for improving nursing care. She experiences a feeling that she is being put on the spot. The story of her conflict with the hospital power structure spills out, and suddenly she realizes that although she has many ideas, they are ill-defined. Are her nebulous perceptions of need for change valid? Suppose her conflicts with the power structure carry over to school? What then?

Still, she senses acceptance in the interview situation, and leaves with the knowledge that, while her ideas need to be consolidated, they are accepted as valid. With some wonder, she recognizes that the confrontation exists mainly in her own mind. This fleeting realization of personal responsibility will have to be repeated, endlessly it seems, before she can accept it with equanimity.

A few weeks later, the first semester finally begins, and Jane meets the rest of the nursing department student body for the first time. Among them, she finds consensual validation of her intuitive need to seek new horizons. Problems revolving around the question of hospital nursing versus nursing in other settings constitute a recurrent theme in their conversations. Having attended associate degree or diploma schools, many students consider their training to have been specifically geared to hospital nursing. Others feel limited because they have worked in hospitals for many years. New directions for nursing have sprouted and grown all around them, while their own roots pushed deeper and deeper into hospital sod. Now, how to get out? That question brought them to Sonoma and the Second Step.

Phil, too, finds some other students with problems similar to his own. The sharing of mutual needs and prospects is quieter for him than for Jane and her new-found friends. There is less of the religious zeal in the sharing, more quiet recognition. In a way, Margie's reasons for taking the Second Step are similar to his own. Both experience a sense of simply doing what is expected. The main difference is that, while on the one hand Margie was accepted into the first baccalaureate program to which she applied, Phil had spent several years corresponding with established colleges and university programs, hoping to penetrate the thicket of application requirements, changing prerequisites, and shortages of academic space.

Jane, Phil, and Margie are lucky. All the qualified applicants for the initial class could be accepted. Students applying for the next classes encounter some new frustrations. The number of applicants increases faster than spaces available. Applicants who qualify for admission are accepted on the basis of chance, and the old feeling of having no control over their own destinies returns to some of those who are rejected. It is not clear to the students what advantage chance has over selection on the basis of when applications are first received—first come, first served. And so, all the concern that the program has for the particular needs of R.N. students cannot overcome the fact that there are more prospective students, more needs, than the program can handle.

Another factor differentiates the admission policy encountered by the members of the first class from that encountered by later students. It is a matter of course requirements. While the experience of the first class is now history, and the situation is not apt to be repeated; that experience is of interest here as a step leading to decisions regarding later policy. At the outset, the requirement for admission to the program was an associate degree in nursing or its equivalent. Graduates of diploma nursing schools received equivalent in nursing units, and after completing the required GE courses were certified as having an equivalent degree. In the event of partial certification where certain requirements of the community college were unfulfilled by a given student, the deficiency could be made up in the process of completing requirements for the Second Step.

Jane feels fortunate that she can make up her general education requirements after admission to Sonoma State. She need not wait another semester while she picks up California history, mathematics, and philosophy to complete her lower division general requirements. There is one drawback to the proposition. It is that the time spent taking history, mathematics, and philosophy interferes with her scheduling certain electives that would strengthen the focus of her upper division work. However, at the time that she is applying and even when the first classes begin, the impact of nine semester units of lower division general education requirements, spread over a two-year program, seems insignificant.

Later applicants who have to make up general education deficiencies before admission will bemoan the fact that even the Second Step is not willing, or able, to accept diploma nurses without some sort of delay. Jane has at least learned, when taking some earlier night classes while the babies were small, that those general education classes deserve their own ration of time and energy. After being out of school for five years, confident in the belief that her education really satisfied her needs, she had taken two semesters of English composition as the first effort toward preparing for working on a bachelor's degree. The effort had been a revelation. It opened doors to new worlds and new perceptions. It laid bare her complacent acceptance of the status quo, and ushered in a new era of examining values and seeking new truths. The effect carried over into her Second Step experience, enhancing the expectation of growth.

Conversely, Margie's status as new graduate precludes the existence of a set of values as uniquely her own as Jane's. Yes, Margie has opinions that differ from those of other nurses of her own age. Some of her expectations derive from her earlier home situation. Some are adopted from the youth culture of which she is a part. None reflect the impact of years of individual decision making, responsibility for current needs, and adjustment to career and family demands that make up Jane's recent experience.

Ultimately, each person's experience molds a certain set of values. Those values weigh the interest invested in each aspect of the Second Step program. Admission requirements are no exception. They merely herald the approach of the experience of being a Second Step student.

RELATING TO THE PHILOSOPHY OF THE SECOND STEP

The entire experience of a Second Step student reflects the philosophy of the program, or reacts to it. The principles of that philosophy infiltrate not only the student's image of the client, but also his image of himself and his interaction with faculty. It would be difficult indeed to come away from the program without a sense of having confronted the issues of the philosophy. Those issues are defined in another chapter. Briefly, they express concern for man's specific individual problems. Man is seen as a biological, psychological, and social being; his ever-changing needs are affected by his culture, particularly as the culture is reflected in his value system. His desire for dignity and self-determination are basic to his needs.

From the outset, the student interprets the philosophy in relation to both his own needs and those of his client. When these concepts are sufficiently well integrated, they can extend to all facets of the educational situation and of his life. As it is with any learning experience, however, the level of integration varies over time. New concepts seem to materialize in geometric progression, until awareness becomes selective, in its own defense. Integration of the program's philosophical base continues throughout the academic experience, and cannot be teased completely away from it. For that reason, it will not be separated here. It will become apparent in the section of this chapter that is related to the student-faculty relationship, however, that students translate the program philosophy largely on the basis of how it is reflected in the activity of faculty members.

THE EXPERIENCE OF BEING A SECOND STEP STUDENT

Three distinct phases make up the experience of being a Second Step student. First, there is a period during which the educational experience is in stark contrast with the recent work setting, primarily in the first year of the program. Second, there is a period in which the developing relationship with faculty dominates. This period overlaps the contiguous portions of the first and second years. Third, there is a period in which a new gestalt forms around the student's emerging view of nursing, generally during the second year. Each phase has its own price and its own reward. Again, the student's background of work and of life experience helps to mold his reaction to each phase of the Second Step program.

Several concepts form unifying links of meaning throughout the curriculum. The two which require the largest investment of student energy are the concept of self-actualization and the concept of the nurse as the agent of change.

The concept of self-actualization appears at first glance to be synonymous with that of self-directedness; a concept which appeals to most nurses with work experience. In the early months in the program, many students think of self-actualization mainly in personal terms. Later, it becomes a goal for clients as well. But in the beginning the student's self-determination is foremost in attention. Students adopt the concept readily. They adopt it in terms of their own understanding of the concept. There is some friction between students and faculty, particularly during the first year of the program, while definitions are being structured. Students often define self-determination as freedom to choose particular classes. Faculty may define it as freedom to apply concepts from required classes to the student's area of interest. Whatever friction occurs can be seen later as necessary and part of the growing experience.

The concept of the nurse as an agent of change also undergoes some alteration in the minds of students as they progress through the program. In the beginning, some students find it very difficult to imagine nurses changing the status quo of patient care in the face of the established policies. Experience changes that mind-set, in most cases. The way in which change comes about will be described in some detail later in this chapter.

The student's life experience provides the background for every step in the process of recasting values and attitudes, both in the area of patient care and in his or her relationships with coworkers and peers. In the context of gestalt formation, the more diverse the background of experience, the greater the potential that the experience will be harmonious with a broad range of happenings in the present. Any contribution to one's diversity of previous experience, then, must increase the probability for more rapid assimilation of new health care concepts and acceptance of client's values as valid.

Contributions to diversity may be related to a progression of events over time, such as the experience of viewing the world as a child, student, wage earner, and parent. Thus a given student can consider events from several perspectives. On the other hand, some students may have knowledge and experience of more than one culture or more than one economic level. Generally, Second Step students recognize the importance of the different experiences of other students. They place considerable value on sharing, both in and out of the formal classroom. Shared experiences involve those who are parents at the present time comparing viewpoints with students of their children's ages. They involve exchange of ideas between psychiatric and medical-surgical nurses, long term care and intensive care nurses, nurses recently involved in nursing and those who have not been active in nursing for several years. The sharing, itself, contributes to the diversity of experience of each student, and enhances the integration of new concepts encountered in every phase of the Second Step experience.

The inevitability of change becomes apparent soon after Jane and Phil enter the Second Step Program when the contrast between their previous work situations and their new educational experience becomes a major issue in their lives. The source of the contrast can almost be narrowed down to two required courses: Community Health Nursing and Interaction and Change.

THE COMMUNITY HEALTH NURSING EXPERIENCE

In Community Health Nursing, the student confronts the contrast between *doing* and *being*. *Doing* characterizes the self-image typical of a hospital nurse. The patient comes to the nurse for help, on the nurse's territory. Acting on one's own initative or on doctor's orders, a nurse makes decisions relative to the patient's needs, and then acts on those decisions; frequently insisting on a certain course of action if the patient resists being cared for.

Being, on the other hand, implies presence, with openness to whatever the moment may bring. In Community Health Nursing, the nurse's authority is subservient to that of the patient. At the same time that the Second Step student begins to perceive a personal need for change, the client reserves the right to refuse to change. Every aspect of the situation seems to erode the nurse's comfortable symbols of authority. Even the familiar nomenclature is gone. The patient, now on his own territory, is a client. Stripped of the familiar trappings of authority, the nurse must learn to *be* instead of to *do*. The frustrating confrontation with the necessity of creating a new self-image signals the onset of culture shock—the problem of being, in an unfamiliar world.

Jane anticipates the community health experience as her major vehicle for learning a new approach to nursing care. The need for dramatic change in the nurse-patient relationship dampens her enthusiasm only temporarily before she manages to shift gears and move deliberately into the experience. Involving the client in the planning and process of care demands recognition of the client's values, and respect for them. Armed with a growing acceptance of different values, Jane finds that conflict or cooperation between client and community is a very real component of the process of care.

Jane's previous experience with patient care provides a valuable comparison for evaluating health status of family members. Also, it enhances the quality of her educational experience. In the community health facility and in her contacts with other community agencies, Jane presents herself as a registered nurse. As a result, her contacts in these agencies relate to her primarily as a registered nurse, secondarily as a student. In the community health facility, she participates fully in outpatient clinics. On occasion, she discovers that her skills in certain areas go beyond those of the staff members with whom she works. Somehow, the resulting bolstering of her self-confidence helps her to accept the need to adopt new ideas in other areas.

Students do have help in finding their own way through the maze of established habits and changing values. Help comes partly in the form of another course which, paradoxically, helps create the perception of contrast between previous work situations and educational experience. The class is called Interaction and Change.

INTERACTION AND CHANGE

Interaction and Change deals with the concepts of group process, self-image, communication, and planned change. As a Second Step requirement, it engenders a variety of reactions among students. At the outset, some who have years of experience in psychiatric nursing see little reason for taking such a class. On the other hand, nurses whose experience has been in medical-surgical settings find this course a rude confrontation with self and one they would prefer to avoid. The fact that the first semester focuses on experiential process and the second semester focuses on theory is another matter of much concern. Most students' previous experience fosters the expectation that theory will be presented before experience is required. However, there is no compromise. Interaction and Change remains a matter of learning first from experience, then from theory.

The experience of Interaction and Change comes at a crucial time in most students' lives, in the first few months of the program. The class itself is sometimes a laboratory, as it turns out, for dealing with feelings triggered by the switch from the work situation to the educational setting. In some cases, problems associated with changes in the family interaction, resulting from the return to school, provide grist for the mill. Whether aroused by school or family related events, the spontaneous feelings of individual students must be dealt with, and one available opportunity is the Interaction and Change class.

I would not suggest that Second Step students experience more emotional upheaval than students involved in the more usual progression of nursing education. I would suggest however, that the problems are different, and recognition of the difference facilitates resolution of the problems.

Perhaps the most challenging prospect for nurses with very many years of experience is that of readjusting their views of how a nurse interacts with patients and others in health care settings. Students who learned in the old school that nurses must remain aloof from the feelings encountered in the helping situation react generally in one of two ways. On the one hand, they may consider that the old method was unworkable, anyway, and they will welcome the prospect of feeling free to experience the emotions that are hidden just beneath the surface. In this case, most problems emerge with the discovery that once certain bits of self are brought to the surface, they must be dealt with and that sometimes the consequences are unexpected. On the other hand, some students may have integrated the concept of contained feelings so well that many emotions are simply not recognized. Change comes about more slowly in such cases, but change remains inevitable.

Experiences that contribute to change include recognition of one's own self-image, improved communication skills, and increased awareness of resistance to change. The impact of these experiences is enhanced by the fact that Interaction and Change class is open to students in departments other than nursing. Frequently, a student with a well-developed image of a nurse is faced with the necessity of comparing that image with the sometimes quite different image conceived in the mind of a student who is not a nurse. Such comparison takes place outside the classroom if it does not happen in the classroom. The effect is to force the nurse's re-evaluation of herself, or to challenge her to reinterpret the image of the non-nurse. It is not my intent to characterize the confrontation of the nurse-image as unwelcome. The process is repeated frequently throughout the experience of the Second Step Program, and is often instigated by the nurse.

Phil takes the opportunity to examine his orientation as a nurse in some depth in an elective class in sociology. He finds the other students in the class curious about nurses, and somewhat antagonistic toward the health care "system." As the only nurse in the class, Phil is able to provide a new view of nurses and the system through a class presentation of the socialization of nurses. In addition to the opportunity to share some of his insights with a group of laymen, he finds the exercise helpful in clarifying some of his own ideas. The opportunity works both ways, of course, and in the same class he is exposed to a variety of other experiences in socialization.

I will not present a litany of the multitude of experiences to which nursing students may be exposed in the context of a liberal arts college. Suffice it to say that the past experience the student brings to each new stage of the process of education increases the understanding of each individual as a nurse. The fact that often he or she is in this situation after having some experience in the health care system enhances his or her ability to re-evaluate the old, integrate the new, and convey to others some understanding of the phenomenon of being a nurse.

RELATIONSHIP WITH FACULTY

The relationship between faculty and students in the Second Step Program is inseparable from the impact of classes such as Community Health Nursing and Interaction and Change and from the fact that students are registered nurses. Several aspects to the student-faculty relationship deserve attention. Probably the most important is the fact that students are treated as peers by the faculty. Closely related to this treatment is the sincere effort on the part of the faculty to encourage students to take part in program committees. Committee involvement is real, as opposed to token involvement reported from other schools.

The opportunity to influence the evolution of the program is only one outstanding feature of committee involvement. Another

196

important aspect is the student's opportunity to observe faculty in relationship to each other. This opportunity provides a laboratory for considering the wisdom of adopting an individual faculty member as role model. Here, the attitudes and techniques employed by faculty in their involvement with students in the classroom can be observed in another significant milieu. It would be difficult to put too much emphasis on the reality of the nursing educator as role model. My personal bias is that students are usually presented a very limited view of the faculty members as persons. Any new perspective is useful. Peer relationship is exceptional. In a program such as the Second Step, the idea of R.N. educator as peer to R.N. student makes sense.

In some ways, faculty is seen by Second Step students as in some way different from faculty they have contacted elsewhere. That is, there seems to be faculty unity, and committment to the program philosophies, to a considerably greater degree than students have noticed elsewhere. At the same time, it is apparent that individual faculty members are comfortable in their agreement. The peer relationship is such that students consider themselves to be in a position to make such a statement, and that is probably part of the mystique of the relationship.

There is patently a mystique to the relationship. Partly, it stems from the problem that students confront in defining the difference between Second Step faculty and faculty elsewhere. Yes, faculty appear to be committed to the philosophy of the program, but are they committed to the philosophy because they are on the faculty, or are they on the faculty because of pre-existing commitment to such a philosophy? I guess the question in my mind has to do with a purely theoretical problem: are there enough potential faculty members out there somewhere to staff enough such programs to satisfy the demand?

It is obvious to students that faculty have their own problems. Because the experience of teaching a lower division student body made up entirely of registered nurses is as new as the experience of being a part of such a student body, faculty also has growing pains. It is not simply sadistic interest that makes faculty problems fascinating to students. The remarkable thing is that in the face of such problems it becomes apparent that faculty members practice what they preach. They use the same problem solving techniques that they offer to students as approaches to difficulties encountered in the field. This is a remarkable re-enforcement of attention to academic lessons. And this common use of problem solving techniques increases the student's sense of a peer relationship with faculty members.

A few weeks into the program, Jane, Phil, and Margie compare notes on their experiences, particularly about faculty attitudes. Jane and Margie are surprised at the sense of being really listened to in conversation with the faculty. Jane, especially, is impressed with the fact that her ideas are treated as really meaningful. She is involved in the curriculum committee, where at first she expected that there probably would be little chance of participation, but where it turned out that she is treated the same as any other committee member. In fact, she is expected to present student opinion, make suggestions, and propose changes. Her ideas are treated with genuine respect.

Jane's suggestion that the committee reconsider the use of the presently required text for one course was discussed in committee. Some suggestions included incorporating more background and discussion in the seminar period, or using an additional optional text for students who thought they would find it helpful. No decision was reached at that meeting. At the most recent meeting, however, all of the ideas were considered in more detail. Some change will very likely come about as a result of Jane's suggestion. At the same time she knows better than ever, now, that when she makes a suggestion it had better be well thought out because she will be held responsible for her participation. Without a doubt, she *knows* that her involvement in the program is taken seriously. The student's sense of involvement in the program, along with student-faculty involvement, matures with progression from junior year activities into the senior year and its preceptorship experience.

SENIOR YEAR PRECEPTORSHIP[1]

A major emphasis in the Second Step Program is the senior year contractual preceptorship—eight semester units of an independent learning experience. This anticipated experience is in some way a factor in most students' decisions to apply for admission to the program. Some enroll in spite of this innovative feature, some are simply resigned to it, some come because of it. But by graduation time, virtually all agree that it is an outstanding learning experience.

The preceptorship serves as the means of concentration on a student's (or, occasionally, a group's) particular area of interest. As a senior year course, it puts to practical use many of the Community Health Nursing and group process concepts introduced at the junior level. In addition, it encourages expansion of health care ideas conceived out of the individual's career and life experience.

A concomitant preceptorship seminar explores concepts of leadership style, the nurse as change agent, identification as a professional in the health care system, nursing autonomy, and personal self-actualization. While the preceptorship takes place in the senior year, planning for it starts well ahead of that time. Because of the difficulties encountered by students in the earliest classes, relative to contract writing and preceptorship selection, a seminar is now offered in the second semester of the junior year where this preplanning can be shared more easily with advisors and other students.

The first step is selecting an area of interest which for most students is the easiest task. Then the challenge grows greater. With the assistance of a faculty advisor, students must draw up a "contract," that is, a statement of purpose, previous related experience, activities to be carried out during the preceptorship, support to be provided by the advisor and the preceptor, objectives, evaluation methods, duration of the study, and the credit to be achieved. This statement also serves as a valuable tool in guiding students through the separate independent courses of study they choose. After the guidelines are clear but before the contract can be completed, students must identify and select a preceptor, modify the contract so that it is satisfactory to both the preceptor and student, and have it signed by an advisor, preceptor, and department chairman.

In a survey to which 25 senior students responded, 13 indicated that a career plan preceded selection of a preceptorship focus and 6 were undecided about career goals at the time of planning the preceptorship. The remaining 6 students who participated in the survey chose not to respond to the question, a fact which may indicate that a clear-cut answer was not always possible. Informal sharing of experiences indicates that if specific career focus is in question at the time of preceptorship planning, that time is an important factor in career decisions. In some instances, the career is well established, and the preceptorship focus is a peripheral interest aimed toward broadening the student's understanding of nursing. Some students recognize entirely new clinical interests as a result of the experience.

Some students elect relatively structured group projects in school nursing or family practitioner programs. The majority, however, prefer to develop individual preceptorships. The first students chose such areas as family planning, emergency nursing, renal dialysis, newborn intensive care, drug abuse treatment, management and staff development, or research.

The precise focus of a preceptorship becomes more fully defined during the contract writing process. Contract writing amounts to setting priorities, clarifying objectives, and organizing a planned experience so that the objectives can be met. Usually, writing the objectives presents unexpected problems. One major problem is that of defining the objectives in behavioral terms so that they have meaning to others as well as to the student. It is at the point of writing the objectives that the need for clarification becomes apparent. With clarification the entire organization of the experience comes into better focus, as the objectives define the strands of learning that they are expected to follow.

When the objectives are clarified and desired activities outlined, the student is ready to begin negotiations with a preceptor. For some, contracting with a preceptor presents no problem. Usually the

process is less complicated when the student and prospective preceptor are acquainted. Another factor that affects the ease of coming
to agreement is how closely the projected activities adhere to traditional nursing activities. It is possible, however, for preceptorships
to be quite imaginative. The possibility of increased time and energy
spent in negotiating with a preceptor is only one of the many hurdles
that have to be cleared in the interest of innovation, but the hurdles
do not rule out the possibility of arranging for an unusual experience. The limiting factor is the student. And by the time students
in the Second Step reach the stage of developing a preceptorship, the
concept of limits has often come to have a new meaning. The new
meaning is an element of the formation of a new gestalt around the
student's view of nursing and of himself.

THE EMERGING VIEW OF NURSING—A NEW GESTALT

The actual experience of the senior year preceptorship is one of
shifting perceptions and redefinition of goals for many students.
The concept of a new gestalt is appropriate in this context. The
term "gestalt" implies perception of a figure (the prominent characteristic of the situation) against a ground (all the perceptions, in
and out of awareness, that relate in any way to the figure). Polster
and Polster's[2] use of the term expands somewhat on the basic concept of gestalt therapy, so that the principle is eminently adaptable
to the preceptorship experience as a life situation.

Basic to the concept of gestalt is the idea of constant shifting of
figure and ground formations. Also, the term embodies the idea of
acceptance and definition of present moment experience in the here
and now, rather than interpretation of their implications in the light
of past experience. A frequently neglected aspect of the implications
inherent in here and now definition of experience is the tenuous
nature of understanding, when understanding is in continuous flux.
The tenuous nature of understanding of the here and now constitutes
both the major difficulty encountered by students in the preceptorship situation and the source of my amazement regarding the ability
of Second Step faculty to deal with the myriad experiences of their
students at any one time. The faculty's ability to deal with the
yeasty proliferation of student ideas, and to deal with them in the
here and now, facilitates student use of these ideas. This attribute
of faculty members is not limited to the preceptorship experience,
but to some students it is most evident there. To most, it is indispensable there.

The concept of preceptorship as a process of shifting gestalt formation is apparent in Jane's experience. The concept can be seen in
discrete portions of the experience and in the experience as a whole.
Jane came to the Second Step with the nucleus of a preceptorship
plan. She wanted to set up a program for making home visits to

families where there was a chronically ill child in the home. Her hope was to be able to help parents examine the problems that arise regarding caring for the child, and to help them work out solutions to the problems. Because to her knowledge there were no nurses doing exactly what she wanted to do, at least in her geographical area, Jane thought it would be best not to seek an R.N. as a preceptor. Much to her surprise, her first serious conversation with a social worker who was willing to consider working with her revealed that a new program related to care of such children in the community included a registered nurse on the staff. After contacting the nurse and discussing both of their concerns about parent teaching, Jane contracted with her to act as preceptor.

Later it occurred to Jane that one of her nursing professors had indicated there was such a person in the community. The idea had been so foreign to her that Jane did not consider it seriously. In her own time, she "discovered" the information, examined it, and included it in the "figure" of her preceptorship as it took form. While on the surface it may seem that the outcome would have been the same if Jane had simply incorporated the information at the time it was first presented to her, such is not the case. The fact of her having the knowledge is quite dissimilar. The resulting gestalt includes a new element, a new image of herself. The new image is herself as an explorer, a conqueror, who has obtained a goal through her own efforts. As such, it alters forever her approach to the world.

Yet, a paradoxical twist finds its way into Jane's thinking. Asked, near the end of the preceptorship experience, whether she would want any changes in the program if she were to do it again, she suggests that it would help if the school would arrange for a kind of professional flea market, where students who are planning their preceptorships could find experts in one or more interest areas and pick their brains. Or perhaps some new elective courses could deal with background information about a variety of issues. Not all students would agree with this approach. Some would. But one of the first graduates commented that once she overcame the desire to be spoonfed and accepted the opportunity to expound and expand, she derived courage and great pleasure from finding her own way through the preceptorship.

Margie was unsure early in the program as to what focus she preferred for her preceptorship. Like most students who came directly from associate degree programs, she felt a need for increased proficiency in acute care skills. Toward the end of the junior year, she decided to concentrate on emergency room nursing, and talked with the emergency department supervisor at the hospital in her home town about being her preceptor. After the first interview, she was unsure again. The sense of urgency she felt in the department at the time of the interview, and the question of whether the supervisor would have time to devote to her amid all the distractions Margie perceived around them, made her wonder if such a situation was right for her. However, the supervisor seemed to think it would work. If only someone could tell her whether this was the right decision! Finally, Margie realized she was frightened by what she perceived as a major decision in her life plan. She made up a list of other nursing areas where a sound knowledge of emergency nursing would be an asset if she later changed her mind about wanting to work in the department. That helped some. But what really contributed to confidence in her own choice was her later decision to work in medical-surgical nursing during the summer before the preceptorship. Returning to school in the fall, she finally felt like a nurse. And all the thought she'd had to give to the preceptorship decision was helpful during the summer experience. Best of all, she would have more courage in her decisions from now on.

Other students find preceptorship planning equally challenging. And the challenge continues throughout the experience. For the nurse who wants to influence change in the health care system, the preceptorship provides a workshop where approaches to change may be practiced, where the urge to attain change can and must be tested against the realities of resistance to change, where this practice and reality testing can be done from a perspective of knowledge and support. For the nurse who is interested in an in-depth study of already established health care approaches, the preceptorship provides access to interaction with qualified professionals and facilities in the community, flexible schedules, and continuing evaluation of progress. Whatever wishes and expectations the student brings to the situation, the concept of new gestalt formation is appropriate to the preceptorship experience.

INFLUENCING THE EVOLUTION OF THE PROGRAM

Individual personal involvement in the preceptorship contributes to the student's sense of self, a factor important to his or her desire and ability to influence the evolution of the Second Step Program. Certainly, his or her influence has been felt from the first weeks since admission. However, the trend throughout the two years of participation is toward mature thought, refined perception, and improved communication skills. Quality of input evolves with this development. Consideration given to the input, on the part of the program, evolves also.

The opportunity for students to be heard on the subject of their reaction to elements of the Second Step Program occurs not by happenstance, but by strategy. Along with the ongoing research program, other formal and informal student input provides information concerning the effectiveness of, and student reaction to, various aspects of the program. Direct student input differs from research data sometimes in its unpredictability, and occasionally in its high level of feeling. As noted above, certain textbooks or other teaching tools may be considered inappropriate by some students in some classes. The relevance of any given activity that is directed toward a particular goal may be challenged. Faculty have the responsibility for weighing the aptness of the challenge as well as the suitability of that which is challenged.

Nor are the challenges immune to change. Students, having reacted to the challenges of the junior year, return with a new set of expectations as seniors. As increasing amounts of information about the program reach the community, prospective applicants incorporate bits of intelligence and later return it to the Second Step in the form of new expectations. Faculty are on the growing edge of the program at all times, interpreting the new expectations into new approaches to the continuing task of keeping the program congruous with changing needs in the community. The Second Step maintains its relevance only as it reacts to the reality of the health care system and the needs of nurses in the community.

REALITY SHOCK REVISITED

Kramer[3] defines reality shock as the reaction of new workers to a situation for which they thought that by virtue of their education they would be prepared, but for which they suddenly find they are not prepared. Kramer asserts that the real problem of the new graduate nurse today is her inability to postulate how to make her visions and skills of the future into present reality. This concept has relevance for the Second Step Program. Second Step provides a solution to the problem, both for neophyte nurses and for nurses whose many years of experience have been less than optimally rewarding because of the residual effect of reality shock.

The solution for the neophyte nurse may be to go directly from the basic program into an advanced program that deals with the problems of ideals versus empirical realities. Such a situation exists for associate degree and diploma nurses who participate in the Second Step before entering the work force. On admission to Second Step, these students already possess the beginning skills of a registered nurse. In the Second Step, they are able to approach resolution of the conflict between professional role conception and bureaucratic role conception that characterizes reality shock. Actual experience in applying professional attitudes and behaviors in the context of the bureaucratic setting and within the context of the educational system, simultaneously, guarantees a realistic outcome. Only in a situation some way divorced from the traditional teacher-student model of nursing education can the reality be expressed. The senior year preceptorship provides this new orientation.

The process is somewhat different for the nurse who enters the Second Step after several years of nursing experience. However,

Kramer offers a role configuration paradigm eminently applicable to that situation.[4] She groups nurses according to their scores on a tool identifying high and low bureaucratic role conception and high and low professional role conception. One group in Kramer's study stands out as most apt to return to school to find a "better" approach to nursing. This group is made up of nurses who score high in professional role conception and low on bureaucratic role conception. Nurses in this group are referred to as lateral arabesquers—they arabesque their way right out of the patient-care situation.

Kramer's lateral arabesquers are students or graduates of generic baccalaureate programs. The lateral move out of the work situation is expected to take them into graduate school or teaching positions. Diploma or associate degree graduates with similar role conceptions may be expected to move into baccalaureate programs. Those who move into Second Step find a realistic approach to the very role conception conflict that foments discontent in the work situation. Their next expedition into the job market can be expected to find Second Step graduates well prepared for the demands put on professionals in a bureaucratic world.

AFTER THE SECOND STEP

Moving out of the Second Step, graduates find that there are still some surprises. Those taking school nursing positions regret that their counseling skills are not considered by administration to be applicable to that area. School budgets seldom allow sufficient nursing staff for that purpose. Those going directly into graduate school may chafe at having somewhat less freedom for academic self-direction than they are accustomed to. It is to be hoped that the unique background obtained in the Second Step has equipped them to live with these problems while finding a way to correct them.

Some positive changes add a new dimension to the work world. Students emphasizing management skills in the preceptorship find that the actual experience they have had prepares them appropriately for the job situation. The preceptorship provides the necessary background for school nursing also, particularly from the standpoint of self-assurance. Attitudes toward job situations and ability to work cooperatively with other personel are frequently cited as areas where positive change occurs as a result of the educational experience.

In graduate school, Second Step alumni agree that the program equips them for asserting themselves in a situation where increased self-direction is expected of them. A large percentage move quickly into teaching assistant or research assistant positions. And, like their counterparts in the job situation, they are quick to praise the preceptorship experience in particular, noting that they profited from it in a way that would be difficult indeed to duplicate in a traditional program.

Nearly all Second Step students come away convinced that the fact that students are all registered nurses is an important factor in the success of the preceptorship. Also, they consider the preceptorship to be the outstanding experience of the program, both from the point of view of the amount of realistic empirical knowledge obtained, and from the point of view of satisfaction derived from personal accomplishment. It is true that every student has to struggle with increased anxieties, uncertainties, and pressures because of the high degree of personal involvement. But accepting responsibility for the educational endeavor and working through the development of one's own ideas prove to be the key to an unusually gratifying experience.

REFERENCES

1. Portions of this section are adapted from Lionberger, H.: The Senior Year Preceptorship. *Nursing Outlook* 23:320, 1975.
2. Polster, E., and Polster, M.: *Gestalt Therapy Integrated.* Brunner/Mazel, New York, 1973.
3. Kramer, M.: *Reality Shock: Why Nurses Leave Nursing.* The C.V. Mosby Company, St. Louis, 1974.
4. Kramer, *op cit.,* p. 79.

CHAPTER 10

The Second Step Research Project

Haywood C. Vaughan, M.S.

INITIAL PLANNING

A research oriented evaluation study was incorporated into the Second Step Program as an integral part of the curriculum. Although originally the specific design for the investigation was left open, there was a commitment to "carefully study" the curriculum and the characteristics of the students. Responsibility for the formulation of the particulars of the evaluation research component was delegated to a research specialist who had no teaching responsibilities in the program. The general plan envisioned the collection of data which could provide answers to such questions as:

1. What characteristics differentiate between professional and technical nursing education and practice?

2. How effective is the approach of building upper division nursing cognitive knowledge on a base of lower division nursing and general education studies?

3. What are student characteristics in the Second Step Program and how do they change?

4. How effective are specific inputs of the curriculum—Contractual Study, Micro-teaching, Health and Culture, Science Principles, Interaction and Change, and Community Health Nursing?

5. What factors determine admission to and success in the program by minority ethnic group members?

6. What student characteristics and experiences relate to withdrawal from the program?

7. How does the graduate of the Second Step Program compare with other registered nurses and generic baccalaureate graduates in the work setting after graduation?

Clearly the scope of the original research plans extended beyond a straight forward experimental or quasi-experimental design intended to measure the program's effectiveness in achieving a set of stated objectives. It was intended that the data should be descriptive by providing baseline data on the students, and predictive by indicating which variables related to success in the program. However, the study needed to serve many other purposes. Because this particular model of nursing education was a new venture without precedent and, indeed, with some opposition in the community of nursing educators, it was hoped that the data would assist in establishing the legitimacy and credibility of the Second Step approach. The formative evaluation dimensions of the study were also crucial. Faculty wanted data on which to base decisions about admission policies and curriculum, and saw the research as a valuable asset and resource in this regard. Finally, since the program began with substantial economic support from both federal and private granting sources, it was imperative that a systematic assessment of its effectiveness be made.

THE ORIGINAL STUDY DESIGN AND ITS SUBSEQUENT ADAPTATIONS

The department began the systematic evaluation upon the arrival of the first class of nursing students. The overall plan for the evaluation rested on the following principles:

1. It was assumed that the best evidence about the effectiveness of the educational program consisted in what the students gained from their experiences in the program. For this reason, the students themselves constituted the primary focus of the research. Their experiences with the curriculum, the faculty, clinical practice, fellow students, and other aspects of the program were examined.

2. The study relied heavily on hard data, for example, tests and questionnaires, because those sources of data were more reliable and "objective" than impressionistic approaches. Oral interviews were introduced during the first year. Anecdotes and participant observation will play an increasingly greater part in the entire evaluation scheme as the work progresses.

3. Comparative approaches were utilized where appropriate. That is, Sonoma students were compared with national norms, with each other, and with students in subsequent classes to determine their relative position on a number of variables. This feature allowed the researchers to learn the extent to which students mastered a body of knowledge and their achievement relative to students in other nursing programs.

4. A longitudinal approach was employed. For instance, although it was helpful to know how students scored on a test after an educational experience, it was even more useful to know the extent to which they changed relative to their scores before that experience. Thus, some instruments were administered to students when they entered the program, and were readministered to them when they

graduated so that changes could be measured. Efforts will be made to identify which aspects of the program were most and least responsible for the various changes measured.

There were many content areas which an evaluative project such as this might study, but in order to provide some focus three major areas were selected: cognitive knowledge of nursing and the related sciences, personal and professional orientations of students in general and as they relate to nursing, and competencies in the practice of nursing.

Cognitive Knowledge about Nursing and the Related Sciences

The nursing faculty and evaluators were interested in obtaining an independent assessment of students' cognitive knowledge about nursing and related sciences which would supplement grade point averages and classroom test results. In the interest of combining feasibility with validity, it was decided to use the existing National League for Nursing Achievement Tests. These tests were immediately available and were already normed for other accredited programs which included baccalaureate, associate degree, and diploma schools. The tests selected were the NLN comprehensive achievement tests in Natural Sciences in Nursing, Maternity and Child Nursing, Medical-Surgical Nursing, and the NLN achievement tests in Psychiatric Nursing and Community Health Nursing. An early analysis of these test results strengthened the view of the faculty that students from the two preparatory sources, the associate degree schools and the diploma schools, were equally well prepared to undertake upper division nursing studies. Additionally, results of these tests administered to students after completion of the first year confirmed the view that our students were progressing satisfactorily when compared with other students in the normative group, and were indeed obtaining a knowledge of facts and principles required of a baccalaureate nurse.

Personal and Professional Orientations

The Second Step Program places a special emphasis on community and family nursing. Professional effectiveness in these areas is substantially influenced by the personal and interpersonal characteristics of nurses. Further, most students attracted to the program were not expected to have had much preparation for working outside the structured hospital setting or much experience with families in communities. They were, therefore, likely to experience several kinds of changing orientations and attitudes about nursing as they went through the two years. For these reasons, a major thrust of the evaluation consisted of a study of the attitudes, values, and personality orientations in general and as applied to nursing in particular.

208

The plan for this phase of the project consisted of a longitudinal study of students as they progressed through the program. At the beginning of the junior year, all students were asked to complete a battery of questionnaires and standardized instruments. At the end of the junior year the students were individually interviewed to obtain information about their experiences, satisfactions, dissatisfactions, changes in their nursing orientations, and changes in themselves. Near the conclusion of the senior year, students were asked to complete another battery of standardized tests as well as a graduation questionnaire which contained items concerning their college experiences, self-perceived changes, benefits derived from various aspects of the program, and future educational and career plans. Finally, students and their employers will be surveyed one year after graduation for information about employment situations and job performance.

It is expected that the data obtained on a longitudinal basis and from different perspectives will provide answers to a variety of questions about the program and its effects on students.

The following are sample research questions:

1. What kinds of students are attracted to this distinctive kind of program?

2. What are the characteristics of students who persist in the program as compared with those who drop out before obtaining a degree?

3. What kinds of changes do students experience in their orientations toward nursing and nursing practice?

4. How do students develop as individuals during their involvement in the program?

5. What educational experiences are associated with different degrees of growth and development?

6. Do students who come with different educational backgrounds concentrate in different nursing specialties, and do those who differ in age, sex, or ethnic background react differently to the Second Step Program?

7. What kinds of educational experiences and achievements are related to successful performance on the job after graduation?

Competencies in the Practice of Nursing

Perhaps the most important focus of an evaluation effort such as this would be to assess the extent to which students demonstrate their competencies in the practice of nursing. The faculty presently rely on the time-honored practice of observing students in the clinical areas of nursing and assigning letter grades based on standards derived from internalized faculty experience and leveled behavioral objectives. This procedure, of course, assumes standardization norms for faculty members who conduct the clinical training.

Several complementary assessment possibilities are being considered: competency based evaluations with definitive standards, rank order evaluations of students by faculty, peer evaluations by students, and an implied proficiency type of evaluation based on supervised practice. The latter plan is currently being observed in the clinical preceptorship of the Family Nurse Practitioner option of the senior year where 20 senior students in four semesters have seen nearly 3000 patients either in supervised or full responsibility appointments.

Unfortunately, the task of defining, developing, and obtaining sound data about these matters is complex and difficult.

THE COMPROMISES

During the first year of the research, a comparative study design was inaugurated with the assistance of the nursing departments of two other California state colleges. These schools have generic nursing programs, and the research staff believed that many useful comparisons might be made between the four year baccalaureate nurse and the Sonoma Second Step nurse. Additionally, students in the Biology Department and in three experimental cluster colleges of the Sonoma campus participated in the study. The same battery of survey instruments was used to gather pretest data on each of these reference programs.

Response rates for all schools were excellent during the first year of the study except for the Sonoma cluster colleges. Unfortunately, a high level of faculty interest could not be sustained outside our own program and resulted in a declining response rate in the second year of the study.

The Sonoma cluster colleges provided an interesting highlight in the data gathering process. Not only were all response rates from these experimental schools extremely low, but several students made formal appointments with the researchers to challenge the practice of asking for data from any person for any purpose.

Despite these obstacles, the researchers felt that judicious grouping of the reference data would permit useful comparisons to be made. Unfortunately, this comparative effort was undertaken with the expectation that additional external funding for this phase of the research project might be forthcoming, but such support was not realized. Thus, the comparative feature of the evaluative research design reaching beyond the Sonoma program remains more a potential than an actual feature of the evaluation.

PRACTICAL ASPECTS OF THE RESEARCH

The researcher frequently encounters a problem of balance between asking for all the information he or she would like to have, and realistically seeking only as much data as needed to meet the research

objectives. There is a point beyond which students are reluctant to
answer questions of uncertain relevance to their lives. Students are
busy people, particularly at the beginning of a new term, and the
time spent in filling out research questionnaires is time lost from
studies, searching for living accommodations, and in the case of many
older students, time away from their families. The researcher must
establish priorities, decide where to compromise in the search for
data, and design instruments to be as concise as possible, keeping in
mind that he or she will return again to the same students for post-
test data. There is a need to insure future acceptance, at least, and
even hope for a warm welcome by students who have become
further professionalized during the intervening years, and who see
the necessity and value of research and see their participation in survey research as a learning experience.

In view of the somewhat non-coincident interests of researcher and
subject, the investigators decided to use a multifaceted approach to
data gathering which utilized specially constructed questionnaires,
standardized tests, and individually conducted interviews. A special
effort was made to personalize the approach to the students, to discuss and explain the value of the project, and to maintain an open-
door attitude in the research office throughout the school year.

At the time of distributing the initial survey packets to the students,
the nature of the research and its general objectives were discussed in
detail by the research staff. The students were invited to participate
in the project as subjects, and their assistance was emphasized as
being a vital part of the program. At the same time, the confidential
nature of their responses was explained, as were the interests and
concerns of the Campus Committee on the Rights of Human Subjects
in Research. Students have responded well to this invitation, and the
participation rate at entry has been on the order of 91 percent.

About 40 percent of the survey materials were usually returned
within two weeks. A personalized follow-up memo was then distributed to individuals who had not returned their packets. The final
effort to obtain the packets was ordinarily made by faculty members
to clinical groups of students with whom they had frequent contact.
The entire data-gathering process was based upon a policy and a
procedure which emphasized the value of research, the advantages of
student input to their own program, and the mutual cooperation of
professionals in advancing the state of the art.

Method of Data Collection

The pretest survey was administered to the three entering classes of
the program as early as the students' schedules would permit during
the registration period. The value of the early administration lies in
the objective of obtaining the students' attitudes, views, and characteristics before these attributes can be affected by exposure to the

211

college. There are also economies of time for both students and staff since the purposes and objectives of the research can be explained in detail and the timed intelligence test can be administered on a group basis. Within a few weeks after registration, the class work has become absorbing and schedules are established with a resultant lessening of interest in filling out research questionnaires.

Data Gathering Instruments

The principal data gathering instrument of the research project is a survey battery composed of a pretest and a post-test. The battery is quite comprehensive and consists of an introductory letter, a consent to participate form, and a three part questionnaire. The questionnaire itself is divided into a General Questionnaire, a Nursing Student Questionnaire, and a Nursing Background Questionnaire. The Omnibus Personality Inventory and the Cattell Culture Fair Intelligence Test round out the pretest. The general questionnaire also incorporates a Nursing Orientation Scale directed toward work-related issues. This scale was developed by Drs. Virginia Olesen and Fred Davis of the University of California, San Francisco.

An oral interview is conducted with each student near the end of the first year. At the conclusion of the second year, the O.P.I. is re-administered and the students fill out the Graduation Survey. A Post-Graduation Survey seeking both qualitative and quantitative information is presently being developed, and will be administered to graduates and their employers one year after graduation.

The survey instruments are packaged so that students can fill in their answers outside class hours, and return the survey questionnaires in complete confidentiality. One exception is the Cattell Culture Fair Intelligence Test, which is administered on a group basis at several scheduled times convenient to the students. This test is ordinarily given in conjunction with some other activity at which a sizable block of students is present. Administration of this test which includes explanation, actual testing time, and a question period requires about 30 minutes. The entry survey package consists of 450 variable items of information which encompass multipart questions, raw scores from the 14 scales of the Omnibus Personality Inventory, and the intelligence test raw score.

The majority of variable items are precoded for immediate keypunching to data cards; however, a few open ended questions are coded later on an ad-hoc basis. Data cards are computer processed using the Statistical Package for the Social Sciences regime, an integrated system of programs especially useful for social sciences research.

The Omnibus Personality Inventory

In order to obtain a detailed baseline of information about the personal characteristics of nursing students, the Omnibus Personality Inventory (OPI) was administered to all students as they entered the program.

The OPI was developed within the Center for the Study of Higher Education, University of California at Berkeley. One of the features of this inventory which makes it of particular value to the Sonoma program is that it was designed to measure attitudes, values, and interests considered to be important in an academic setting.[1] The scales of the inventory were chosen by the authors for their relevance to academic activities and for measuring distinctions between students. While measuring broadly the areas of normal ego functioning and intellectual activity, the grouping of various scales provides an assessment of general or social-emotional maturity, a range of intellectual concerns or activities, and information about such traits as flexibility, impulsivity, and emotional well being.

Four of the scales serve as primary criteria for an Intellectual Disposition Category, with two additional scales providing supplemental criteria. The primary scales of Thinking Introversion, Theoretical Orientation, Estheticism, and Complexity are followed by the secondary scales of Autonomy and Religious Orientation which, as a group, provide an index of an intellectual-scholarly disposition.

The OPI was administered to all students as they entered the program and again when they graduated nearly two years later. The personal characteristics of students are considered by the research staff to be important independent variables, and many of the changes students undergo during the program are indicated by the pre-test and post-test use of this instrument.

The Cattell Culture Fair Intelligence Test

The standardized intelligence test provides a useful and easily obtained measurement of mental ability. Although the concept of intelligence may be subject to various interpretations, the I.Q. as traditionally determined is a correlate of academic success and may have a valid role to play as an independent variable in our future studies of professional success and work-related competencies. Since measurements of I.Q. are relatively easy to obtain and are based on widely accepted population norms, the I.Q. datum of intellectual functioning was selected as a fundamental independent variable.

Since one objective of the program is to increase the numbers of ethnic minority students holding baccalaureate degrees, it was appropriate to utilize test instruments designed to eliminate or reduce cultural bias in measurement whenever possible. The Cattell Culture Fair Intelligence Test, Scale 3, Part A[2] was chosen as part of the

213

entering battery of tests to provide a measurement of general intelligence that is relatively free of cultural contamination, and which can be administered on a group basis. The Culture Fair Test contains four subtests which are individually timed and administered consetively. The subtests deal with competencies in the areas of series, classifications, matrices, and conditions which are summed to provide a single raw score. These raw scores may be transformed to standard score I.Q.s comparable to those of the classical Stanford-Binet Intelligence Test.

The Oral Interview

The research team interviewed all members of the junior classes as they finished their first year in the program. The purpose of this structured interview was to seek out the student's experiences with the college, the nursing curriculum, and the faculty. Important parts of the interview were the student's perceptions of changes which may have occurred in his or her role as a nurse, as a professional, and as a person after one year in the program.

These oral sessions were quite informal and were usually held outdoors under a tree or at a table in the quadrangle. The individual interviews followed an established format and were conducted by members of the research staff or by psychology students at the college who were hired and trained for the work. These students interviewers were found to be quite competent, and they saw the interviewing process as a valuable learning experience in keeping with their career interests.

One unanticipated consequence of the oral interview that occurred often enough to be noteworthy was the catharsis opportunity it provided for some students. Quite often, the interview questions caused the student to recapitulate, perhaps for the first time, the year's joys and pleasant experiences, as well as the frustrations and hard work. When these ventilating sessions occurred, the interviewers were especially alert for succinct and cogent expressions which offered the rich, qualitative detail so important in capturing the essence of a student's feelings about the program and about himself.

FINDINGS AND UTILIZATION OF THE RESEARCH

The questionnaires, standardized tests, and oral interviews provided a large amount of information about each student. These data in turn furnished a broad view of each class as well as a composite view of the three classes that have entered the program thus far. Oral interviews were conducted with all classes after one year in the program, and graduation information is in hand for two classes that have finished the two year program.

214

Early formative use of the research data provided faculty with a general background about their students. This took the form of information about age, work experience, G.P.A.s, personality characteristics, and other important variables which were usually expressed as means, ranges, percentages, and as other descriptive statistics. As additional data such as students' reactions to specific parts of the curriculum were compiled, these data were furnished as memoranda or presented in faculty meetings as specific feedback to the educational process.

Another important use of the data occurred during the self-evaluation study in preparation for National League for Nursing Accreditation. Demographic data, test scores, and characteristics of students from the various preparatory sources were compared to illustrate the composition of the classes and to substantiate choices made in curriculum development. These analyses indicated that students from diploma programs and students from the community colleges were equally well prepared to undertake upper division study, and that there were few important differences in cognitive abilities between students from the two types of preparatory schools.

Results of NLN Achievement Tests given to junior students are shown in Table 1. When compared with test results of a normative group of students in baccalaureate programs, the class means were at the 50th percentile on the Natural Sciences test, the 56th percentile[on the Maternity Child Nursing test, the 75th percentile on the Psychiatric Nursing test, and the 47th percentile on the Comprehensive Medical-Surgical Nursing test. The dominant impression gained from this comparison is that the students entering this program have knowledge in these several areas that closely approximates that for students who are enrolled in other baccalaureate programs.

It may be argued that this is a misleading comparison; that the students, for example, who entered this program at the junior level should be compared with students in associate degree programs. When this comparison is made, the Sonoma students score relatively higher on each test, as may be seen also in Table 1. Their scores are well above average for each of the three tests for which normative information is available.

These data indicate that the students are better prepared to undertake this upper division program than most graduates of lower division programs. Indeed, it is likely that the students who have entered the Second Step Program and wish to obtain a B.S. degree are higher achieving students than those who terminate their formal education at the associate degree. It is also apparent that they are, as a group, at least comparable to students in other baccalaureate programs, since their scores generally range around the mean for students of four year programs.

The results of the senior students in the NLN Commnity Health Test are shown in Table 2. When compared with the norms derived

Table 1. NLN Achievement Test results for junior students,
September 20, 1973

Test name	Score BD norms*	Mean percentile AD norms†
Natural sciences		
Facts and principles	56	76
Application	46	66
Total	50	73
Maternity child nursing		
Normal obstetrics—newborn	40	64
Sick children	70	82
Total	56	76
Psychiatric nursing		
Facts and principles	53	78
Practice	61	65
Total	75	57
Comprehensive medical-surgical nursing		
Part A	42	—
Part B	45	—
Knowledge	47	—
Application	47	—

*Percentile norms are based on the performance of 490 students in 15 accredited baccalau-
reate degree programs.
†Percentile norms are based on the performance of 410 students in 15 accredited associate
degree programs.

from a large group of baccalaureate students, the seniors scored well
above average on each of the three tests. These results indicate that
on the average they have mastered three major bodies of knowledge
about nursing to a greater extent than the comparison group of
students in four year programs.

Together, these sets of data confirm several curricular assumptions
of the program. First, entering students do have a body of knowledge about nursing which can serve as a basis for undertaking upper
division work. Second, students who complete the junior year of
the program are more knowledgeable than students in comparable
baccalaureate programs. And third, these data lend support to the
assumption that senior students have a fund of knowledge upon
which individualized and specialized preceptorships may be built.

Other early results of the research effort may be informative. The
analysis of the classes upon entrance revealed that the students were
an extraordinarily diverse lot. Their intellectual abilities, personality profiles, attitudes toward health care, and educational prefer-
ences were about equally as varied. In short, the data support the

Table 2. NLN Achievement Test results for senior students, October 4, 1973

Test name	Mean percentile score*
Family health	61
Community health	74
Science and general information	63
Total	69

*Percentile norms are based on the performance of 490 students in 19 baccalaureate programs.

Nursing Department faculty's belief that students have traveled many different routes, distances, and directions in their profession and have gained widely varied life experiences prior to entering their program. Indeed, they are probably the kinds of students seeking innovative nursing programs across the country.

The implications of this diversity of students have been pointed out to the faculty, along with some suggestions for ways of providing educational experiences which are appropriate to the different students. The senior preceptorship is a particularly useful device for trying to individualize instruction, and the community health practicum and various seminars are also more likely to be useful teaching strategies than are more uniform lecture procedures with this group.

The interviews held with students at the end of the junior year revealed several insights about their first year in the program. A brief summary and a few salient points may be appropriate here. First, the vast majority of students seemed to be acquiring new nursing roles. For instance, 124 of the 135 students interviewed said they had become more competent and confident in dealing with families and working in the community setting; more than two thirds said their concept of themselves as nurses had changed and broadened; and about 90 per cent said they work more effectively with their patients than they did before. Second, 105 out of the 135 said they felt they had grown as persons during the year, including developing broader interests, becoming more understanding and tolerant toward other people, and developing greater self-awareness.

Despite the fact that students reported making these professional and personal gains, they had quite mixed reactions to various aspects of the program. When asked "How do you feel about the overall curricular structure of the department?" the majority of the nurses expressed general satisfaction although several offered a variety of minor suggestions. The community health course was said to be the most valuable part of the first year program by many students, most of whom specifically mentioned the clinical experience with families in the community. Curiously, the lecture portion of the same course was often mentioned as the least valuable part of the program. Apparently, the classical pedagogic challenge of making classroom materials relevant to the practice of nursing was only partially met with the first class. However, the second and third classes found considerably more relationship between classroom and clinic. Changes made in the classroom presentations were in part due to short loop feedback of formative research data.

Because the philosophy of the program places a heavy emphasis on the diversity of student experiences, interests, abilities, and learning styles, the research staff was interested in student experiences in this area. Students were asked, "Do you feel your individual needs and learning styles have been taken into consideration in your work this year?" Again, of the 135 students, 74 students answered in the affirmative, 45 in the negative, and the remainder in a mixed fashion. In the same vein, the researchers were interested in discovering how such a diverse group of students interacted and what they learned from each other. Fully 111 of the 135 students affirmed that other students contributed much to their education. Indeed, it appears that the students, all of whom are registered nurses, most of whom have worked professionally, and who have various life experiences, provide an important learning resource of this particular program.

The first class of a school, like the first child, has a number of advantages and disadvantages which following classes do not share. Therefore, students in the first class were asked to comment on the experience of being in the original class. Twelve thought it was more of an advantage to be in the first class, 12 thought it more of a disadvantage, and the remainder reported both advantages and disadvantages. The advantages centered on the challenge and pioneering quality of the new program, the greater willingness of the new faculty to help students, and the opportunity to see problems of a planned program emerge and be dealt with. The major disadvantages cited were the newness of the faculty to the program with resulting discrepancies in faculty expectations of student performance and the lack of learning resources and facilities. These difficulties are doubtless at least partly responsible for the less than enthusiastic response of the early students to the classroom part of the community health course. Some of these problems have been corrected simply because the faculty have had time to work closely together and develop more resources and facilities.

The Omnibus Personality Inventory administered to all students as they entered the program in September, and again when they graduated in May, nearly two years later, revealed interesting data. Comparisons of scores for individual scales of the OPI have been made for all three classes, and the entry-exit comparisons are available for the first two classes of graduates.[3]

OPI scores for Sonoma nursing students have been compared with scores from the normative sample of students from 37 institutions of higher learning located in 14 states (Fig. 1). The scores for Sonoma nursing students were found to be notably higher than the norm in the scales for Autonomy and Personal Integration. The rather high Autonomy score indicates that our students show an independence of authority greater than that shown by the normative sample of entering college freshmen. It may also suggest than an historically held view of nurses as passive and docile may not be entirely warranted, especially in the case of older nurses with work experience. The relatively high Personal Integration score indicates few attitudes that characterize socially alienated persons; it indicates that our students feel they are understood by other people, and they are about as happy as others seem to be.

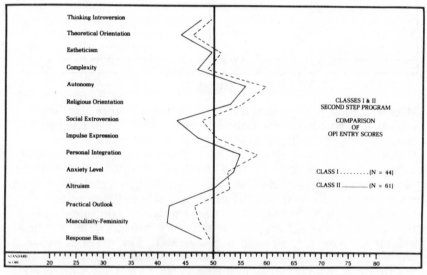

FIGURE 1.

On the other hand, our students in all three classes fall below the college norm on the scale of Social Extroversion. They tend to find less enjoyment in large gatherings of people and enjoy doing independent work. The relatively high score in Autonomy, and the relatively low score in Social Extroversion may support the faculty view that the preceptorship model of the senior year has considerable relevance for nurses in upper division baccalaureate education.

We have obtained a large amount of exit data from the senior posttest for the first class of graduates from the program. A preliminary analysis of these data shows that those students changed in a number of desirable ways during their two years at Sonoma (Fig. 2). They became more professional when compared with generally accepted criteria of professionalism such as autonomy, organization, and the

219

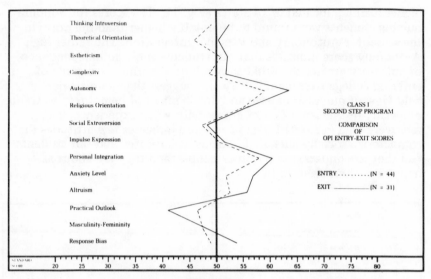

FIGURE 2.

effects of their professional skills. They became more altruistic, ethical, and trusting in relationships with others. They changed in the direction of finding a greater appeal in ideas than in facts, and in discussing philosophical problems. There was a general increase in the scores of six scales of the OPI which constitute the intellectual disposition category. The first class of students to graduate showed a distinct increase in their intellectual and scholarly interests.

At this phase of the evaluation of the program, additional questions, such as those above, concerning the extent to which the program realizes its purposes will be researched. Yet, previous experience suggests that finding reliable answers to such questions is only the first step in an effective evaluation effort. It is also important to consider ways in which the program may be modified so that its purposes may be more effectively realized. Above all, it is essential that the findings and implications from the research evidence be communicated to administrators and teachers in the department so that they may make decisions that are based on factual data. Additional ways are being sought to make the evaluation a more integral part of and a source of continual improvement in the program.

RESIDUAL ISSUES AND STRATEGIES FOR THE FUTURE

It is apparent from the evaluative research conducted thus far that many goals of the Second Step Program have been attained. A large amount of data have already been collected, and new classes of students are providing other indications that the faculty's initial views

220

of the curriculum and the nursing student body are essentially sound. Comparisons with other normative groups confirm Second Step Program assumptions that nurse-students can benefit from open curricula and independent study.

Students who have gained their basic technical education in various lower division programs are progressing equally well in an upper-division baccalaureate program situated in a small liberal arts college. Students who came from widely diversified backgrounds which often included years of experience in the order and discipline of the hospital are competent to undertake courses of study which emphasize individual planning, development, evaluation, and the lonely pursuit of an indistinct goal. Indeed, the students are meeting the expectations of the faculty, and are changing as professional nurses and as persons in many ways which were expected and in other ways which were not anticipated.

A great deal of work is currently underway which addresses both the formative and the summative aspects of the evaluative research. Activities are being carried out to further some of the preliminary findings, and a large number of variables now in the files remain to be investigated.

The original comparative aspirations of the study have not been forgotten. This dimension of the research will be resumed as soon as problems of time and resources are overcome. Several other upper division nursing programs have already indicated an interest in participating in such a study.

The thrust of the present evaluative research effort has been to combine specially developed surveys and standardized tests with interview techniques to elicit data in the most effective way, and to analyze the findings for the benefit of the program. Future efforts of the research staff will aim toward developing a model for the preparation of baccalaureate nurses to meet new challenges in education and health care delivery. The staff also plan to examine critically the methodology of evaluating this program as an approach for the evaluation of other baccalaureate nursing programs. We hope that such a model and such a methodology may be useful to other educators planning a similar upper division program.

REFERENCES

1. Heist, Paul and Yonge, George: *Omnibus Personality Inventory, Form F, Manual.* The Psychological Corporation, New York, 1968, pp. 1-7.
2. Cattell, Raymond B., and Cattell, A.K.S.: *Culture Fair Intelligence Test, Scale 3, Forms A and B, Handbook.* Institute for Personality and Ability Testing, Champaign, Ill., 1959, pp. 1-18.
3. Reproduced by permission. Copyright 1962, 1968 by the Psychological Corporation, New York. All rights reserved.

BIBLIOGRAPHY

Cattell, Raymond B., and Cattell, A.K.S.: *Handbook for the Culture Fair Intelligence Test.* Institute for Personality and Ability Testing, Champaign, Ill. 1959.

Chronbach, Lee J., and Gleser, Goldine C.: *Psychological Tests and Personnel Decisions.* University of Illinois Press, Urbana, Ill., 1965.

Chronbach, Lee J.: *Essentials of Psychological Testing.* Harper and Row, New York, 1970.

Heist, Paul, and Yorge, George: *Omnibus Personality Inventory Handbook.* The Psychology Corporation, New York, 1968.

Nie, Norman, Best, Dale H., and Hull, C. Haddlai: *Statistical Package for the Social Sciences.* McGraw-Hill, New York, 1970.

Runyan, Richard P., and Haber, Audrey: *Fundamentals of Behavioral Statistics.* Addison-Wesley, Reading, Mass., 1968.

Senter, R.J.: *Analysis of Data.* Scott, Foresman, Glenview, Ill., 1969.

CHAPTER 11

Curriculum Evaluation Research

Holly Skodol Wilson, R.N., Ph.D.

Evaluation, writes a well known researcher, is an elastic word that stretches to cover judgments of many kinds.[1] Nursing faculties talk about evaluating students' clinical performances, evaluating each other's teaching effectiveness, and evaluating a textbook or learning module for possible adoption. What all these uses of the word have in common is the notion of judging merit. Someone is examining a phenomenon (a person, a thing, an idea, or a program) against some explicit or implicit criteria.

In this chapter I will be talking about evaluation of one particular kind of phenomenon—educational curricula. All educators are involved in evaluating the effectiveness of their work. Many, however, are dissatisfied with the quality and usefulness of the appraisals they make and welcome help in improving them. This chapter is a response to that need. I have set out to offer an orientation to the full scope and function of curriculum evaluation, some basic considerations of design and methodology, and an examination of the social-psychological intricacies of action research. I believe that evaluation is an integral part of any innovative curriculum intent upon achieving its goals. Hopefully, this chapter will impart some of the reasons why.

SOME BACKGROUND DATA

I am proposing that curriculum evaluation is particularly important in the development and establishment of innovative programs. The Open Curriculum idea as implemented in CSCS's Second Step model represents one of the most prominent innovations in nursing education of the 1970s. In many ways, it was initiated in a context of traditions in baccalaureate nursing education which were at best curious about its feasibility and in some cases clearly opposed to its basic premises. The pangs of moving nursing education out of the apprenticeship model in service-oriented hospital schools of nursing into institutions of higher learning were still fresh in the memories of many leaders in the profession. Some of them viewed the notion of equating diploma education with lower division collegiate education with scepticism if not direct disapproval.

Furthermore, research and writing on the subject of differentiation between technical and professional nursing argued that the two were qualitatively different kinds of practice implicitly challenging the assumption that one, technical nursing, is the appropriate basis for the other, professional nursing.[2]

Despite social mandates to provide upward mobility within nursing, the Second Step model was faced with proving its viability. Curriculum evaluation research offered one approach to gaining support for the ideas and basic premises in the sense that it held the promise of demonstrating that the innovative program model was indeed effective in preparing a professional, baccalaureate nurse.

Without previously tested precedents to rely on, faculty in the Second Step Program viewed curriculum research as having an additional, more immediate value. It could offer some basis for making rational choices about day to day implementation decisions. Questions were many and cogent. Should more emphasis be placed on attitudes about self, role, and identity than on specific nursing content? Should curricula be different for diploma versus associate degree graduates? What criteria could be used to admit students likely to succeed in upper division studies? Should a specified period of work experience be required of the applicants for admission? Faculty accustomed to relying on their own experience and intuitive judgment turned to a curriculum evaluation study to provide them with additional direction on practical questions such as these. Curriculum evaluation was seen as one means by which to understand and manage something new.

EVALUATION: WHAT IS IT?

Despite its widespread popularity, the term evaluation is loosely defined. One finds a variety of statistical records, inventories, testamonials, and experiments all classified as curriculum evaluation studies. Such studies range from the "is everybody happy" approach to complex research designs.

In my own perspective, evaluation designates a process of appraisal which involves accepting certain values and using a variety of data collection tools as the basis for making judgments of worth.[3] Evaluation is a way of thinking—a disciplined inquiry that results in a story. It tells what happened. It tells of the merits and shortcomings of a program. As a bonus it may even offer generalizations for the guidance of subsequent educational programs. Evaluation refers to a process of making judgments of value. Yet what passes

224

in reality for such a process is a mixed bag at best, and chaos at worst.

Distinctions Between Evaluation and Evaluation Research

In this chapter I make a distinction between "evaluation" and "evaluation research." The former is used in a general way which implies some rational basis for making judgments of merit, but does not require any systematic procedure for marshaling and presenting the evidence to support the judgments. Following Suchman's lead, I retain the term evaluation research to refer to a disciplined inquiry in which the methods of scientific research are pressed into service to make an evaluation.[4] In its research guise, evaluation establishes clear and specific criteria for success. It collects evidence systematically and compares it with the criteria which were set. It then draws conclusions about the effectiveness, the merit, the success of the phenomenon under study. Doing *evaluation research* rather than *evaluation* increases the possibility of "proving" rather than "asserting" the worth of an educational program. As Weiss points out, the research process takes more time and costs more money than offhand evaluations that rely on intuition, opinion, trained sensibility, testimonials, and inventory lists, but it provides a rigor that is particularly important under certain cricumstances.[5] These circumstances include (1) when the outcomes to be evaluated are complex and hard to observe, (2) when the decisions that follow are important and expensive, and (3) when the evidence is needed to convince other people about the validity of the conclusions.

Evaluation research applies the methods of social science. Everything we know about design, measurement, and analysis comes into play in planning and conducting an evaluation study. What distinguishes evaluation research is not method or subject matter, but the purpose for which the research is done. Weiss has synthesized some additional differentiating characteristics.[6]

1. Evaluation is intended for use. Evaluation is a form of applied research the major objective of which is not the production of new theory, but rather the application of knowledge in program decision-making.

2. The questions that evaluation considers are shaped by program concerns. Unlike the basic researcher who formulates his own hypotheses, the core of the study reflects the administrative and programmatic interests. The most common evaluation hypothesis is that the program is accomplishing what it set out to do.

3. In addition to the scientific aspect of evaluation research, it also has an ethical dimension. The role of values is clearer in some stages of the evaluation process than in others. The program's objectives are based on value assumptions. Judgment against criteria is basic to evaluation research and differentiates it from other kinds of research.

According to Williams and Williams, the statement and assessment of program goals is therefore essential to program evaluation.[7] Initially, values guide the selection of these objectives and ultimately dictate what value or disvalue is attached to the results found.

4. Evaluation research takes place in an action setting where the most important thing that is going on is a program serving people. The methods and tools of scientific research must be applied in an action context that is often structurally and social-psychologically inhospitable to them. Researchers who embark on evaluation research with preparation only in research methods often bog down in the complexities of the action setting. The judgmental quality of evaluation means that the merits of the program are being weighed and the possibilities for friction and role conflict are obvious. I will have more to say about this later.

5. The evaluation researcher has multiple allegiances. He or she has responsibilities to contribute to curriculum decision making and change. He or she also has an obligation to remain unbaised and objective in applying the methods of social research. Finally, there is also the obligation to develop knowledge within the profession. Although dilemmas posed by these multiple allegiances may make the lot of an evaluation researcher look unduly harsh, compensations are found in the opportunity to blend scientific knowledge and social action in the improvement of programs which benefit people.

There are some important similarities between evaluation research and other brands of research that bear mentioning. Like other research, evaluation attempts to describe, to understand the relationship among variables, and to trace out causal sequences. Because it studies a curriculum that intervenes in people's lives with the intention of causing change, evaluation can sometimes make direct inferences about causal links that lead from program inputs to outcomes. Evaluators use the whole repertoire of research methods to collect information—interviews, questionnaires, tests of knowledge and skill, inventories, observation, content analysis of documents, and psychometrics. The classical design for evaluation studies has been the experimental model. This approach involves measurement of the relevant variables for at least two similar groups— one that has experienced the program being evaluated and one that has not. But many other research designs are used in evaluation studies—case studies, post-program surveys, longitudinal studies, correlational studies, and so on. I will discuss the scientific decisions later in the chapter.

WHY EVALUATE?

Faculty and administrators decide to evaluate a program for many different reasons. Government agencies often require that a program

226

evaluate its effectiveness for continued financial support. Professionals decide to evaluate due to a realization that resources are limited and that allocation of them must be discriminating.

Another source of pressure is the need of educators to make intelligent and responsible choices among alternatives that are available. Most often people are seeking answers to pressing questions about a curriculum's future. Should it be continued? Should it be expanded? How can we help a teacher to choose wisely? Does the curriculum promote the learning expected of it? Does it really work? What changes should be made in its operation or design?

Questions of evaluation have gained salience from social forces which have emphasized the outcome of the educational process in terms of student learning and on the educational process itself. It is no longer satisfactory to speak only of inputs—what teachers are teaching and what the program offers. Attainment of program objectives must also be assessed through observation of curriculum outcomes. This shift in emphasis is particularly apparent in open curriculum models which attempt individualized instruction in order to achieve identified competencies.

Covert Purposes

There are occasions when an evaluation study has different roles to fulfill. These are best understood at the social-psychological level. Evaluation research may be commissioned as a way to postpone a decision to revise a curriculum. Sometimes evaluation is used to make what appears a highly successful program more visible for public relation purposes. Such motives are not necessarily less than legitimate. Often there is a need to justify a program to the public who pays the bills, or an administrator may be seeking organizational support for a new program in which he or she believes. Generating support for a new program is a common motive for embarking on an evaluation study. Sometimes the decision to carry out evaluation research stems from sources outside the program itself. Many federal grants, for example, require an evaluation component for demonstration projects receiving funds.

Evaluation, then, is a rational enterprise occasionally undertaken for less rational or at least covert reasons. Obviously it is beneficial for an evaluator to determine the real purposes of intent in undertaking the study. Most writers comment that the most rewarding study is one undertaken "in an organization where there is a real commitment to using the results of the evaluation to improve future decision-making."[8]

Overt Purposes

When an evaluation study is undertaken for the purpose of learning how well the program is meeting its objectives, an evaluation study can deal with the following issues:

1. Identifying goals or objectives to be evaluated.
2. Discovering whether and how well the objectives are met.
3. Determining reasons for specific successes and failures.
4. Analyzing problems with which the program must cope.
5. Determining which outcomes are due to the program and which are due to some other cause or factor.
6. Ascertaining some indication of the durability of the effects of the program.
7. Studying the relative success of alternative techniques.
8. Redefining the means for attaining the objectives and even redefining the goals in the light of some of the research findings.[9]

Herzog offers the following questions as those worthy of consideration in a quality research effort:[10]
1. What kind of change is desired?
2. By what means is the change brought about?
3. What is the evidence that the changes are due to the means employed?
4. What is the meaning of the changes found?
5. Were there unexpected outcomes as well?

Although authors on the subject of the overt purposes for undertaking an evaluation study use different language to describe them, the preceeding list evidences some common themes. Among them are that the curriculum evaluator needs to start by examining and assessing the objectives which guide the investigation. Furthermore, not only must the outcomes be measured but some link should be attempted between these outcomes and specific features of the curriculum. Finally, the design ideally ought to strive to control for possible alternative factors which may have resulted in the identified outcomes.

HOW TO EVALUATE

I am proposing that the scientific method is one of the most powerful of all approaches yet devised to obtain answers to the kinds of questions raised above. Describing the scientific method is not an easy task. In fact, it is a somewhat risky venture in view of the literature indicating that even our most esteemed scientists fail to agree on the details of how a scientist operates. Yet there is a basic structure present in most conventional views of the process of scientific inquiry.[11]
1. A problem or question is identified and carefully stated.
2. Hypotheses or propositions are formulated.
3. Data are collected.
4. Data are analyzed to draw conclusions.
5. The conclusions are assessed in terms of the original questions.

It is most important to note that the foregoing steps need not be followed in a rigid sequence. Most scientific inquiries involve a shuttling back and forth between different phases of the process. This is particularly true in the action setting of evaluation research.

At first glance it might appear that all that is necessary for a curriculum evaluation is to combine specific course evaluations to obtain a general picture of the effects of the total program. This strategy does not work well for several reasons. Evaluations made by different teachers are often not comparable. Also, a curriculum evaluation and assessments of student achievement done in specific courses to assign the students their grades are done for different reasons. Each has, as its referent, a different set of objectives. Many times the instruments and data obtained from them used to assess student performances in courses are incomplete for a full curriculum evaluation. A curriculum evaluation instrument may reflect an attempt to measure outcomes of educational significance not connected with specific instructional objectives. An example of this idea in the evaluation of a Second Step model might be the curriculum evaluator's interest in measuring the degree to which a professional identity is supplanted for that of a technical nurse when such an objective is not directly identified in any single course. This kind of outcome is an example of what Trow calls profound as opposed to proximate aims.

> Some outcomes of education are easily measured. . . .But whatever their objective importance, they may be inadequate measures of more enduring outcomes of the educational experience. They are poor measures of the success of a liberal education in refining sensibilities or the enhancement of an individual's capacities for enjoying life and making fruitful contributions to it. . . . In large part, these qualities of mind and spirit do not show themselves during the college years, but may be laid down then as potentialities that bear fruit in later life and career. . . . In a word, then, the most important and truly valued outcomes of education are extremely difficult to assess.[12]

He goes on to urge the curriculum evaluator to avoid confining his or her study to the most obvious and easily measured outcomes of education, such as achievement of course objectives.

> There are ways to explore changes in basic values and attitudes of students . . . to explore changes in life plans and the conditions which give rise to them; to attempt to study such subtle matters as creativity and independence of mind and judgment.[13]

Just as curriculum evaluation cannot be equated with a combination of course evaluations, similarly it must be distinguished from teacher performance evaluation. It is hardly reasonable to expect teachers to be objective in assessing program success if their own survival in the system depends on the results of the evaluation.

Analysis of these considerations in curriculum evaluation leads inescapably to the need for a systematic design or plan in response to the question: "How to evaluate?" The design or plan for an evaluation study should include the following:

1. Consideration of why one is evaluating—for what purposes and how will the results be used.

2. What does one want to know? Choices must be made about what is being assessed. What are the objectives that will provide areas for data collection?

3. How is the evaluation to be carrried out? What instruments and procedures will be used? Who will conduct the study? Will the evaluators be internal or external to the study?

4. What is the sampling plan? From whom will information be needed and at what points in time?

5. What system will be used for recording and storing the data?

6. What plans are possible for checking out the objectivity, reliability, comprehensiveness, validity, and relevancy of data?

7. What kinds of comparisons can be made?

8. What plans exist for obtaining consultant help and data processing services?

9. What ways are there for summarizing findings so that they can be used for decision-making and program improvement?

10. Finally, what will the task assignments and time schedule be?

The preceding list offers a relatively useful and comprehensive list of guidelines for planning an evaluation project.

WHEN TO EVALUATE

Stufflebeam considers evaluation useful to decision makers throughout the entire life of a program.[14] He denotes four specific times when evaluation studies can provide particularly worthwhile information. These are the context, input, process and product phases of a program. Provos also looks at the developmental stages of a program and sees evaluation as relevant in all of them.[15] The general argument advanced by Tripodi and others posits that evaluation should and can take place throughout all stages of a program's life—asking different questions at the different stages.[16]

Formative and Summative Evaluation

One of the most useful distinctions introduced into the discussion of when to evaluate and for what purpose is made by Scriven in his work on formative and summative evaluation.[17] Formative evaluation produces information that is fed back during the development of a curriculum to help improve it. It serves the needs of the faculty developers and implementors. Summative evaluation is done, on the other hand, when the curriculum is finished by a class of learners. It provides information for making decisions about over-all program effectiveness. Summative evaluation measures outcomes. Many programs are never "finished" in the sense that the curriculum no longer requires adaption and modification. The issue posed to the summative evaluator is how can we hold the program steady?

The Shifting Program

Curriculums always seem to be in a state of revision. If a program has altered its course, what does the evaluator do? Does he or she continue on as if studying the old program, never knowing what it was that led to the outcomes? If the original evaluation is dropped and a try made to start anew, the baseline data may be lost. In either case, the evaluator has no assurance that the same kind of shift will not take place again.

Some authors recommend that when innovative programs are being evaluated, the researcher should be in control of the whole operation. Then the program would be conducted with the evaluation require-ments in the forefront and random changes fended off. Freeman and Sherwood go so far as to suggest that the curriculum evaluator stand over the original curriculum "like a snarling watchdog" to prevent program faculty from altering it.[18] Mann concludes that programs are too complex and variable in operation to provide fair tests of program principles.[19] He gives up on evaluating in action settings and recommends taking programs back to the laboratory for evalua-tion and study of small segments of the program. Weiss and Rein believe that it is better in action programs to discard the investigation of goal achievement altogether.[20] They purport that the researcher will learn more from a careful analysis of what is actually going on.

Holding the program steady, let alone controlling it, is beyond the authority of most evaluators in settings I have seen. There are limits to what the evaluator can do to hold back the tide of change, modi-fication, and adaption in a curriculum. Yet to surrender to the com-plexities and retreat to the laboratory seems like a cop out.

To cope with the evaluation program in flux, Suchman has proposed a four stage developmental process.[21] He differentiates a pilot phase when program development proceeds on a trial and error basis, a model phase when a defined program strategy is run under controlled conditions, a prototype phase when the model program is subjected to realistic operating conditions, and an institutionalized phase when the program is an ongoing part of an organization. It is only during the model phase that the program must be held stable for summative evaluation. At other stages, rigorous formative study suffices and variation in input is not only tolerated but expected.

Alas, such a rational course of program development is rare and ultimately the evaluator in most instances must make the best of program shifts in the absence of such clear demarcation of program phases. Formative evaluation is less problematic amid a program in process and flux. Nevertheless, study of development does not supplant evaluation of outcomes. Critical as it is to learn more about the dynamics of operation, it is still important to find out the effects of educational programs on people. Certainly the discovery of new models of educational evaluation need to focus on ways in which the study of program process can be combined with the study of program outcomes.

WHO SHOULD DO THE EVALUATION STUDY

There is a long tradition of controversy about whether in-house or outside evaluations are preferable. Weiss concludes that neither has a monopoly on the advantages.[22] Some of the relevant considerations she identifies as having bearing on this decision are: (1) adminstrative confidence, (2) objectivity, (3) understanding of the curriculum, (4) potential for utilization of findings, and (5) autonomy.

Administrators and program faculty must have confidence in the professional skills of the evaluation staff. Sometimes nursing faculty are only impressed by credentials and reputations of academic researchers who are professional evaluators. They fear that evaluation research conducted by members of the teaching faculty would somehow be second rate. Conversely, a faculty may view outside evaluators as too remote from the program realities to produce information which they will consider useful. Competence is of course the biggest factor in ensuring confidence and deserves emphasis in this choice.

Objectivity is another crucial variable. It requires that evaluators be insulated from any possibility of biasing their data or its interpretation by a desire to make things look good. Safeguarding the study against even unintentional bias is often easier when outside evaluators are used.

One area in which outsiders may be at a disadvantage is that of knowledge of what the program is all about. However, it is not impossible for outside evaluators to find out about the program if they make the effort and are given access to sources of information.

Using the results of an evaluation study often requires that evaluators take an active role in moving from research data to interpretation of the results in a policy context. Often evaluation staff who are themselves faculty members are better able to get a hearing for recommendations based on research results.

Evaluators who are members of a program faculty generally take the basic assumptions and often even the organizational arrangements of the program as "givens" and conduct their evaluation within that context. The outside evaluator who may be at a disadvantage on some of the preceding points may be able to exercise more autonomy and take a different perspective.

These considerations must all be balanced against each other. There is no one best for every program. The factors have to be weighed and decisions about who should conduct the evaluation made on the basis of how the advantages line up and what is practically possible.

In California State College, Sonoma's Second Step Program, a research team composed of a nurse researcher with part time teaching responsibilities and a research associate with competencies in methodology and freedom from the role of faculty member provide a desirable blend of objectivity, autonomy, and understanding of an influence on the curriculum. The social-psychology of this structural arrangement will be taken up when discussing the action setting.

FORMULATING THE QUESTION AND MEASURING THE ANSWER

As with all research, a curriculum evaluation study begins with some effort to determine what the evaluator is going to study. The most apparent formulation of the research question in curriculum evaluation is: "To what extent is the curriculum reaching its goals or objectives?" Does a Second Step model prepare professional nurses as well or better than a generic baccalaureate program? Which components of the respective programs are having more success? How well is the program being studied achieving specified results with different groups of learners who possess different characteristics?

Despite these variations, the basic notion is the same. There are goals or terminal objectives, there are planned activities or a curriculum aimed at achieving these goals, and there is a measure made of the extent to which the goals are achieved. Formulating evaluation questions sounds relatively simple. All the curriculum researcher has to do is:

1. Find out the program goals.
2. Translate the goals into measurable indicators of goal achievement.
3. Collect data on the indicators for those who participated in the program and for an equivalent control group who did not.
4. Compare the data on participants and controls with the goal criteria.

Suchman has conceptualized the evaluation process in the model in Figure 1 which particuarly emphasizes the importance of values in the whole process.[23]

He points out that what seems elementary on the surface, turns out in practice to be a very demanding and complex endeavor. The clear cut definition of program objectives and even the identification of responsible program activities is not an easy task. He proposes that the evaluator's responsibilities in relation to program goals alone include consideration of all of the following:

233

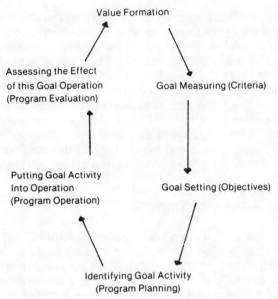

Value Formation

Assessing the Effect
of this Goal Operation
(Program Evaluation)

Goal Measuring (Criteria)

Putting Goal Activity
Into Operation
(Program Operation)

Goal Setting (Objectives)

Identifying Goal Activity
(Program Planning)

FIGURE 1. The evaluation process. (From Suchman[4])

1. What is the nature of the objective's content? Is the program trying to change knowledge, attitudes, and/or behavior?

2. Who is the target of the program? At which groups is the program aimed? Is the curriculum trying to reach some groups, for example nursing students, directly and other target groups, such as patients, indirectly?

3. When is the desired change to take place? Is the curriculum looking for an immediate effect or is it building toward some postponed effect? How long does one expect the effects to last? Is the curriculum aimed toward permanent or transient changes?

4. Are the curriculum objectives unitary or multiple? Are the changes to be the same for all learners or do they vary for different groups?

5. What is the desired magnitude of effect? Does a particular proportion of effectiveness have to be attained before the curriculum is considered successful?[24]

All of the above questions play some role in determining which of the often hazy, ambiguous and multiple possible objectives the evaluator selects as a basis for study. It is not uncommon to find that official goals are merely a long list of pious and even incompatible platitudes. The evaluation researcher must aim to get a real sense of what the program is trying to accomplish. The experienced evaluator also searches for the hidden agenda, the covert goals of the program which may not be articulated. Ultimately, whether the curriculum developers have done it or whether the evaluator

234

collaborates in formulating them, curriculum goals must be stated in clear, unambiguous, and potentially measurable terms.

Once the goals of the program are clearly, specifically, and behaviorally defined, the next step is to decide which of them to evaluate. Part of this decision is made on the practical basis of money, time, and access. Frequently, a compromise must be made between what ought to be studied and what is easier to study. Almost all programs have multiple objectives. There are long range, short range, broad, narrow, subsidiary, immediate, intermediate, and ultimate objectives. An evalutor must decide which set of possible objectives will provide the focus for the study. Table 1 summarizes the three different levels of objectives identifiable in the Second Step nursing curriculum.

Herzog identifies three types of evaluation studies.[25] "Ultimate evaluation" refers to a determination of the final success of a program in eliminating or reducing the social problems at which it is aimed. "Pre-evaluation research" deals with the intermediate problems that need to be solved before one can attempt ultimate evaluation, such as the development of reliable and valid classification of the problem, the definition of action goals, and the perfection of tools and techniques. Short term evaluation is limited to seeking specific answers to concrete procedures in terms of immediate utility. Such students attempt no generalizations beyond the limits of the data.

YARDSTICKS OR CRITERIA

Once the final selection of goals is accomplished, the evaluator must deal with the question of which yardsticks indicate success. Is a tiny change sufficient? Is no change also viewed as success because it is better than retrogression? Weiss proposes that a comparative stance be taken on this issue, wherein the evaluator compares the program with itself at various points in time or compares the program under investigation with an alternative program model designed to meet relatively similar objectives.[26] Suchman goes one step further and offers five categories of criteria according to which success or failure of a program may be evaluated. These are: (1) effort, (2) performance, (3) adequacy of performance, (4) efficiency, and (5) process.[27] The categories are interrelated and each is taken up briefly below.

1. Evaluations based on the "effort" have as their criterion of success the quantity and quality of activity that takes place. The focus is on inputs of energy regardless of output. It answers questions like "What did you do and how well did you do it?" The National League for Nursing Accreditation self-evaluation documents tend to focus on this criterion.

2. Performance or "effect" criteria measure the results of effort rather than the effort itself. Clearly, a curriculum can be rated "A" for effort yet can be a failure in terms of performance criteria.

Table 1. California State College, Sonoma's Second Step
Program objectives

Ultimate objectives of the program
1. To increase upward mobility for registered nurses holding A.D. degrees.
2. To increase the number of California nurses holding B.S. degrees.
3. To increase the number of male nurses holding B.S. degrees.
4. To increase the number of ethnic minority nurses prepared at the B.S. level.
5. To decrease the per capita cost of nursing education to both the student and the institution.
6. To provide baseline information on the characteristics and interests of registered nurse students upon entering and leaving the program as a preliminary study to further research on the characteristics of B.S. education and practice.

Immediate goals of the program
1. To prepare the student to organize and utilize the concepts, principles, and theories of the related sciences in such a way as to derive meaning for the practice of nursing.
2. To prepare the student to assess each client situation in relation to its placement on the health-illness continuum.
3. To prepare the student to define the multiple variables which operate to produce any given client situation.
4. To prepare the student to utilize the problem solving process to conceive and initiate intervention measures and apply criteria to explain, justify, predict outcomes, and evaluate those measures.
5. To prepare the student to recognize and participate in changes within a dynamic society and in health care systems.
6. To prepare the student to pursue the quest for personal and professional growth and development.

Intermediate program objectives
To produce a nurse who:
1. Has a broad knowledge of the health-illness continuum and the factors which affect clients, families and communities as they move on the continuum.
2. Uses a systematic problem-solving approach in assessment and analysis of health problems, and in planning, implementing, and evaluating nursing interventions.
3. Examines the process of change as it pertains to self, clients, and systems.
4. Formulates a philosophy of professional nursing practice.
5. Has self awareness and understands the nature of self-actualization.
6. Realizes the importance of nursing research and demonstrates a willingness to incorporate new knowledge within his or her framework of practice.

---

3. Adequacy of performance refers to the degree to which effective performance is adequate to the total amount of need. This criterion needs to be tempered by a realistic awareness of what is possible at a given state of knowledge and with available resources. The concept of increments of progress toward idealized long range objectives needs to be built into this criterion.

4. The criteria of efficiency addresses the question of whether there is a better way to attain desired results. Efficiency is concerned with the evaluation of altenative paths or methods in terms of costs—in money, time, personnel, and public convenience.

5. Process may also offer a criterion. An evaluation study may limit its data collection and analysis simply to determining whether or not a program is successful without examining the whys and wherefores of this success or failure. However, an analysis of process can have both administrative and scientific significance. Making sense of the evaluation findings is the central reason for adding a concern with process to the evaluation study. Otherwise one is left with the descriptive results of the evaluation without any explanations. An expansion of this dimension of curriculum evaluation research is planned for California State College, Sonoma's Second Step Nursing Program. A project proposal has been funded by the National Institute of Health, Division of Nursing, to undertake a case study of the "Sonoma Experience" using field methods. This study will collect and analyze qualitative data with heuristic potential for developing explanations and conceptualizations of a process, the specifics of which have already been described in earlier chapters. Our proposed study will move beyond exclusive focus on goal achievement to include consideration of (1) attributes of the program itself, (2) experiences of the students in the program, (3) an analysis of the situational context within which the program takes place, and (4) the different kinds of outcomes produced by the program.

MEASURING THE OUTCOMES

After the specific goals have been identified as the focus for a curriculum evaluation study, and some sense of the yardsticks agreed upon, the evaluator's next step is the development of indicators of program outcomes which represent the dependent variables in a research oriented study.

The development of measures or instruments to provide indicators of outcomes is a demanding phase of the evaluation process. It is usually worth a fair amount of searching to locate instruments that have already proved workable rather than to always try to create new ones. Several handbooks of well piloted measures have been published for research and merit consulting by the curriculum evaluator.[29]

Sometimes the curriculum evaluator is able to find no instruments directly relevant to the foci of his or her study. In these cases, energy must be devoted to developing new measures. Devising questions, test items, and forms often looks so easy that it comes as a surprise to discover the complexity of considerations of reliability or validity which need attention in developing original measures. Items often must be pre-tested and revised several times around before it is clear that they are bringing the desired information.

Adequate indicators of success in evaluation, like adequate measures of other concepts in research, benefit from multiple measurement. By using a number of measures to get different slices of data, it is possible to limit irrelevancies and develop a more inclusive picture of program outcomes. In discussing curriculum evaluation, Cronbach argues for measures of classroom behavior, attitudes, and the subsequent careers of learners in addition to assessment by tests or questionnaires.[30]

Types of Measures

Measures that are useful for evaluating outcomes of a curriculum can deal with attitudes, values, knowledge, behavior, productivity, budgetary allocations, and many other items. Most evaluations tend to concentrate on changes in program participants—in the case of our study, the students—although effects could also be examined in clients, organizations, and agencies offering nursing services, as well as the community at large.

Measuring effects on learners is customarily concentrated on attitudes, values, personality variables, knowledge, and skills, each of which may be directly relevant to program goals. Most curricula intend to change overt behavior as well but evalutors tend to rely heavily on attitudinal data and self-reports from individuals rather than attempting the more difficult and time-consuming direct behavioral observation. With our proposed extension into process-oriented curriculum evaluation research, we will move into the behavioral realm through the use of participant observation methods of data collection.

Specifying the Program

Making decisions about appropriate indicators of outcome relies ultimately on the evaluator's attempt to specify precisely what the curriculum is attempting to accomplish. This decision is clearly related to the identification of program goals. The evaluator must also conceptualize and describe what the program really is. A nursing curriculum, for example, is a complex undertaking. There are often marked internal variations in operation from day to day and from faculty member to faculty member. It behooves the evaluator to describe and analyze the program input. If he or she has no idea of what the program really is, he or she may fail to ask the right questions. In many cases it is necessary to look for more than just the attainment of goals that are verbalized. Unless there is some coherent definition of the program, the evaluator does not know to what to attribute outcomes that are observed. Unless the evaluator provides a conceptualization and description of the program there is also little basis for decision-making in innovation or modification. A possible outline for capturing the essence of a program is proposed by Weiss.[31] She suggests that the evaluator include the type of service offered, its conceptual emphasis, the type of staff, the setting, and the organizational context. It is important to look at variations within a program in order to clarify the meaning of "the program" and to establish which features of the program work and which do not. Program input variables for Sonoma's Second Step are reflected in the other accompanying chapters of this volume. In addition, characteristics of students may also be classified as input variables. A great deal of energy in CSCS's nursing evaluation research study has focused on identifying characteristics of learners in the program. These include sex, age, socioeconomic status, race, attitudes toward the program, expectations of it, degree of support from family and others, and so forth.

The final output data for evaluation research can be collected from a variety of sources using a whole repertoire of research techniques. The limits are only determined by resources available and the ingenuity and imagination of the researcher. Possible sources include: interviews, questionnaires, observations, ratings, psychometric tests, institutional records, tests of knowledge and skills, projective tests, diary records, documents, and so forth.

DESIGN OF THE EVALUATION

Once the evaluator knows what is to be studied the next step is to devise how to study it. A plan must be developed to select the people to be studied, the timing of the investigation, and the selection of procedures for collection of data. One can aim for a highly controlled experiment or one of the less formalized quasi-experimental designs. One can focus on one curriculum or look at the outcomes of a number with the same basic goals.

Experiments

The classic design for evaluations, in the literature if not in practice, is the experimental model. This model compares experimental and control groups. Measures are taken of the criteria variables before the program starts and after it ends. Differences are computed and the curriculum is deemed a success if the experimental group has improved more than the control group.

The controlled experiment is often quite difficult to achieve in action settings. In the case of our research, possible controls were widely scattered and reluctant to invest the time and effort to cooperate with evaluation research which offered them little in return. Experimental designs have also come under criticism not only because of their problems with feasibility, but also because they may be counterproductive to the program itself. An experimental design

239

requires holding the program constant rather than facilitating its continual improvement. It is also only useful for making decisions after a curriculum has run full cycle and is not used during planning and implementation. With imaginative use of available methodology such as comparative study between a subunit which remains stable and another encouraged to continually improve, repeated periodic measures of outcomes, and other innovations of design and analysis, some of these shortcomings can be overcome. They key consideration is one of fitting the research design to the purpose of the study. The experimental design is an elegant way to find out how well a particular program achieves its goals. If the faculty wants to know other things as well—how to develop a new program, how to secure its acceptance, or how to continually improve the implementation of a program—rough estimates of program effectiveness while it shifts and changes may be a preferable distribution of resources for the research. The essential requirement for the true experiment is the randomized assignment of people to programs. Since curriculums are rarely run for the convenience of the evaluators, turning to quasi-experimental designs may offer a more fruitful approach.

Quasi-Experimental Designs

Quasi-experimental designs have the advantage of being practical when conditions prevent experimentation. They have a form and logic of their own. Among them are the time-series or longitudinal design which involves a series of measures at periodic intervals during the program and after the program ends. This design is reflected in our research in the Second Step Program.

Another design is the nonequivalent control group. Here there is no attempt to randomly assign participants to the program being evaluated and the control program as there would be in an experiment. Instead, available groups with similar characteristics are used as controls. Nonrandomized controls are generally referred to as comparison groups. Before and after measures are made for both groups and compared.

While the experimental design has prestige, power, and symmetry, quasi-experimental designs such as these two have the overriding virtue of feasibility. They can produce results that are sufficiently convincing for many practical purposes.

Nonexperimental Designs

Nonexperimental designs are those most commonly used in evaluation research. There are three popular ones: before and after study of a single program, after only study of program participants, and after only study of participants and nonrandom controls. The inherent weakness of these designs is that they fail to control for the many rival explanations—the notion that observed changes may have been caused by something other than the program. At their best they can be full of detail and imagery, provocative and rich in insight. For many of the formative purposes of evaluation they are likely to be adequate.

Clearly, our evaluation research study, taken up in Chapter 11, reflects such a design decision. A one group pre-test and post-test design has definite advantages over a one shot after approach. It allows one to measure change objectively but makes it difficult to attribute the change to the program being evaluated. Modifying the one group pre-test/post-test to include the possibility for a longitudinal approach in which data is collected at a variety of points during and after the program does, even with all its weaknesses, provide for ongoing and continuous evaluation studies. With a longitudinal case study, the evaluator can check on the progress of the program toward its objectives and, at the same time, use earlier measures as a form of self control and basis for comparisons later. Such an approach seems particularly appropriate when dealing with a longer term developmental curriculum such as the Second Step rather than a short term discreet educational program such as driver training. It provides for a great deal of feedback into the program and contributes potentially useful data for decision making.

THE SOCIAL PSYCHOLOGY OF CURRICULUM EVALUATION: SOME PRACTICAL APPROACHES

A prominent theme in this chapter is that evaluation research, because it takes place in a real social world and because of its connection with value judgments, is more than a mere methodological enterprise. It is a social-psychological process in its own right. Additionally, as an appendage to an ongoing curriculum focused on educating students, an evaluation study has to adapt itself to the program environment and disrupt it as little as possible. Certainly the complexity of social psychology associated with evaluation research has been suggested in my discussions of covert purposes for evaluation research and variables used to make decisions about who should do the evaluating.

Obviously, some interference will take place. For one thing, data have to be collected. Frequently, however, evaluators ask for more information than they will use. A clear focus for the study enables evaluators to lower their demands for data, thus lessening their intrusiveness.

The evaluator works on the turf of another profession. Differences in the roles of evaluator and faculty member can be sources of friction between them. Basically, a teacher has to believe in what she or he is doing and the researcher has to question it. The difference in perspective can create tension. There are several characteristics of evaluation research that can cause conflict.

Data Collection

The request that the researcher have access to people's time for filling out questionnaires or participating in interviews often is viewed as taking time away from the tasks at hand.

Status Rivalry

Teaching faculty on occasion resents what they perceive as the preferential status and schedule of a researcher. They slave away and do the day-to-day heavily scheduled work of teaching the curriculum while the evaluator is granted a schedule suited to contemplation and writing which often yields rewards through publication and professional recognition. At times, the researcher may even be charged with milking the program for opportunities to further his or her own career.

There is an imposing catalog of conflict sources but with good communication and careful planning the two can work together more comfortably. Several conditions seem to contribute to this happy arrangement.

Support from Administrators

A department chairperson or dean who is committed to an evaluation study and its eventual use in decision making is essential to getting and maintaining cooperation from the faculty. He or she can provide incentives, recognition, and rewards for faculty who help rather than hinder the evaluation project as well as see to it that the researcher has adequate resources for the study.

Involvement of Faculty in the Evaluation

Involving the faculty in the evaluation study has further payoffs. A clear benefit is that they gain understanding of what evaluation research is all about and get a sense of how they can make use of the findings. A second benefit is that they have information and ideas to contribute. The contributions of the faculty often enrich the evaluator's understanding of his or her study and enable him or her to make the study more relevant to the program's needs. In the Second Step Program we have attempted to bring the evaluation research into the mainstream of program operations in a number of ways.

We have created opportunities to feedback useful information to the faculty at regular intervals. When the faculty confronted

242

dilemmas about identifying criteria for admission of students, the research staff was able to offer characteristics which correlated with academic success in the program and those which did not. When the faculty struggled with questions concerning curriculum revision, the evaluators synthesized students' testimonials regarding their experiences in the program and their points of critique. This kind of practical information feedback can work to gain faculty's support and cooperation with the evaluation endeavor even though it may seem bothersome and esoteric at times. We have also sought to integrate the process of research into the curriculum itself by offering an introductory course in research and providing an opportunity for senior students to develop senior preceptorships in nursing research under the guidance of the research staff. This strategy involved bringing the curriculum evaluator's expertise in the research process to bear on actual implementation of the curriculum, thus bridging some of the barriers between the emphasis of faculty and that of research staff.

SUMMARY AND CONCLUDING VIEWS

Evaluation research is a basic ingredient of scientific program management. To the extent that operational programs such as curriculums are closely linked to the attainment of some desired objective rather than to the perpetuation of their own existence, they will make constant use of evaluation studies. The list of possible functions that evaluation studies may perform for programs is substantial and varied.

Suchman adds to this list of legitimate purposes an equally impressive list of the ways in which evaluation studies can serve covert functions.[32] The curriculum evaluator is faced with assessing the purpose the study is to serve and designing strategies accordingly. Although, like all research, choices of methodology must rest upon the logic of scientific inquiry, evaluation research is a social-psychological enterprise wherein the evaluator must find the best possible compromise between the demands of science and the conditions of the action setting. Sensitivity to this unique property of research in the action setting and imagination and ingenuity in the innovation of models of research suited to it may prove an even greater challenge to the evaluator than employing the methodological skills necessary to conduct an evaluation study itself. With all its limitations, evaluation research still has the potential for bringing greater rationality to curriculum decision making.

Open curriculum models have been characterized as resulting from pressures on nursing education to change. However, such pressures to change also confront resistance to change. Evaluation research has the potential for resolving these conflicting pressures. It provides data as to what is taking place and information on which judgment to make as to the effectiveness of a new approach. As Hecht has pointed out:

Open curriculum is not an isolated movement within nursing education and practice, but raises basic questions and issues concerning the effectiveness of the current system. Evaluation planning should be no less comprehensive if these questions are to be answered, if the pressures to change are to be meaningfully balanced to the betterment of the nursing profession.[33]

The ultimate purpose of evaluation research is, after all, not so much to *prove*, but to *improve*.

REFERENCES

1. Weiss, Carol: *Evaluation Research.* Prentice-Hall, Inc., Englewood Cliffs, N.J., 1972, p. 1.
2. Waters, Verle, et al. Technical and Professional Nursing: An Exploratory Study. *Nursing Research* 21:124, 1972.
3. Stake, Robert E.: Toward a Technology for the Evaluation of Educational Programs. *AERA Monograph Series on Curriculum Evaluation No. 1.* Tyler, Ralph W., Gagne, Robert M., and Scriven, Michael (eds.). Rand McNalley and Co., Chicago, 1967, p. 5.
4. Suchman, Edward A.: *Evaluation Research.* Russel Sage Foundation, New York, 1967, p. 20.
5. Weiss, *op. cit.*, p. 2.
6. *Ibid.*, pp. 6-8.
7. Williams, Frank C. and Williams, Carolyn A.: Values and Evaluative Research in Health Care: A Conceptual Analysis, in Leininger, Madeline (ed.): *Health Care Dimensions.* F.A. Davis Co., Philadelphia, 1974, pp. 61-77.
8. Weiss, *op. cit.*, p. 30.
9. *Ibid.*, pp. 16-17.
10. Herzog, Elizabeth: *Some Guidelines for Evaluative Research.* U.S. Department of Health, Education, and Welfare, Social Security Administration, Children's Bureau, Washington, 1959, p. 2.
11. Sawin, E.I.: *Evaluation and the Work of the Teacher.* Wadsworth Publishing Co., Belmont, California, 1969, p. 37.
12. Trow, Martin: Methodological Problems in the Evaluation of Innovation, in Wittrock, M.C. and Wiley, D.E. (eds.): *The Evaluation of Instruction.* Holt, Rhinehart and Winston Inc., New York, 1970, p. 297.
13. *Ibid.*, p. 298.
14. Stufflebeam, D.S.: Evaluation as Enlightenment for Decision Making. Reprinted in *Improving Educational Assessment,* ASCO, NEA, Washington, D.C., 1969.
15. Provos, M.: *Discrepancy Evaluation.* McCutchan Publishing Company, Berkeley, Calif., 1971.
16. Tripodi, T., Tellin, P., and Epstein, I.: *Social Program Evaluation: Guidelines for Health, Education, and Welfare Administrators.* Peacock Publishers, Itasca, Illinois, 1971.
17. Scriven, Michael: The Methodology of Evaluation in Tyler, Ralph W., Gagne, Robert M., and Scriven, Michael (eds.): *Perspectives of Curriculum Evaluation.* AERA Monograph Series on Curriculum Evaluation No. 1. Rand McNalley and Co., Chicago, 1967, p. 5.

18. Freeman, H.E., and Sherwood, C.C.: Research in Large-Scale Intervention Programs. *Journal of Social Issues* 21:11, 1965.
19. Mann, John: "The Outcome of Evaluative Research," *in Changing Human Behavior.* Charles Scribners Sons, New York, 1965, pp. 191-214.
20. Weiss, Robert S. and Rein, Martin: The Evaluating of Broad-Aim Programs: A Cautionary Case and a Morel. *Annals of the American Academy of Political and Social Science* 385:118, 1969.
21. Suchman, Edward A.: Action for What? A Critique of Evaluative Research, in O'Toole, Richard: *The Organization, Management, and Tactics of Social Research.* Schenkman Publishing Co., Cambridge, Mass., 1970.
22. Weiss, *op. cit.*, pp. 20-21.
23. Suchman, *Evaluative Research*, p. 34.
24. *Ibid.*, pp. 39-41.
25. Herzog, *op. cit.*, pp. 79-80.
26. Weiss, *op. cit.*, p. 32.
27. Suchman, *Evaluative Research*, pp. 61-67.
28. *Ibid.*, p. 67.
29. See for example, Oscar Buros: *Mental Measurements Yearbook*, ed. 6. Gryphon Press, Highland Park, N.J., 1965; and ____: *Personality Tests and Reviews.* Gryphon Press, Highland Park, N.J., 1970.
30. Cronbach, Lee J.: "Evaluation for Course Improvement." *Teachers College Record* 64:672, 1963.
31. Weiss, *op. cit.*, p. 45.
32. Suchman, Edward A.: Action for What? A Critique of Evaluative Research. *The Organization, Management, and Tactics of Social Research, op. cit.*
33. Hecht, Kathryn A.: A Framework for Evaluation: Philosophy, Basic Principles and Viewpoints. Paper presented at the Open Curriculum Project Conference on Evaluation, Nov. 7-8, 1974, New York. Sponsored by the National League for Nursing, p. 19.

SELECTED BIBLIOGRAPHY

Abramson, D.A.: Curriculum Research and Evaluation. *Review of Educational Research* 36:388, 1966.
Agency for International Development: *Evaluation Handbook.* Government Printing Office, Washington, D.C., 1971.
Alken, Marvin C.: Evaluation Theory Development. *Evaluation Comment* 2:2, 1969.
American Association for the Advancement of Science, Commission on Science Education: *An Evaluation Model and its Application.* Washington, D.C., 1965.
American Institutes for Research: *Evaluative Research Strategies/Methods.* American Institutes for Research, Pittsburgh, 1970.
Aronson, Sidney H., and Sherwood, Clarence C.: "Researcher Versus Practitioner: Problems in Social Action Research." *Social Work* 12:89, 1967.
Asten, A.W.: Criterion-centered Research. *Educational and Psychological Measurement* 24:807, 1964.
Baker, Robert L.: Curriculum Evaluation. *Review of Educational Research* 39:339, 1969.
Barton, Allen N.: *Studying the Effects of a College Education.* Edward H. Hazer Foundation, New Haven, 1959.
Bateman, Worth: Assessing Program Effectiveness: A Rating System for Identifying Relative Program Success. *Welfare in Review* 6:1, 1968.
Benedict, Barbara A., et al: The Clinical-Experimental Approach to Assessing Organizational Change Efforts. *Journal of Applied Behavioral Science* 3:347, 1967.

Bloom, B.S.: Learning for Mastery. *Evaluation Comment* 1:1, 1968.

Brunner, Edmund: Evaluation Research in Adult Education. *International Review of Community Development* 17-18:97, 1967.

Buros, O.K. (ed.): *The Sixth Mental Measurements Yearbook.* The Gryphon Press, Highland Park, New Jersey, 1965.

Buros, O.K. (ed.): *Tests in Print.* The Gryphon Press, Highland Park, New Jersey, 1961.

Caldwell, N.S.: An Approach to the Assessment of Educational Planning. *Educational Technology* 8:5, 1968.

Campbell, Donald T.: Considering the Case Against Experimental Evaluations of Social Innovations. *Administrative Science Quarterly* 15:110, 1970.

Caro, F.G.: Approaches to Evaluation Research—A Review. *Human Organization* 28:87, 1969.

Caro, F.G. (ed.): *Readings in Evaluation Research.* Russell Sage Foundation, New York, 1971.

Cherney, Paul R. (ed.): *Making Evaluation Research Useful.* American City Corporation, Columbia, Md., 1971.

Crenbach, Lee J., and Suppes, P.: *Research for Tomorrow's Schools: Disciplined Inquiry for Education.* Macmillan, New York, 1969.

Daily, Edwin F., and Morehead, Mildred A.: A Method of Evaluating and Improving the Quality of Medical Care. *American Journal of Public Health* 46:848, 1956.

Davis, James A.: Great Books and Small Groups: An Informal History of a National Survey, in Hammond, P.E. (ed.): *Sociologists at Work.* Basic Books, New York, 1964, pp. 212-234.

Educational Evaluation: *New Roles, New Means, 68th Yearbook of the National Society for the Study of Education,* ed. Ralph W. Tyler. National Society for Study of Education, Chicago, 1969.

Evaluation Educational Programs: A Symposium. *Urban Review* 3:568, 1969.

Flech, Andrew C.: Evaluation as a Logical Process. *Canadian Journal of Public Health* 52:185, 1961.

Glass, Gene: *The Growth of Evaluation Methodology,* AERA Monograph Series on Curriculum Evaluation, No. 7. Rand McNally Corp., Chicago, 1973.

Hastings, J. Thomas: Curriculum Evaluation: the Why of the Outcomes. *Journal of Educational Measurement* 3:27, 1966.

Herzog, Elizabeth: *Some Guidelines for Evaluative Research.* U.S. Department of HEW, Washington, 1959.

Heyman, H.H., and Wright, Charles R.: Evaluating Social Action Programs, in Lazarsfeld, Paul F., et al. (eds.): *The Uses of Sociology.* Basic Books, New York, 1967, pp. 741-782.

Hecht, K.A.: *Evaluating Open Curriculum Programs on Nursing: A Planning Discussion.* Presented at the Education Conference, Council of State Boards of Nursing, San Francisco, June 1974.

Klineberg, Otto: The Problem of Evaluation Research. *International Social Science Bulletin,* 7:346, 1955.

Lindvall, C.M., and Cox, Richard C.: *Evaluation as a Tool in Curriculum Development: The IPI Evaluation Program.* AERA Phonograph Series on Curriculum Evaluation, No. 5, Rand McNally Corporation, Chicago, 1970.

Provus, Malcolm: Evaluation of Ongoing Programs in the Public School System, in Tyler, Ralph W. (ed.): *Educational Evaluation: New Roles, New Means,* 68th Yearbook of the National Society for the Study of Education. National Society for Study of Education, Chicago, 1969, pp. 242-283.

Provus, Malcolm: *Discrepancy Evaluation.* McCutchen, Berkeley, 1971.

Rippey, R. (ed.): *Studies in Transactional Evaluation.* McCutchen, Berkeley, 1971.

Scriven, M.: "Goal-free Evaluation," in House, E.R. (ed.): *School Evaluation.* McCutchen, Berkeley, 1973.

Stake, Robert E.: The Countenance of Educational Evaluation. *Teachers College Record* 68:523, 1967.

Scriven, Michael: The Methodology of Evaluation: Perspectives of Curriculum Evaluation, Ralph Tyler et al. (eds.). AERA Monograph Series on Curriculum Evaluation, No. 1, Rand McNally Corporation, Chicago, 1967, pp. 39-83.

Stufflebeam, D.L.: Toward a Science of Educational Evaluation. *Educational Technology* 8:5, 1968.

Stufflebeam, D.L., et al. (ed.): *Educational Evaluation and Decision Making.* Peacock Publishing, Itasca, Ill. 1971.

Suchman, Edward A.: *Evaluation Research: Principles and Practice in Public Service and Social Action Programs.* Russell Sage Foundation, New York, 1967.

Tyler, Ralph W.: Assessing the Progress of Education. *Science Education* 6:239, 1966.

Walberg, H.J. (ed.): *Evaluating Ed. Performance: A Sourcebook of Methods, Instruments, Examples.* McCutchen, Berkeley, 1974.

Weiss, Carol H.: *Evaluation Research.* Prentice-Hall, Englewood Cliffs, New Jersey, 1972.

Worthen, Blaine R., and Sanders, James R.: *Educational Evaluation: Theory in Practice.* Charles A. Jones Publishing Co., Worthington, Ohio: 1973.

Index

ACHIEVEMENT test results for
students, 216-217
Active learning, 36-37
strategies for, 37-56
Administrators, evaluation and, 242
Admission(s)
conceptual framework for, 64-69
criteria and procedures of, 60-61
evaluation data for, 65-80
rationale for, 61-64
entry data on students and, 69-76
exit data on students and, 76-78
institutional requirements for,
66-67, 76
issues and problems of, 59-60
prerequisite nursing requirements
for, 66, 75-76
program characteristics and, 67-69,
78-80
Adult learning
planning for, 34-37
strategies for, 37-56
theory of, 23-28
Advisor in preceptorship study,
88-89, 93-94
Age of students, 21, 70
Andragogy, 23, 34-35
Articulation
direct, 62-64
issues and problems of, 59-80

BIOGRAPHICAL data on students,
65-66
use of, 69

CALIFORNIA system of higher
education, 14-15
Career areas of students, 74-75
Career mobility
admission policy and, 59-60
curriculum and, 2-3

Cattell Culture Fair Intelligence
Test, 212-214
Change process in learning, 49-51
Children of students, number of, 72
Cognitive structures, alteration of,
27-28
Colleague relationships of nurse
practitioner, 128-134
Community health nursing, student
experience of, 194
Conceptual framework for program,
12-31
Cross-cultural learning model, 154-160
application to nursing of, 160-164
Curriculum
conceptual framework for, 11-31
design of, 33-34
setting in, 14-21
students and learning theory in,
21-28
subject in, 29-31
for family nurse practitioner, 109-120
individualization of, 57
liberal arts in, 5
liberation of, from stereotypes of
ethnicity and femininity,
141-166
open, 164-166
pressures for, 1-9
organization of, strategies for, 37-56
planning of, faculty group processes
and, 171-172
preceptorship study in, 82-85,
90-91, 101-103
student influence on, 2-3
Curriculum decisions, developing a
conceptual framework for,
11-31
Curriculum evaluation research, 223-224
design and methodology of, 228-230,
233-235, 239-241

Curriculum evaluation research—*Cont.*
  evaluators in, 232-233
  identifying program goals in, 235-
    237, 238-239
  measurements in, 237-239
  program changes and, 231-232
  project in. *See* Curriculum evaluation
    research project.
  purposes of, 226-228
  scope of, 224-226
  social psychology of, 241-243
  timing of, 230-232
Curriculum evaluation research project,
    206. *See also* Curriculum
    evaluation research.
  comparative study in, 210
  data collection in
    instruments for, 212-214
    methods of, 211-212
  design of, 207-210
  findings and utilization of, 214-220
  focus of, 208-210
  initial planning of, 206-207
  practical aspects of, 210-211
  residual issues and strategies for
    future in, 220-221

DATA collection in curriculum evalua-
    tion project, 211-214
Direct articulation, 62-64
Discovery teaching, 51-53

EDUCATION in redefinition of sex
    roles, 146-147
Educational background of students, 22
Entry data on students, 65-67
  use of 69-76
Ethnic background of students, 21, 71
Ethnicity stereotypes of, liberating
    the curriculum from, 141-166
Evaluation
  design and methodology of, 228-230
  evaluators in, 232-233
  formative and summative, 230-231
  program changes and, 231-232
  purposes of, 226-228
  scope of, 224-226
  social psychology of, 241-243
  timing of, 230-232
Evaluation project. *See* Curriculum
    evaluation research project.
Evaluation research, 225-226
Evaluators, 232-233
Exit data on students, 67
  use of, 76-78
Experience
  alienation from, 166

learning and, 25
Experimental design in curriculum
    evaluation research, 239-240
Expository teaching, 54-55

FACULTY
  evaluation and, 242-243
  for nurse practitioner education
    joint appointments of, 135-138
    preparation of, 134-135
  group and interpersonal processes of,
    170-185
Faculty-student relationship, 56,
    196-198
  learning and, 24
Family nurse practitioner. *See* Nurse
    practitioner.
Femininity, stereotype of, liberating
    the curriculum from, 141-166
Financial support of students, 22,
    72-73
Formative evaluation, 230-231

GROUP and interpersonal processes of
    faculty, 170-185

HEALTH care needs, curriculum
    design and, 18-19
Health care delivery system, curriculum
    design and, 19-21
Health professions, access to, 150-151
History of baccalaureate education for
    RNs, 3-9

INSTITUTION, educational, curric-
    ulum design and, 14-17
Integrative threads in curriculum
    organization, 38-45
Interaction and change course, student
    experience of, 195-196
Interpersonal and group processes of
    faculty, 170-185

LEARNING
  by discovery, 51-53
  cross-cultural model for, 154-160
    application to nursing of, 160-164
  in culturally diverse situations, 151-
    160
  strategies for organization of, 33-57
  through preceptorship study, 82-103
  variations of modes of, 55-56
Learning principles in Second Step
    Program, 28
Learning readiness, 26
Learning theory in curriculum design,
    21, 23-28

MARITAL status of students, 23, 71-72
Modes of learning, variation of, 55-56

NONEXPERIMENTAL design in curriculum evaluation research, 240-241
Nurse practitioner, 84-85, 105-106
  baccalaureate preparation of, 105-134, 139
  curriculum development for, 109-120
  faculty joint appointments for, 135-138
  faculty preparation for, 134-135
  characteristics of, 112-116
  process of role change for, 120-122
  evaluation study of, 122-128
  relationship to other nurses of, 128-130
  relationship to physicians of, 128, 130-134
Nursing
  access to profession of, 150-151
  conceptualization of, 29-31
  sexual and cultural diversity within, 164-166
  student's emerging view of, 200-202

OBJECTIVES of program, 235-237, 238-239
Omnibus Personality Inventory, 212-213, 218-220
Open curriculum, 164-166
  pressures for, 1-9
Oral interview in curriculum evaluation project, 214, 217-218

PERSONALITY inventory results for students, 218-220
Powerlessness, sex discrimination and, 144-147
Preceptor, 86-97, 93-94
  for family nurse practitioner preceptorship, 119-120
Preceptorship study
  advisor in, 88-89, 93-94
  background and rationale of, 82-85
  characteristics of, 85-86
  evaluation of, 99-101
  for family nurse practitioner, 107-109
  curriculum content of, 116-120
  objectives of, 89
  preceptor in, 86-87, 93-94
  recommendations for planning of, 101-103
  seminar in, 98

student in, 90, 198-200
  student contract in, 91-98
  total curriculum and, 90-91
Prerequisite requirements, 66-67, 75-76
Problem-solving approach, 27
Process as content, 36-37
  in curriculum design, 47-51
Professional nurse, 82-85, 150-151
  definition of, 29-31
Program characteristics, admission policy and, 67-69, 78-80

QUASI-EXPERIMENTAL design in curriculum evaluation research, 240

RACE of students, 71
Reality shock, 203-204
Residence of students, 21-22
Returning to school, 188-189
  reasons for, 23
Role change(s)
  education and, 146-147
  for nurse practitioner, 120-122
  evaluation study of, 122-128
Role of women, redefinition of, 146-147

SELECTION of students, 63-64. See also Admission.
  for nurse practitioner preceptorship, 112
Self-diagnosis of learning needs, 24-25
Self-directed study, 53-54
Sequence and continuity in curriculum organization, 45-47
Service area of CSCS, 17-18
Setting
  characteristics of, 15-17
  curriculum design and, 14-21
Sex of students, 22, 70-71
Sociocultural milieu, curriculum design and, 17-18
Stereotypes of ethnicity and femininity, liberating the curriculum from, 141-166
Strategies for organizing learning, 33-57
Student(s)
  achievement test results for, 216-217
  biographical data on, 65-66
    use of, 69
  career areas of, 74-75
  characteristics of
    curriculum design and, 21-23
    in nurse practitioner program, 112-116

Student(s)—*Continued*
  cognitive knowledge about nursing
    of, 208
  competencies in practice of nursing
    of, 209-210
  educational background of, 75-76
  entry data on, 65-67, 69-76
  exit data on, 67, 76-78
  experience of, 187-189, 192-193
    in community health nursing, 194
    in interaction and change course,
      195-196
  in preceptorship study, 198-200
  in preceptorship study, 90
  influence on program of, 202-203
  initial responses of, 189-191
  personal and professional orienta-
    tions of, 208-209
  personality inventory results for,
    218-220
  relationship to program philosophy
    of, 191-192
  selection of, 63-64. *See also* Admis-
    sion.
    for nurse practitioner preceptor-
      ship, 112
  view of nursing of, 200-202
  view of program of, 187-199, 203-
    205
  work experience of, 203-205
  years away from school of, 73

  years of nursing practice of, 73-74
Student control of learning, 37
Student-faculty relationship, 56,
    196-198
  learning and, 24
Study contract in preceptorship study
  components of, 91-96
  examples of, 96-98
Subject, curriculum design and, 29-31
Success indicator criteria data on
    students, 77-78
Summative evaluation, 230-231
Systems model as conceptual frame-
    work for admissions, 64-65

TEACHER
  as cultural agent, 147-150
  role of, 26
Teaching
  by discovery, 51-53
  by self-directed study, 53-54
  cross-cultural model for, 154-160
    application to nursing of, 160-164
  expository, 54-55
  in culturally diverse situations,
    151-160
  strategies for, 37-56
Transfer of knowledge in culturally
    diverse situations, 151-160

WORK experience of students, 22

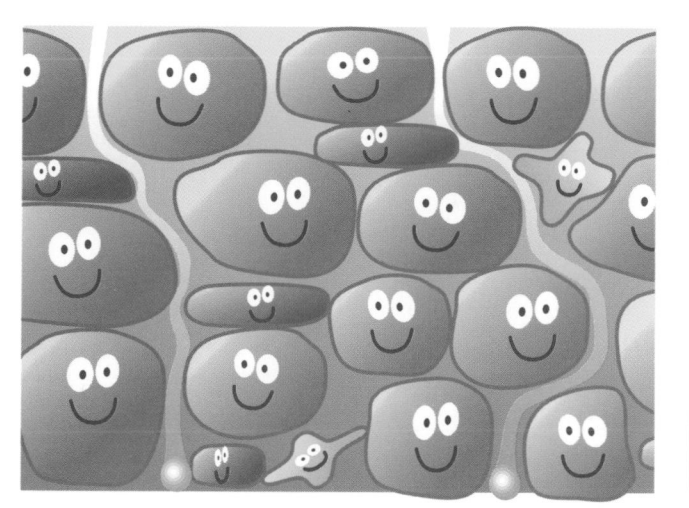

Les sols

Activités scientifiques et technologiques
Cahier de l'élève

Auteurs
Saryl Jacobson, Robbie Olivero, Judy Onody

Comité de rédaction
Peter Williams, Ray Bowers, Denis Cooke

Illustrations
Pottery Chan

Direction éditoriale
Claude Tatilon

Traduction
Claude Tatilon, Manuela Tatilon

Révision du texte
Nadia Medawar

GTK Press

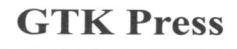

Toronto

GTK Press
18, promenade Wynford, bureau 109
Don Mills, ON, Canada M3C 3S2
Téléphone   : (416) 385-1313
Télécopie   : (416) 385-1319
Courriel   : star@gtkpress.com
Site web   : www.gtkpress.com

Comité de rédaction
Peter Williams
Ray Bowers
Denis Cooke

Auteurs
Saryl Jacobson
Robbie Olivero
Judy Onody

Maquette de la couverture et illustrations
Pottery Chan

Direction éditoriale
Claude Tatilon

Traduction
Claude Tatilon
Manuela Tatilon

Révision du texte
Nadia Medawar

Remerciements
Photographies et images utilisées avec autorisation. PhotoDisc : formation des roches, orignal en hiver (p. 2) ; une poignée de terre (p. 6) ; champ de colza (canola), champ de maïs (p. 9) ; champs (p. 14) ; flanc de montagne, forêt coupée à blanc (p. 17) ; orignal, canards, pollution (p. 18) ; tournesols, carottes (p. 25) ; enfant en train de balayer (p. 34) ; verrerie (p. 41). Corel Photos : lacs, collines (p. 2) ; érosion (p. 18). Denis Cooke : racine pivotante, racine fibreuse (p. 25). Broderbund : façonnage d'une poterie (p. 41). Corel Clipart Images : images prédessinées.

Kids Can Press Ltd : « Au pays des racines », d'après « Under The Ground » de Rhonda W. Bacmeister, extrait de *Poems For All Seasons* (David Booth, copyright © 1990).
Farrar, Straus and Giroux : « Les vers de terre », d'après « Earthworms » de Valerie Worth, extrait de *More Small poems* (copyright © 1976).

Données de catalogage avant publication (Canada)
Jacobson, Saryl
    Les sols. Cahier de l'élève

(Activités scientifiques et technologiques ; 35)
Traduction de *Soils. Science & technology*
    student journal.
Pour les élèves de la 3ᵉ année de l'élémentaire.
ISBN 1-55317-035-0

    1. Sols — Ouvrages pour la jeunesse. I. Olivero, Robbie
II. Onody, Judy III. Williams, Peter IV. Bowers, Ray
V. Cooke, Denis VI. Titre. VII. Collection.

S591.3.J3214 2001   578.75'7   C2001-900282-3

Imprimé et relié au Canada. Contient du papier recyclé.

Table des matières

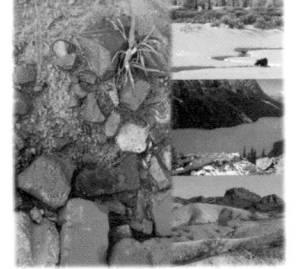

Travaux pratiques **1**

Ce que cache le sol
p. 2

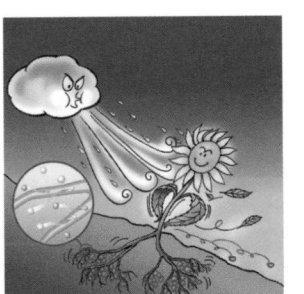

Travaux pratiques **6**

Différentes façons de prendre racine
p. 22

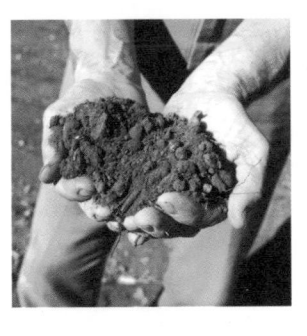

Travaux pratiques **2**

Un bon terrain
p. 6

Travaux pratiques **7**

Une vie souterraine grouillante
p. 26

Travaux pratiques **3**

Une matière absorbante
p. 10

Travaux pratiques **8**

Un nettoyage naturel
p. 30

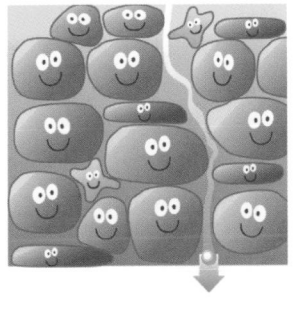

Travaux pratiques **4**

L'action de l'eau
p. 14

Travaux pratiques **9**

La fabrication d'un composteur domestique
p. 34

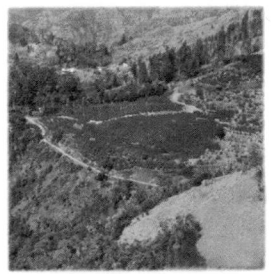
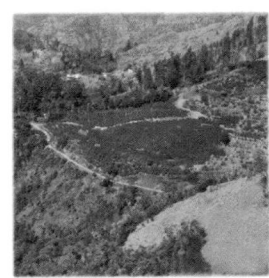

Travaux pratiques **5**

Le filtrage
p. 18

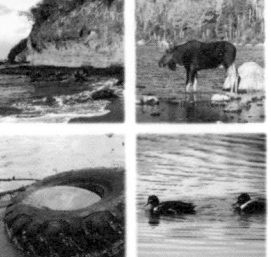

Travaux pratiques **10**

Des matériaux très utiles
p. 38

Tu es super !! 42

Le sol est formé par :

☆ l'éclatement des roches sous l'action de la pluie et du gel,

☆ les débris des êtres vivants (des plantes et des animaux) qui vivent et meurent dans les roches désagrégées.

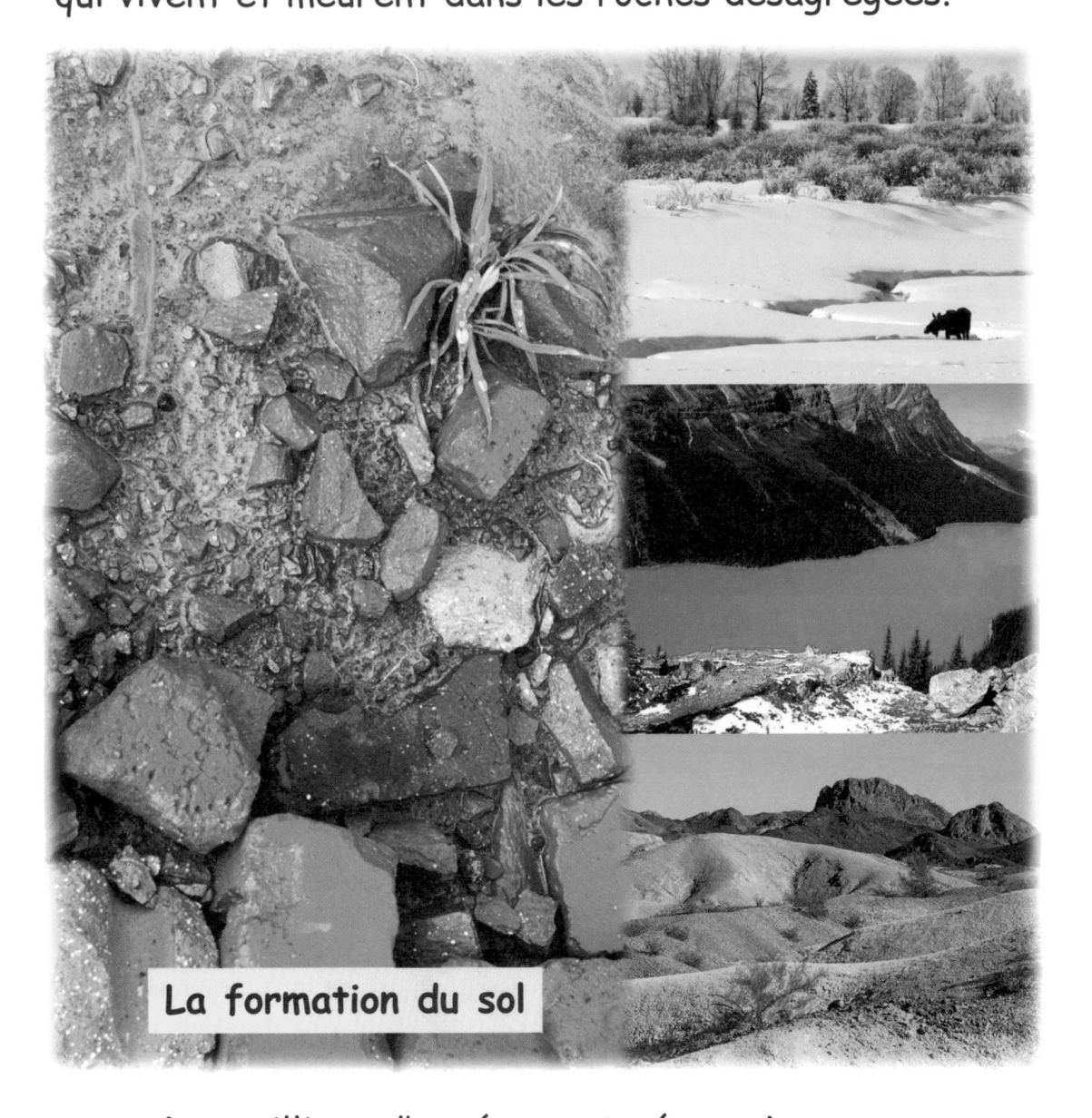

La formation du sol

Des millions d'années sont nécessaires pour la formation d'une petite quantité de sol.

Échantillons de sol

Dessine les êtres vivants que tu as trouvés dans l'échantillon de sol.

Dessine et décris les différentes parties trouvées dans l'échantillon de sol.

De toutes les couleurs

Dessine le contenu de chaque bocal après l'avoir laissé déposer toute la nuit. Colorie chaque couche.

Sol de surface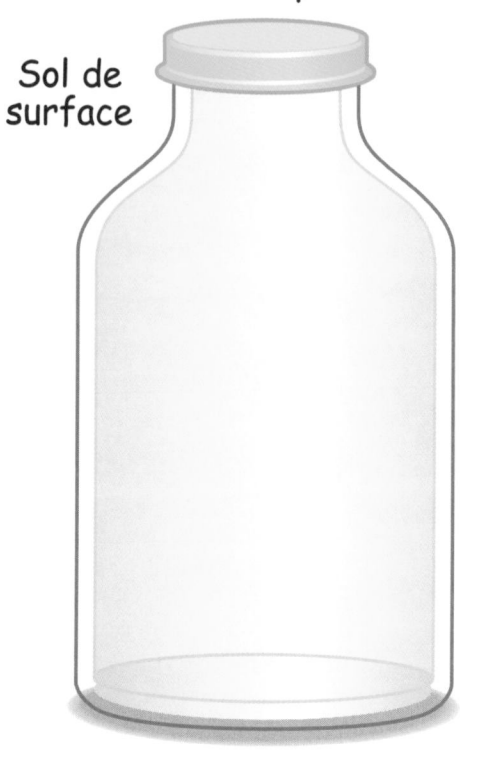

Sol plus profond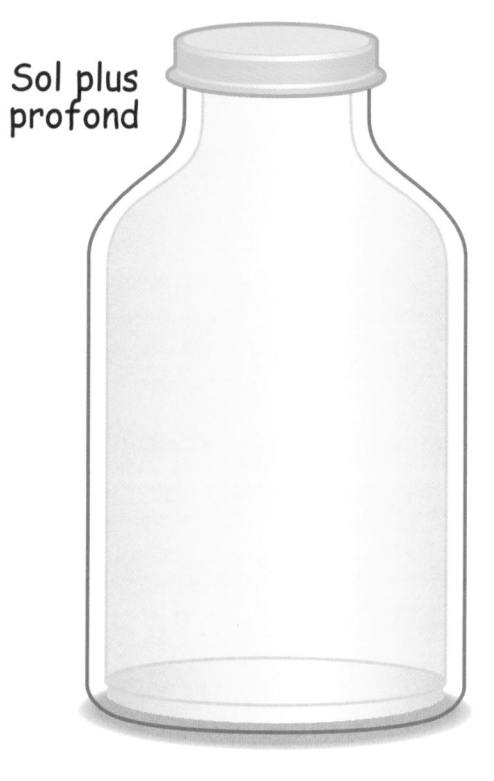

Couche sur couche

1. Nous avons trouvé _____ flottant sur l'eau.

2. Au-dessus du sol, l'eau était _____.

3. Complète le tableau pour chaque couche que tu as examinée :

couches	couleur	taille des particules	texture
première (en haut)			
deuxième			
troisième			

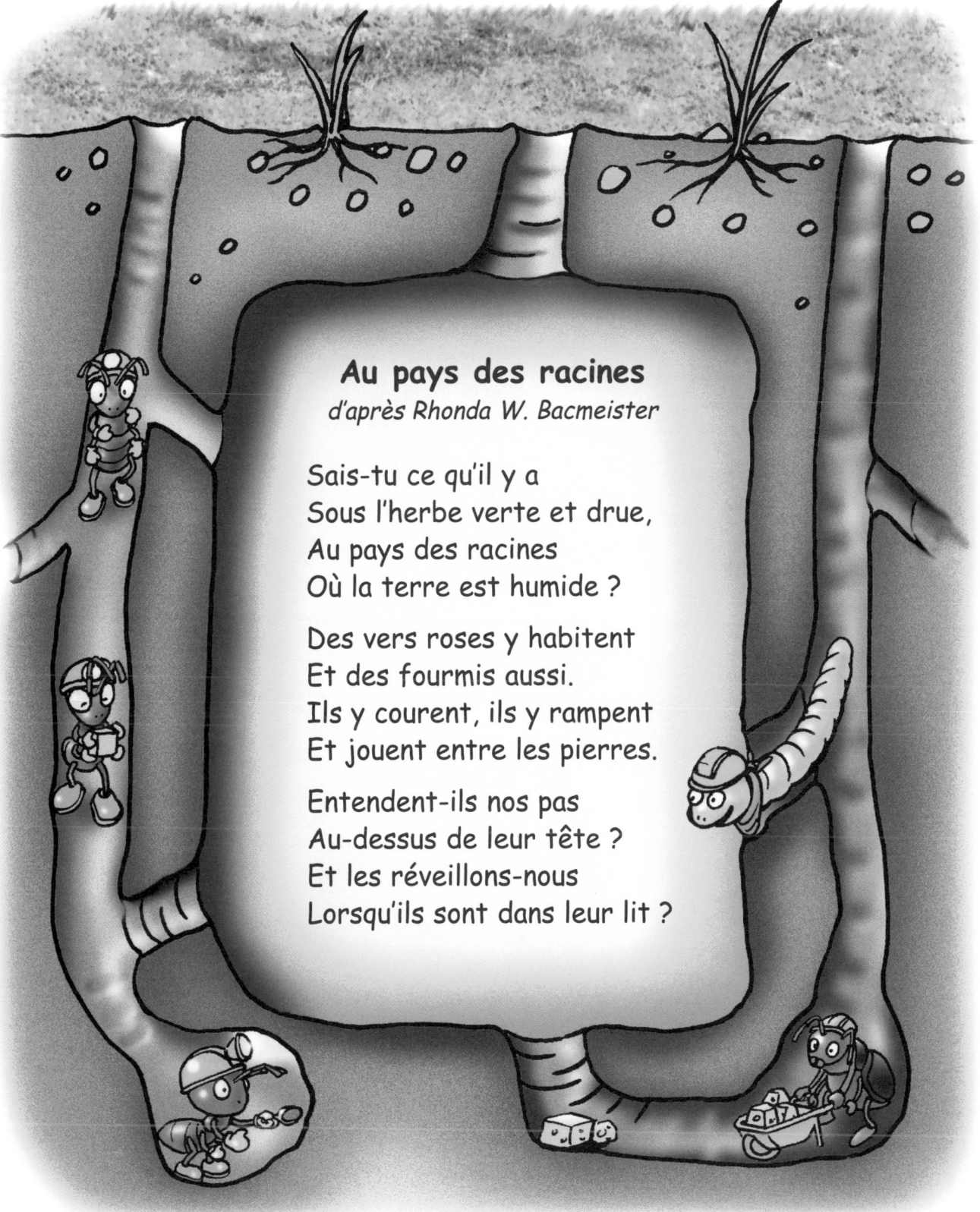

Au pays des racines
d'après Rhonda W. Bacmeister

Sais-tu ce qu'il y a
Sous l'herbe verte et drue,
Au pays des racines
Où la terre est humide ?

Des vers roses y habitent
Et des fourmis aussi.
Ils y courent, ils y rampent
Et jouent entre les pierres.

Entendent-ils nos pas
Au-dessus de leur tête ?
Et les réveillons-nous
Lorsqu'ils sont dans leur lit ?

2 Un bon terrain

Il y a de nombreux types de sols.
Les sols sont faits en partie de particules de roche.

Le type de sol dépend de la taille de ces particules.

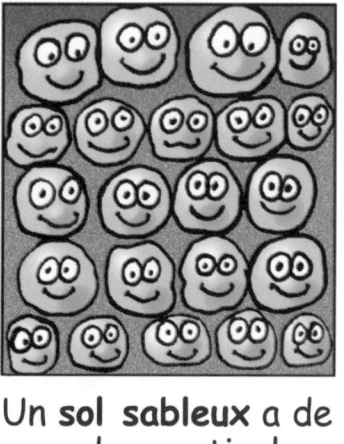

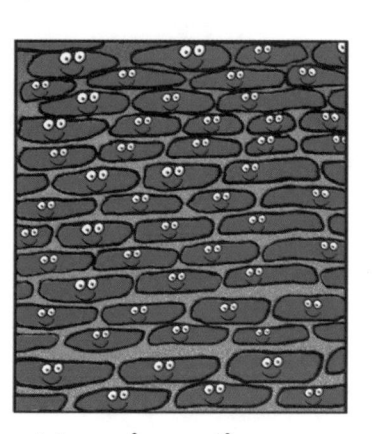

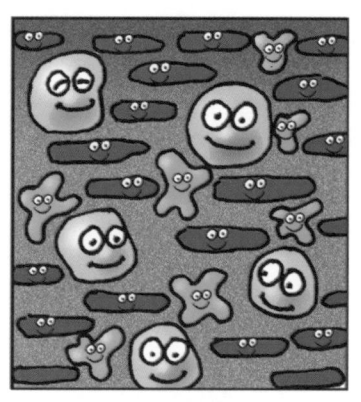

Un **sol sableux** a de grandes particules.

Un **sol argileux** a de petites particules.

Un **sol limoneux** est un mélange de sable, d'humus et d'argile.

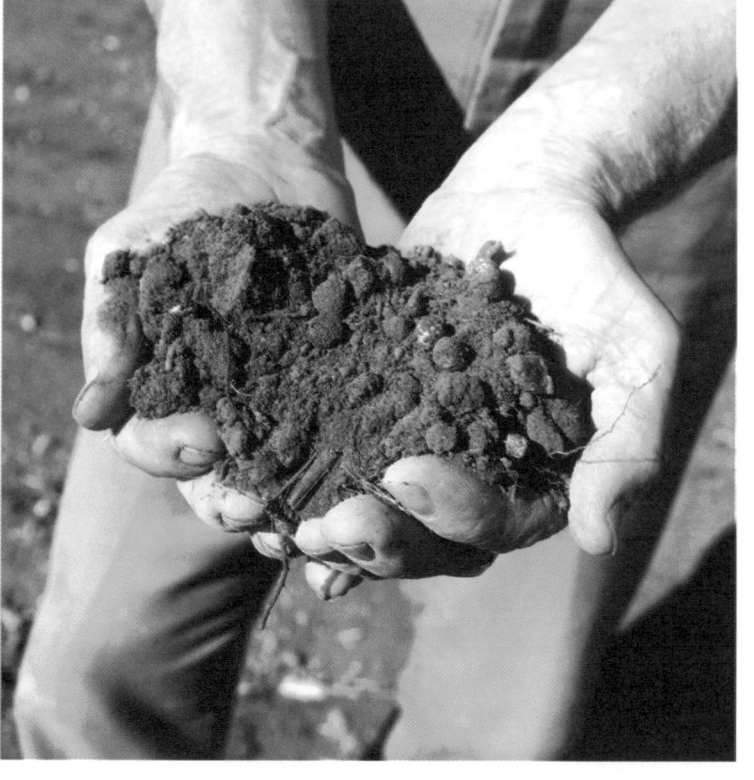

La plupart des sols contiennent de la **matière organique**, qui provient de la décomposition de débris végétaux et animaux. Parfois, la matière organique est appelée **humus**. Le **limon** est le sol qui convient le mieux à la plupart des plantes.

Compare la taille des particules.

Dessine les particules que tu as trouvées dans chaque type de sol.

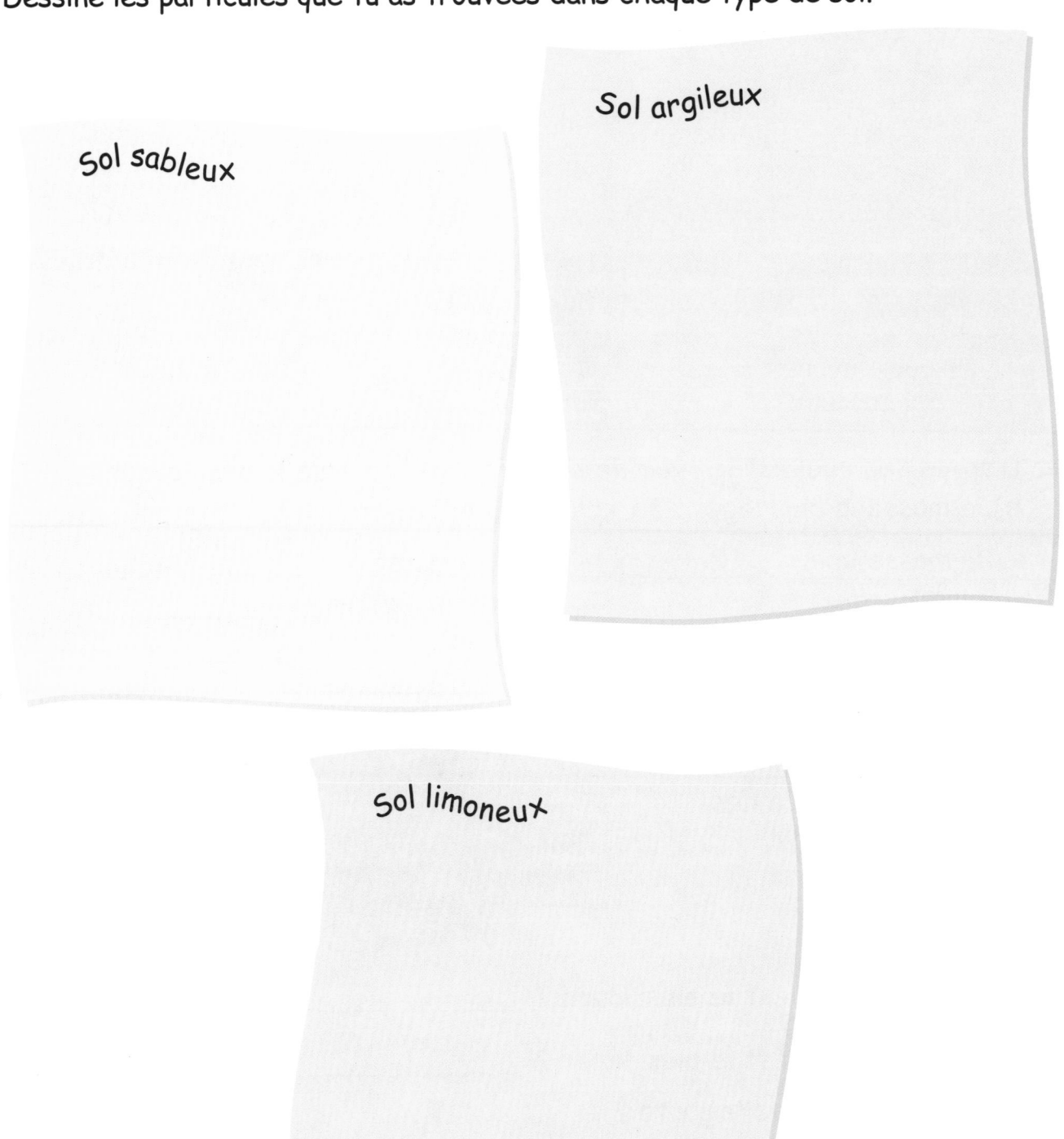

Sol sableux

Sol argileux

Sol limoneux

C'est du solide !

1. Mesure la même quantité de chacun des trois types de sol et mets-les dans des verres en plastique. Dessine le sol qui se trouve dans chaque verre.

| Sol sableux | Sol argileux | Sol limoneux |

2. D'après toi, quel est le type de sol qui a : a) la masse la plus lourde ; b) la masse la plus légère ? Explique ta prévision :

la masse la
plus lourde _____

la masse la
plus légère _____

_____

3. Utilise une balance à deux plateaux pour comparer la masse des échantillons de sol.

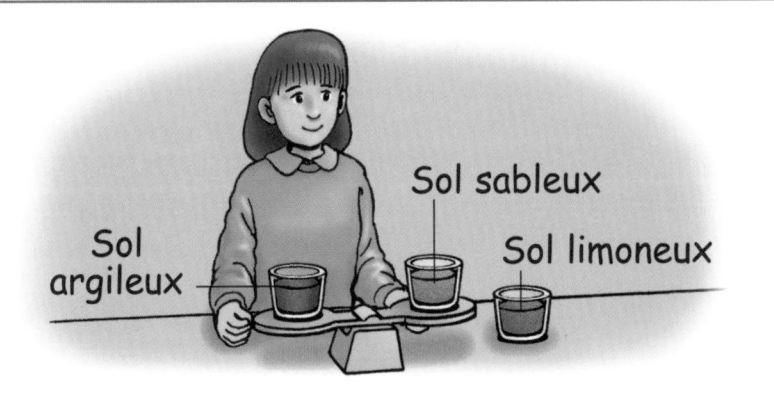

4. Quel type de sol est le **plus lourd** ? _____

   Quel type de sol est le **plus léger** ? _____

5. Ta prévision était-elle juste ?

_____

6. Explique pourquoi un type de sol a une masse plus lourde que les autres.

_____

_____

À propos... de types de sol

Il y a de nombreux types de **SOLS**.
La plupart des sols contiennent de l'humus, qui provient de la décomposition de débris végétaux et animaux.

Le **LIMON** est un mélange de **SABLE**, d'**ARGILE** et d'**HUMUS**.

Un bon sol sableux contient surtout du sable et de l'humus. Certaines plantes poussent mieux dans ce type de sol. Le sol sableux est souvent appelé « sol léger ».

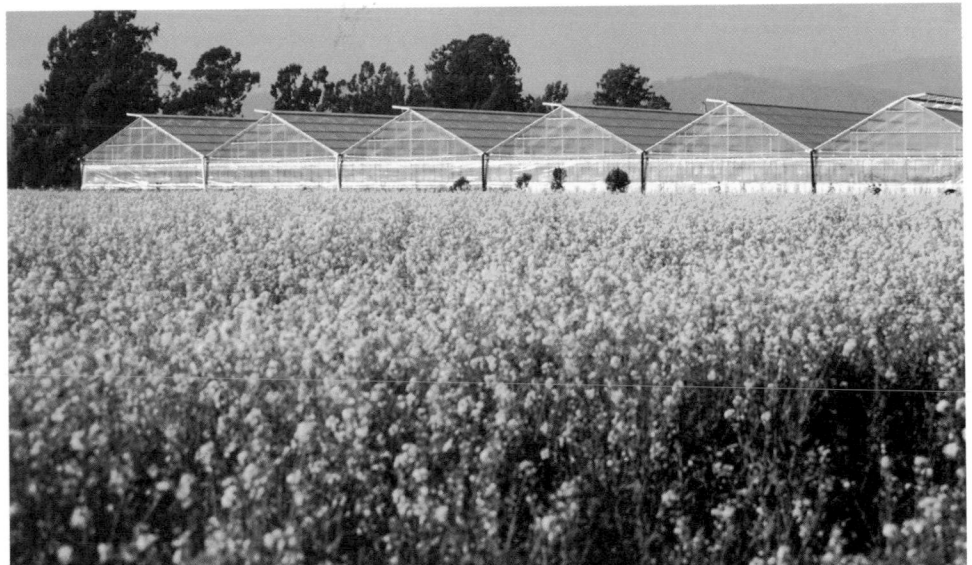

Le canola (ou colza) pousse bien dans un sol sableux.

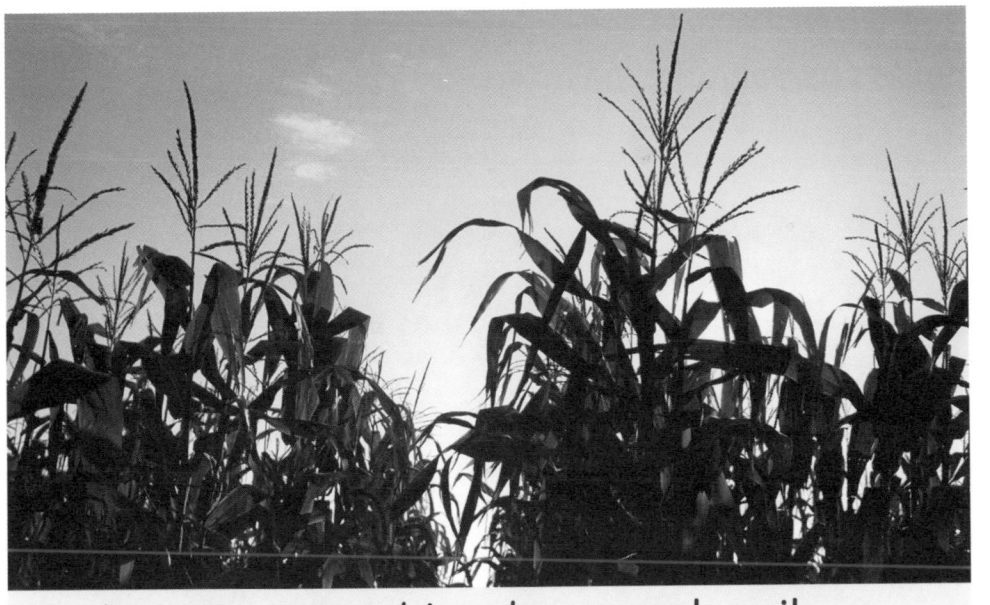

Le maïs pousse bien dans un sol argileux.

Un sol argileux contient surtout de l'argile et de l'humus. Certaines plantes poussent mieux dans ce type de sol. Le sol argileux est souvent appelé « sol lourd ».

3 Une matière absorbante

Un sol sableux présente de grands espaces entre ses particules.
L'eau peut passer librement à travers ce type de sol.
C'est pourquoi il ne retient pas bien l'eau et sèche rapidement.

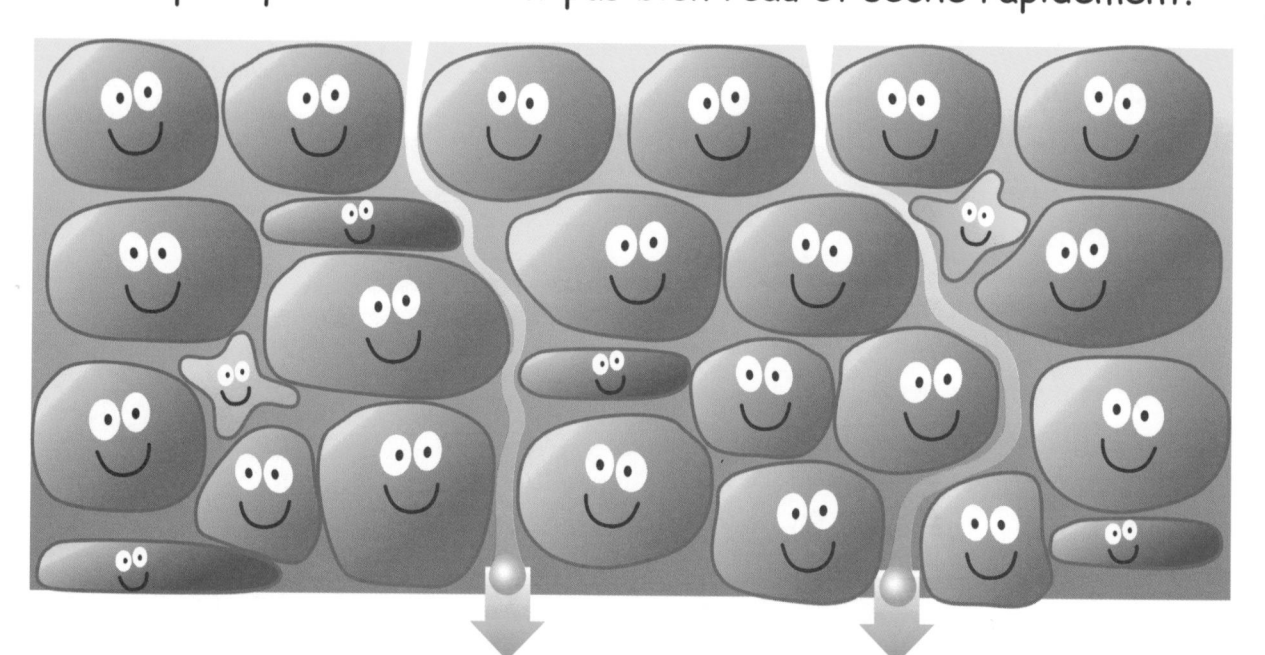

Un sol argileux, au contraire, présente de petits espaces
entre ses particules.
L'eau ne s'écoule pas rapidement à travers ce type de sol.

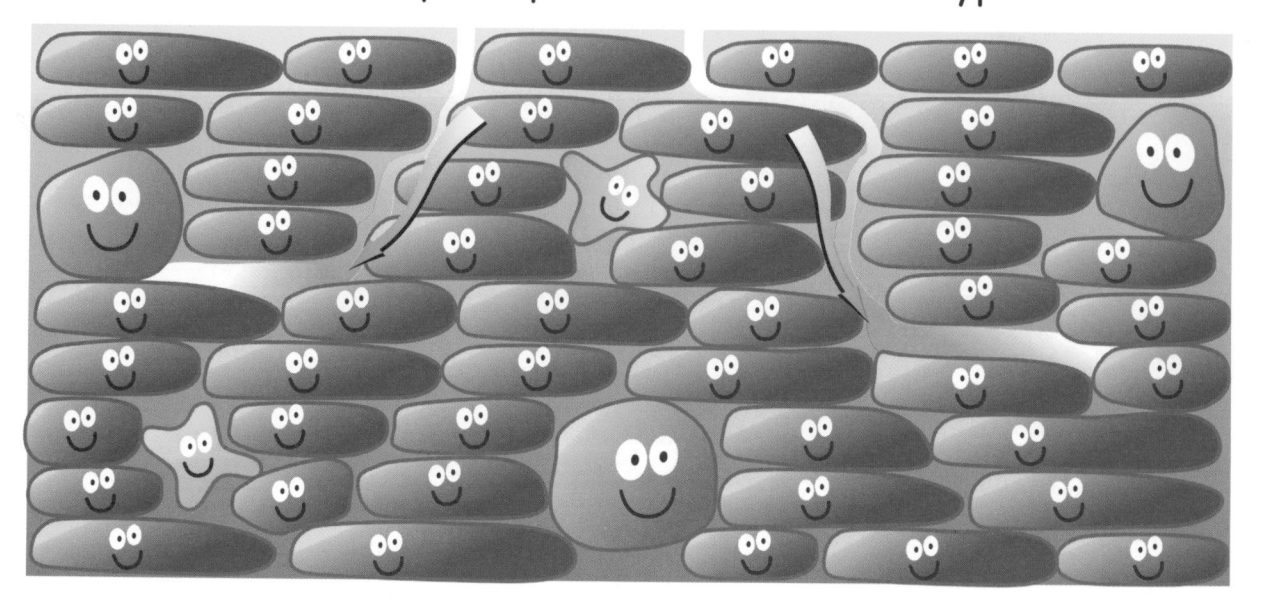

Le drainage des eaux

1. Fais le croquis d'un de tes testeurs d'absorption d'eau.

2. D'après toi, quel type de sol est le plus absorbant ?

_____

3. Explique ta prévision.

_____

4. Note les résultats de tes tests :

	Sol sableux	Sol argileux	Sol limoneux
Eau qui entre	ml	ml	ml
Eau qui sort	ml	ml	ml
Eau absorbée	ml	ml	ml

5. Ta prévision était-elle juste ? Explique ta réponse.

_____

Des « tartes » de boue

Voici à quoi nos « tartes » ressemblent.

Tarte de sable	Tarte d'argile	Tarte de limon

1. D'après toi, quelle tarte sera la plus ferme après avoir séché ? Explique ta prévision.

_____

2. Qu'est-il arrivé, le lendemain, à chacune des tartes ? Sont-elles encore fermes ou se sont-elles effritées ? Ta prévision était-elle juste ?

_____

_____

3. D'après toi, que faut-il pour qu'une « tarte de boue » reste ferme ?

_____

_____

À propos... de mots cachés

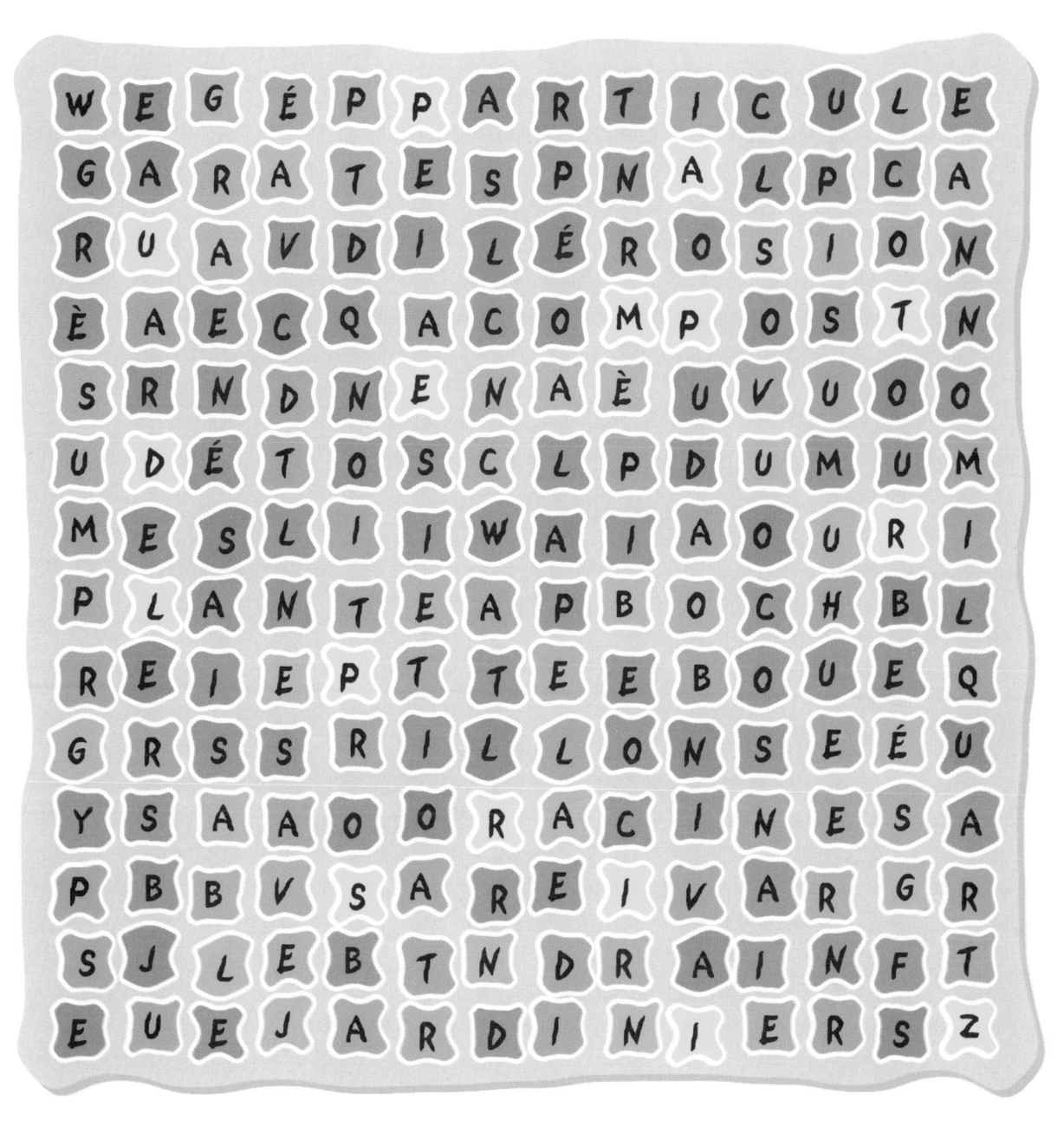

Encercle les mots suivants :

absorption   particule   érosion   tourbe
jardiniers   compost   racines   gypse
boue   plante   gravier   vase
limon   eau   sable   humus
capacité   quartz   grès   ver

Le sol doit toujours avoir un peu d'eau pour permettre aux plantes de grandir et aux petites créatures de vivre.
Mais, parfois, un excès d'eau peut causer de graves problèmes.

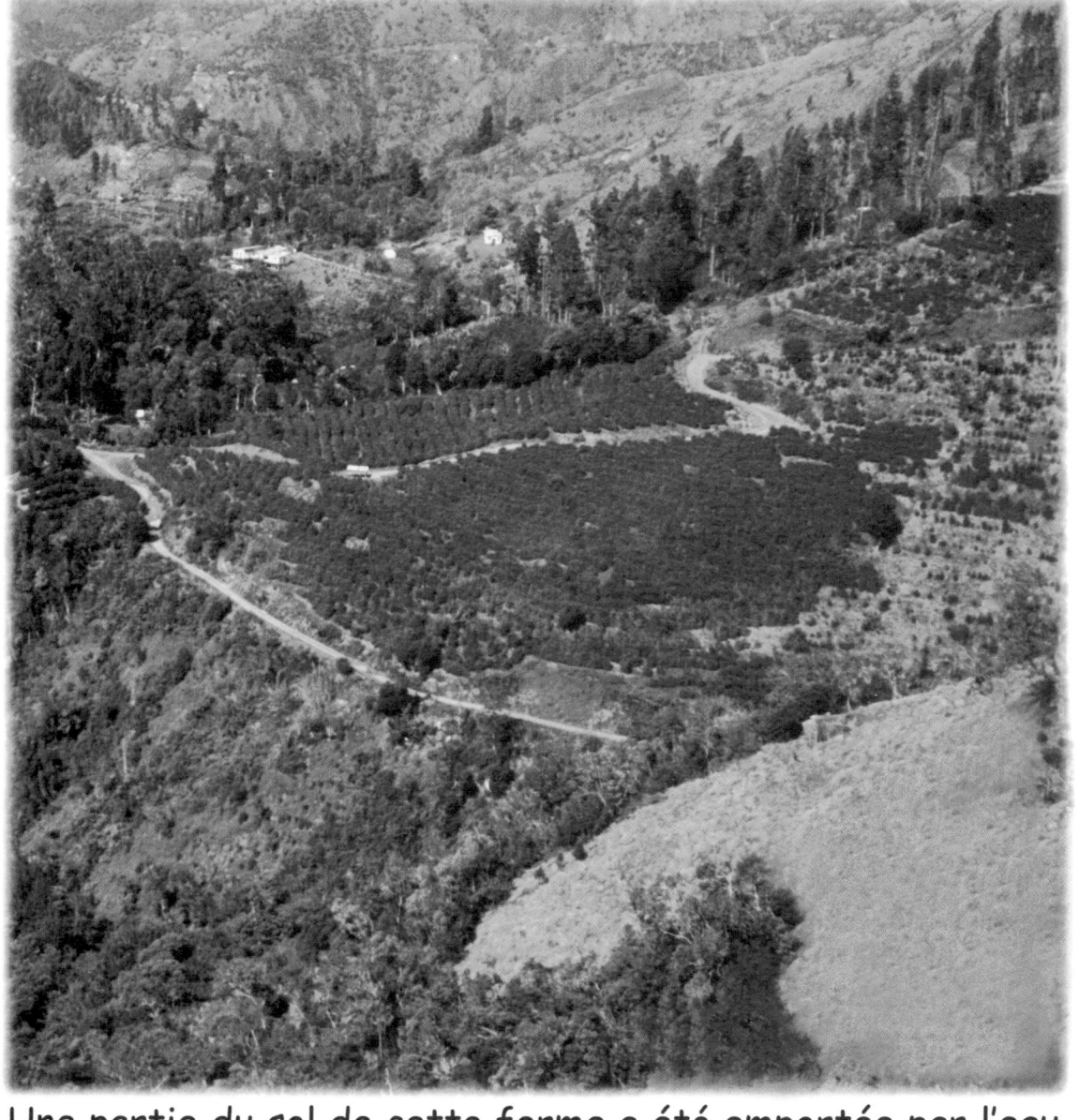

Une partie du sol de cette ferme a été emportée par l'eau de pluie. L'usure du sol causée par l'eau est appelée érosion.
Comment l'érosion peut-elle affecter les plantes et les animaux qui se trouvent dans le sol ?
Que peut faire le fermier pour éviter cette calamité ?

Trop d'eau !

Voici comment placer les deux boîtes de sol.

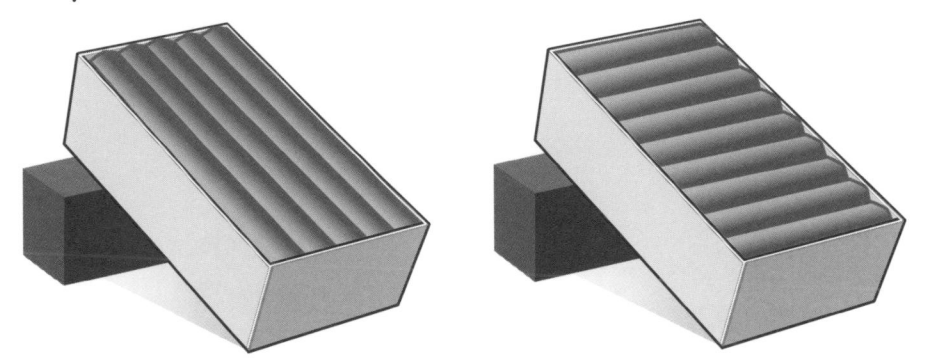

Fais des croquis pour montrer ce qu'il est arrivé au sol qui se trouvait dans les boîtes après l'arrosage.

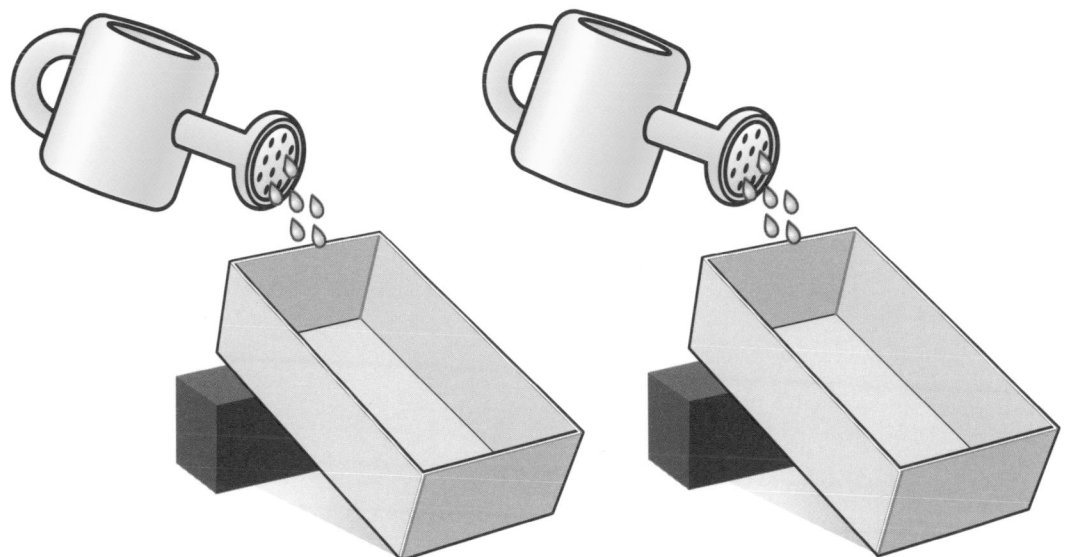

Dans quelle direction doit-on orienter les sillons pour mieux protéger le sol de l'érosion ?

_____

_____

Explique pourquoi.

_____

_____

Comment les fermiers doivent-ils labourer leurs champs et planter leurs graines dans des champs vallonnés ?

_____

_____

Comment combattre l'érosion

Place les deux boîtes comme sur les dessins et arrose-les avec un arrosoir.
Utilise la même quantité d'eau pour chacune.

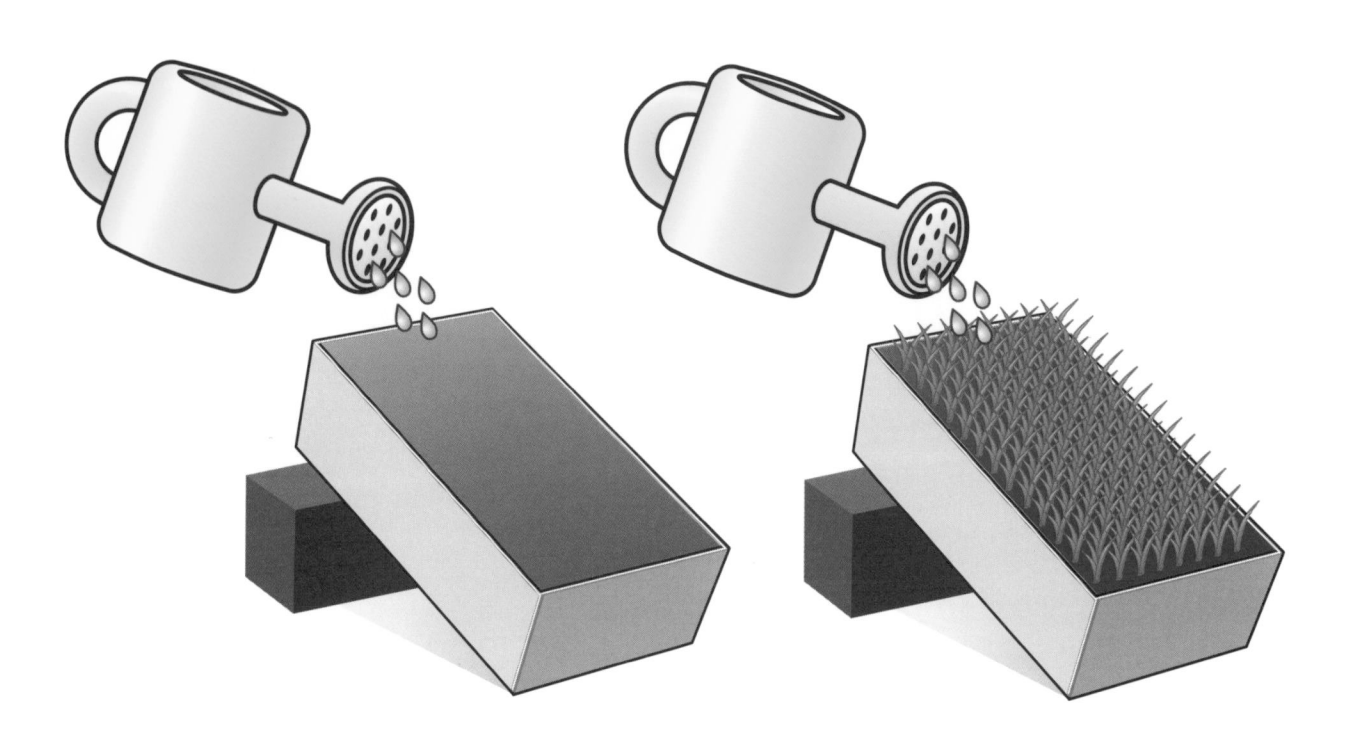

Note ce qui arrive au sol de chaque boîte.

_____

_____

Explique pourquoi l'herbe a produit cet effet.

_____

_____

Que peuvent faire les fermiers pour éviter l'érosion des champs vallonnés ?

_____

_____

À propos... d'érosion

Les racines des plantes empêchent le sol de glisser.

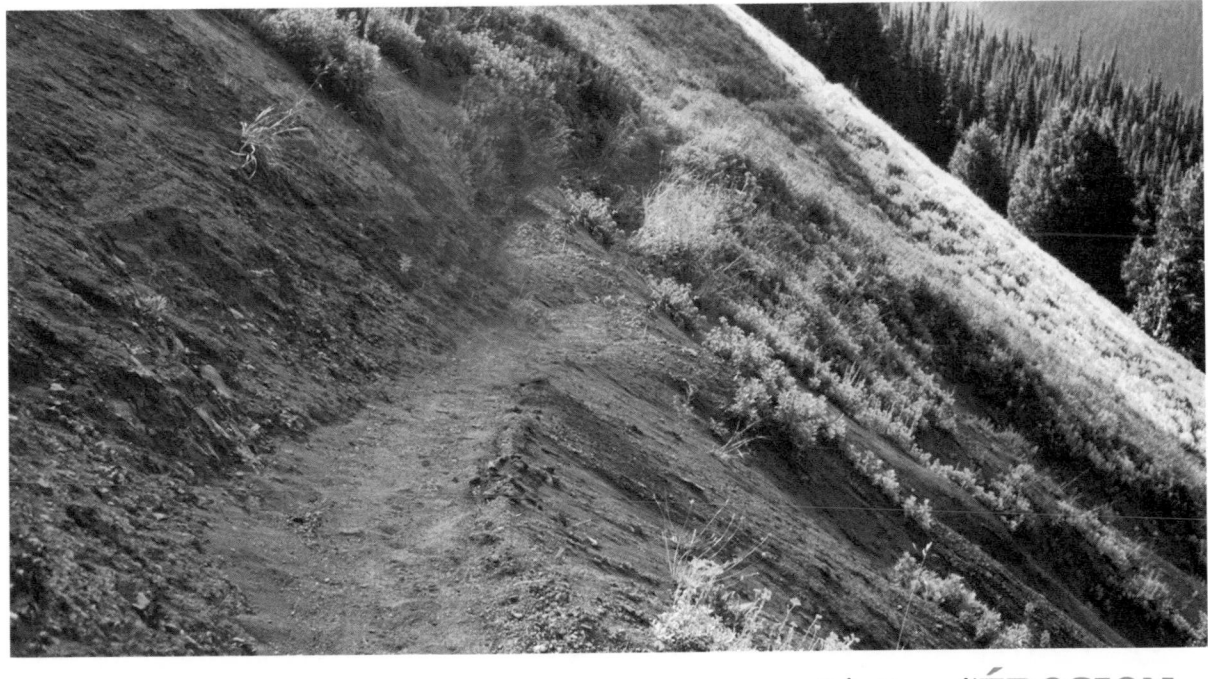

Les arbres et les arbustes permettent d'éviter l'ÉROSION
du sol de nos forêts.

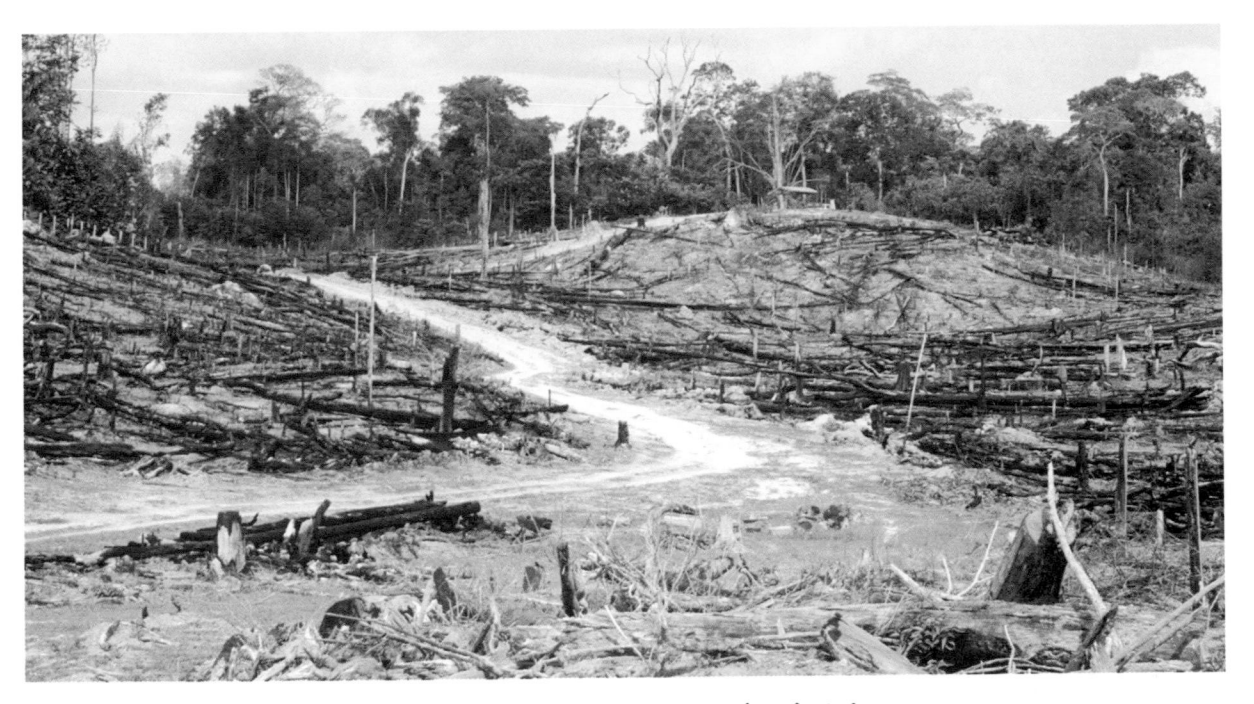

Si une forêt est « coupée à blanc »,
la pluie peut provoquer un glissement du sol.

5 Le filtrage

L'eau des lacs, des rivières et des puits
a normalement besoin d'être filtrée ou
traitée chimiquement avant qu'on puisse la boire.

De quelles façons, d'après toi, l'eau peut-elle être « salie » ?

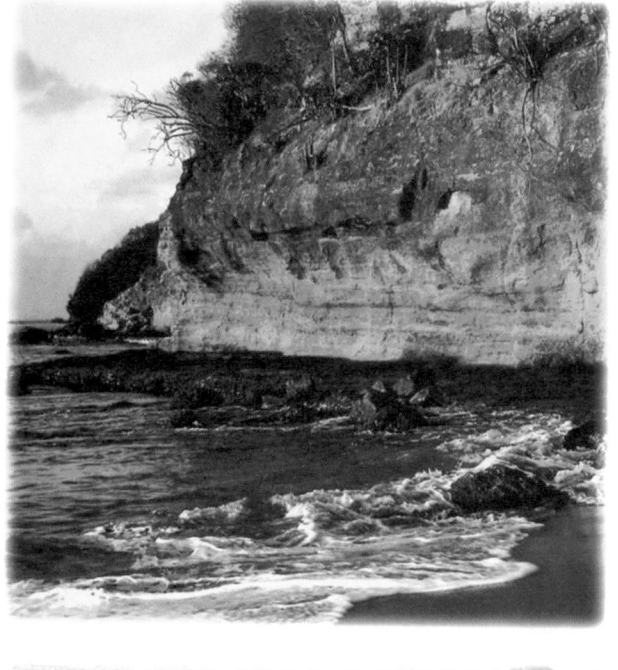 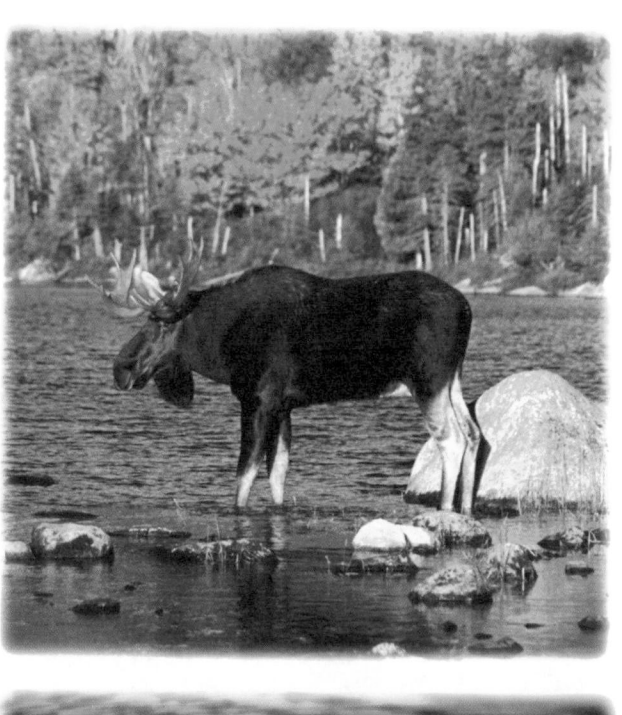

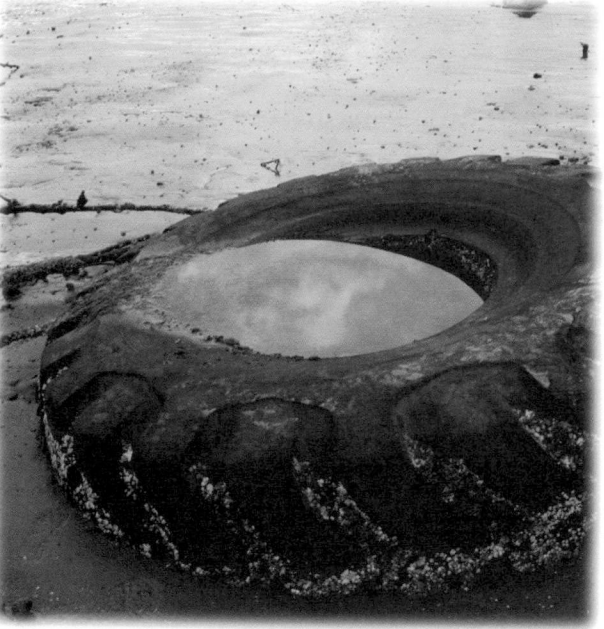 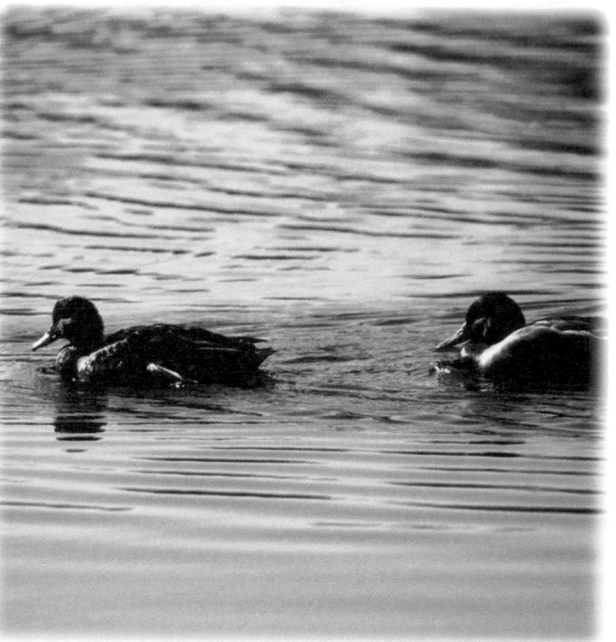

Le filtrage de l'eau

Différents matériaux provenant du sol peuvent aider à filtrer l'eau.

Dessine le filtre à eau que tu as construit et légende les différentes couches.

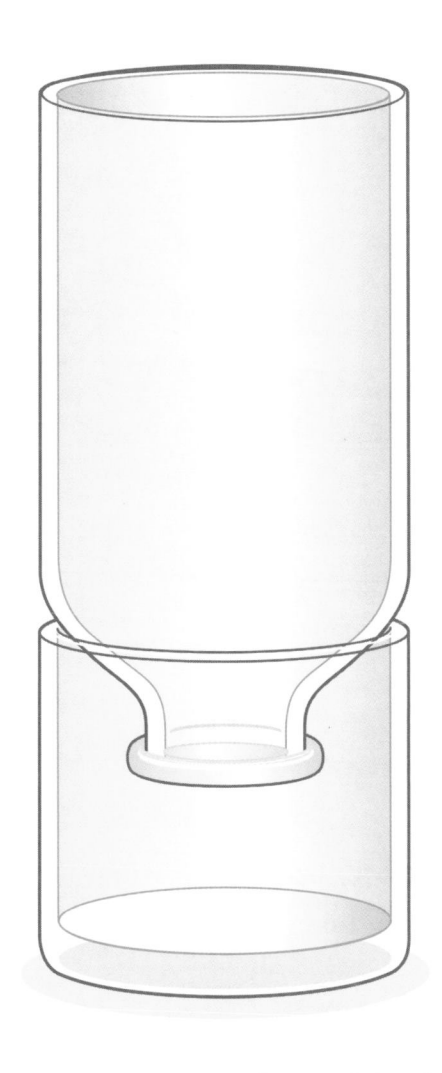

Quelle est la différence d'aspect entre l'eau filtrée et l'eau non filtrée ?

Explique comment le filtre a produit cet effet.

Pourquoi l'eau filtrée n'est-elle pas encore assez pure pour être bue ?

Colorants chimiques

Dans une tasse graduée, ajoute 5 à 10 gouttes de colorant alimentaire à 500 ml d'eau. Verse lentement l'eau colorée dans ton filtre.

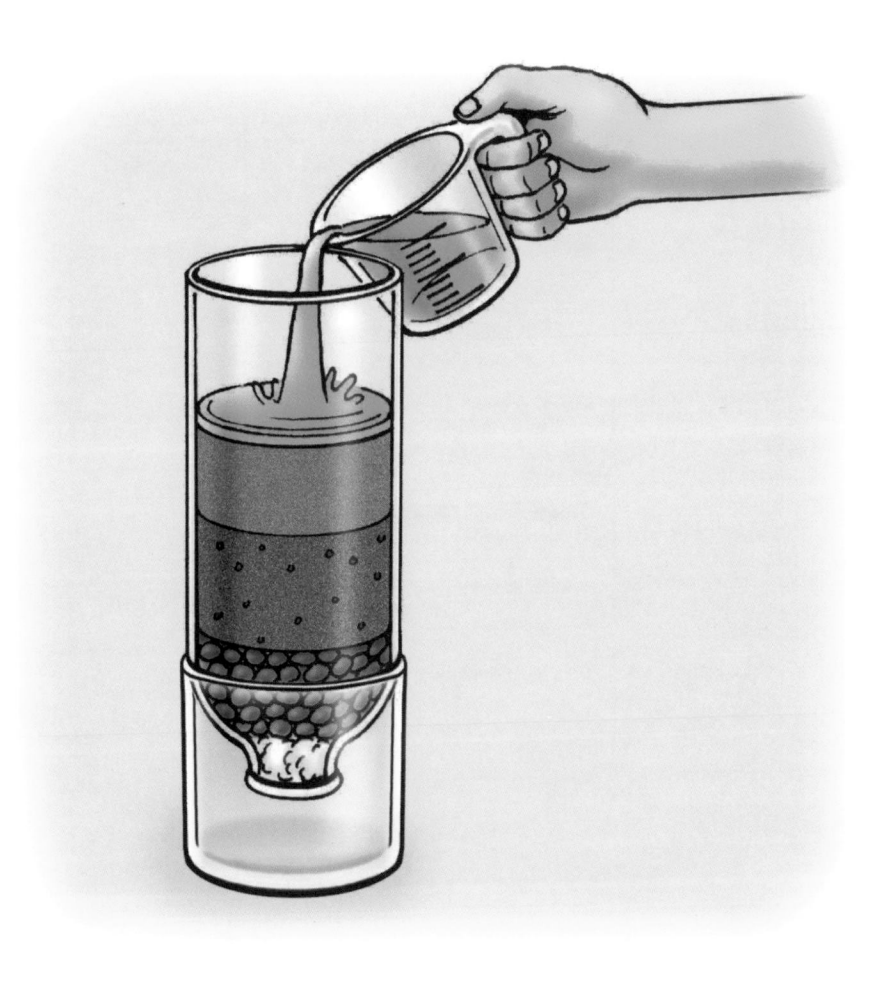

Le colorant alimentaire est un produit chimique qui se dissout dans l'eau. Que lui est-il arrivé lorsqu'il est passé à travers le filtre ?

_____

_____

Qu'est-ce que cette expérience t'apprend sur les produits chimiques qui se trouvent dans l'eau ?

_____

_____

À propos... de filtrage

Avant d'être bue, l'eau des villes et des villages doit être **FILTRÉE** et traitée pour être débarrassée des produits chimiques nocifs et des petits organismes qu'elle peut contenir.

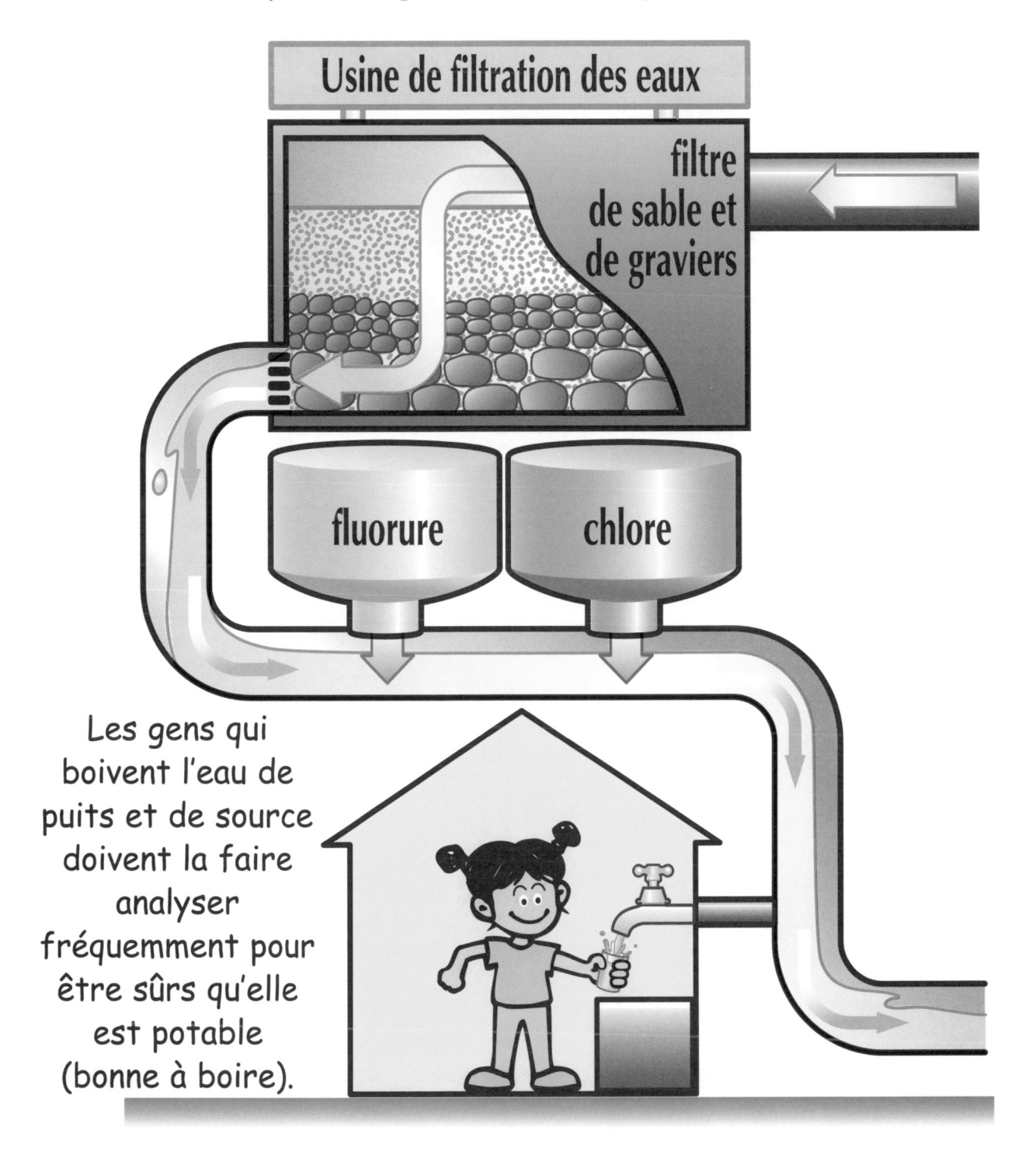

Usine de filtration des eaux

filtre de sable et de graviers

fluorure

chlore

Les gens qui boivent l'eau de puits et de source doivent la faire analyser fréquemment pour être sûrs qu'elle est potable (bonne à boire).

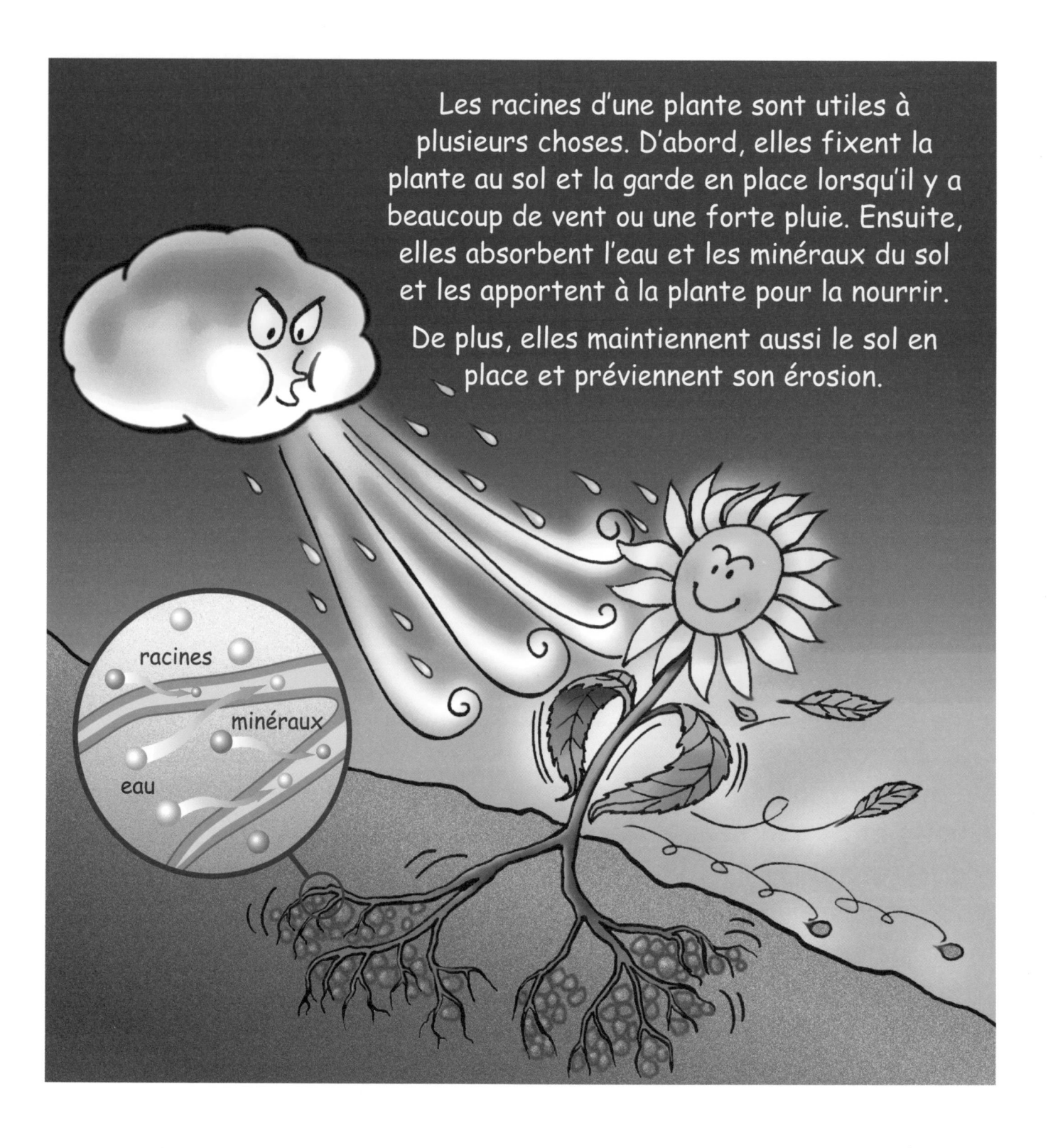

Les racines d'une plante sont utiles à plusieurs choses. D'abord, elles fixent la plante au sol et la garde en place lorsqu'il y a beaucoup de vent ou une forte pluie. Ensuite, elles absorbent l'eau et les minéraux du sol et les apportent à la plante pour la nourrir.

De plus, elles maintiennent aussi le sol en place et préviennent son érosion.

Un solide support

Fais le croquis d'une racine pivotante et d'une racine fibreuse.

racine pivotante	racine fibreuse

D'après toi, quel type de racine fixe le mieux la plante au sol ? Explique ta réponse.

_____

Les racines pivotantes peuvent emmagasiner beaucoup de nourriture pour les plantes. Quelles racines pivotantes as-tu déjà mangées ?

_____

La protection du sol

Dessine le sol après l'avoir délicatement sorti des gobelets en papier.

Sol ensemencé	Sol non ensemencé

Explique ce que tu observes.

_____

_____

Bon sol, mauvais sol

1. D'après toi, quel va être le meilleur sol pour faire pousser l'herbe ? Explique ta prévision.

_____

2. Quelles sont les graines qui ont germé les premières ? _____

3. Quelle est l'herbe qui a poussé le plus haut ? _____

4. Fais le croquis de l'herbe dans chacun des trois sols.

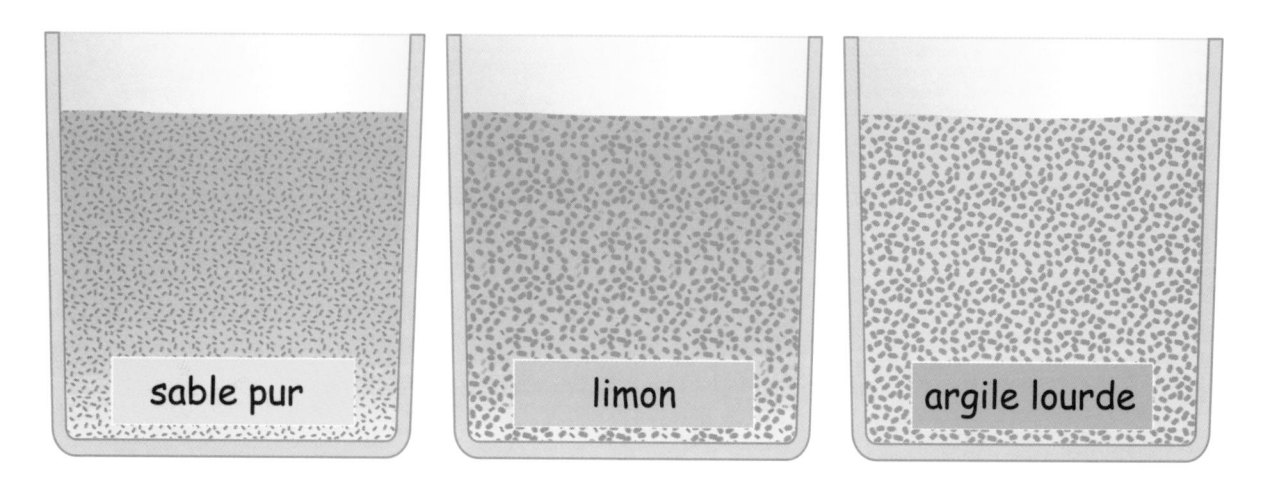

sable pur   limon   argile lourde

5. Après quelques semaines, quelle est l'herbe qui a l'air d'être la plus vivace ?

_____

6. Comment les différents sols ont-ils influé sur la croissance des plantes ?

_____

_____

7. Ta prévision était-elle juste ? Explique pourquoi. Si non, explique pourquoi.

_____

À propos... de racines

Il y a deux grands types de **RACINES**.

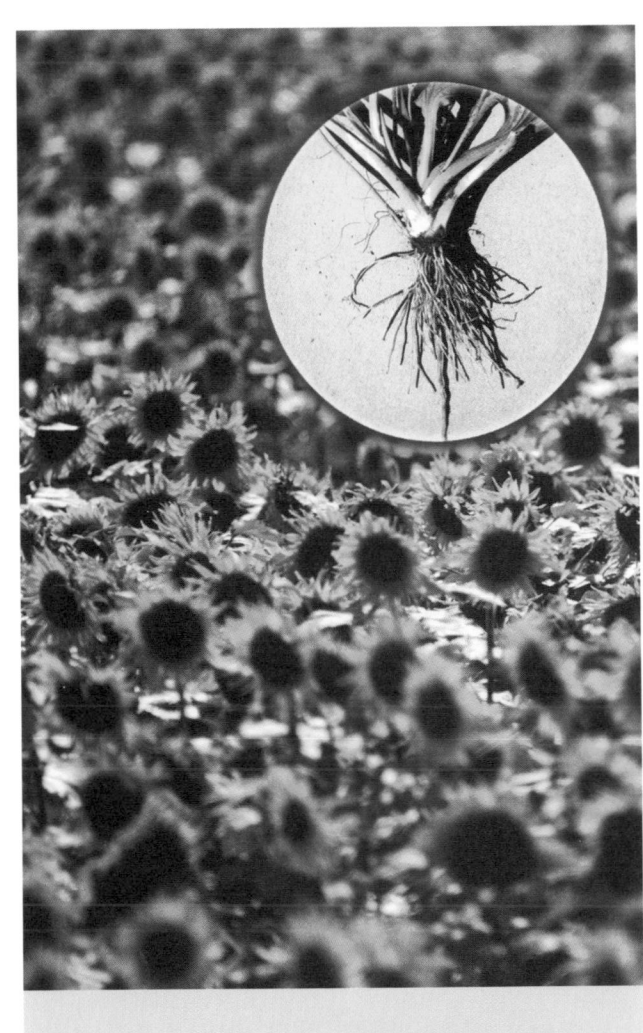

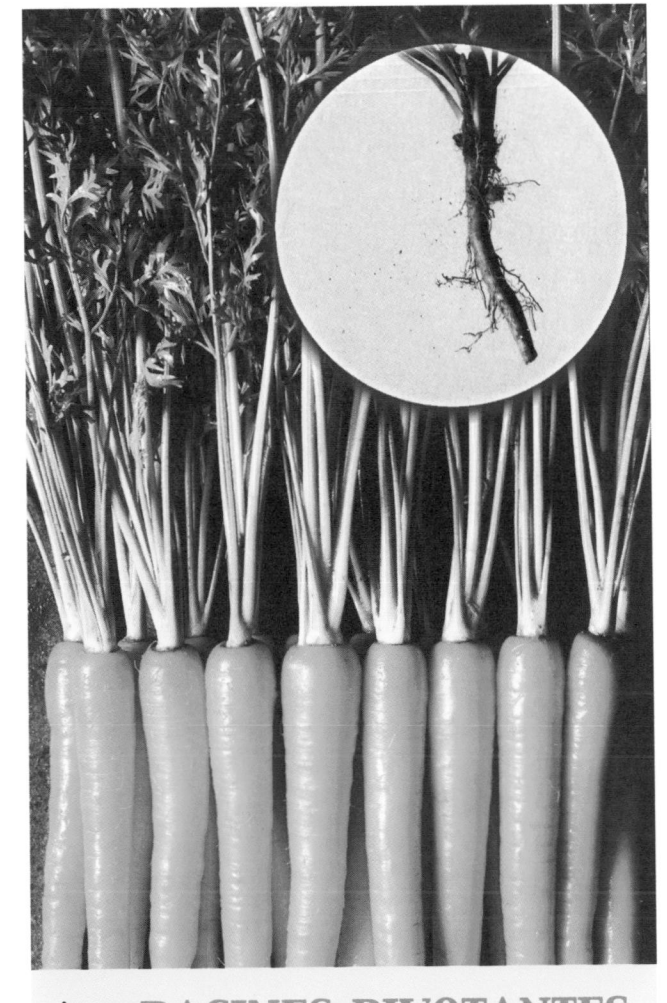

Les **RACINES FIBREUSES** s'étendent dans toutes les directions. Les tournesols, les laitues et les marguerites possèdent des racines fibreuses.

Les **RACINES PIVOTANTES** descendent plus profond dans la terre et peuvent emmagasiner de la nourriture. Les betteraves, les rutabagas et les carottes possèdent des racines pivotantes.

7 Une vie souterraine grouillante

Il y a des milliers d'êtres vivants sous la surface du sol.
Certains y vivent en permanence,
tandis que d'autres vivent à la fois dans le sol et à sa surface.

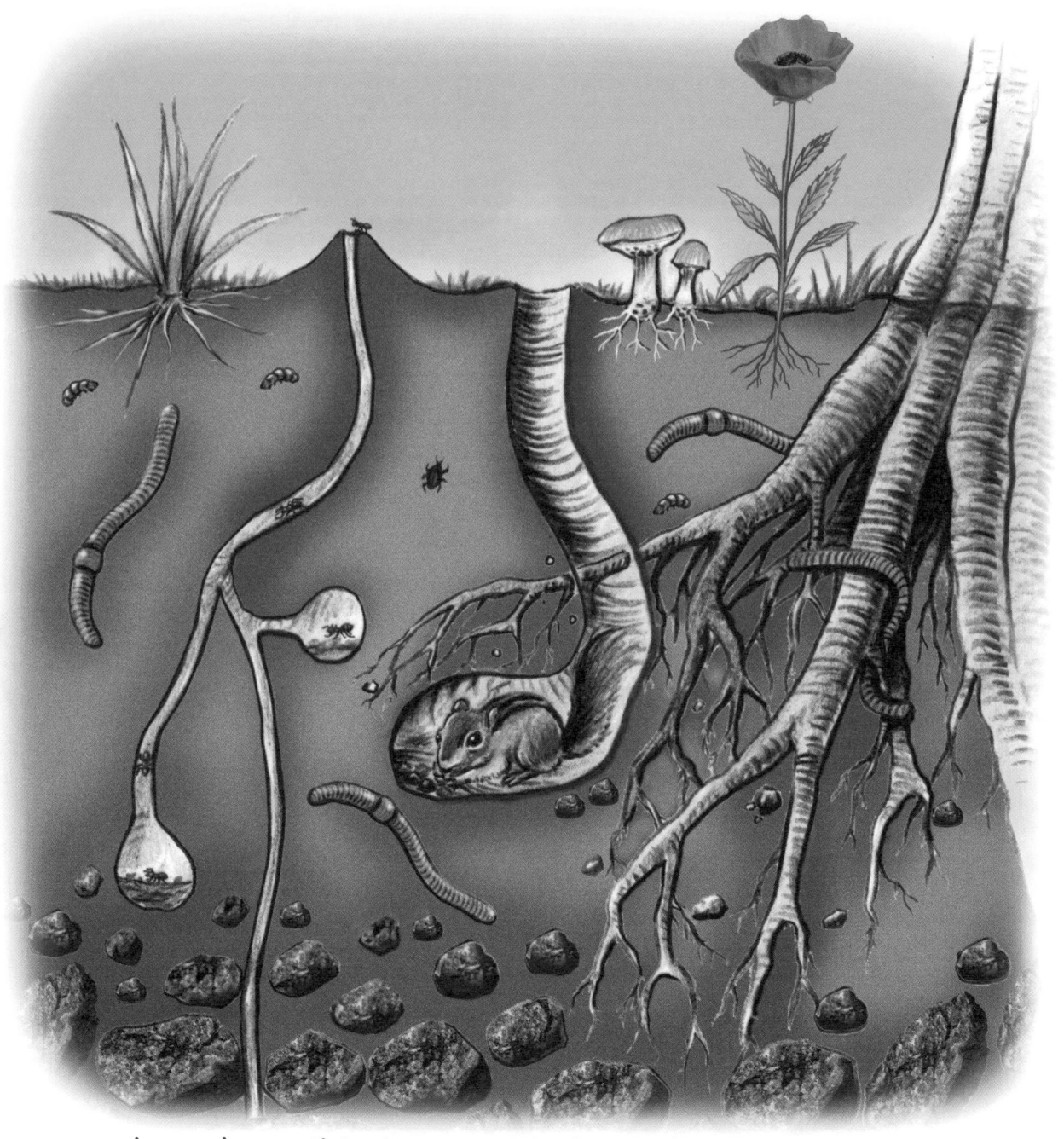

Le sol est-il indispensable à ces êtres vivants ?

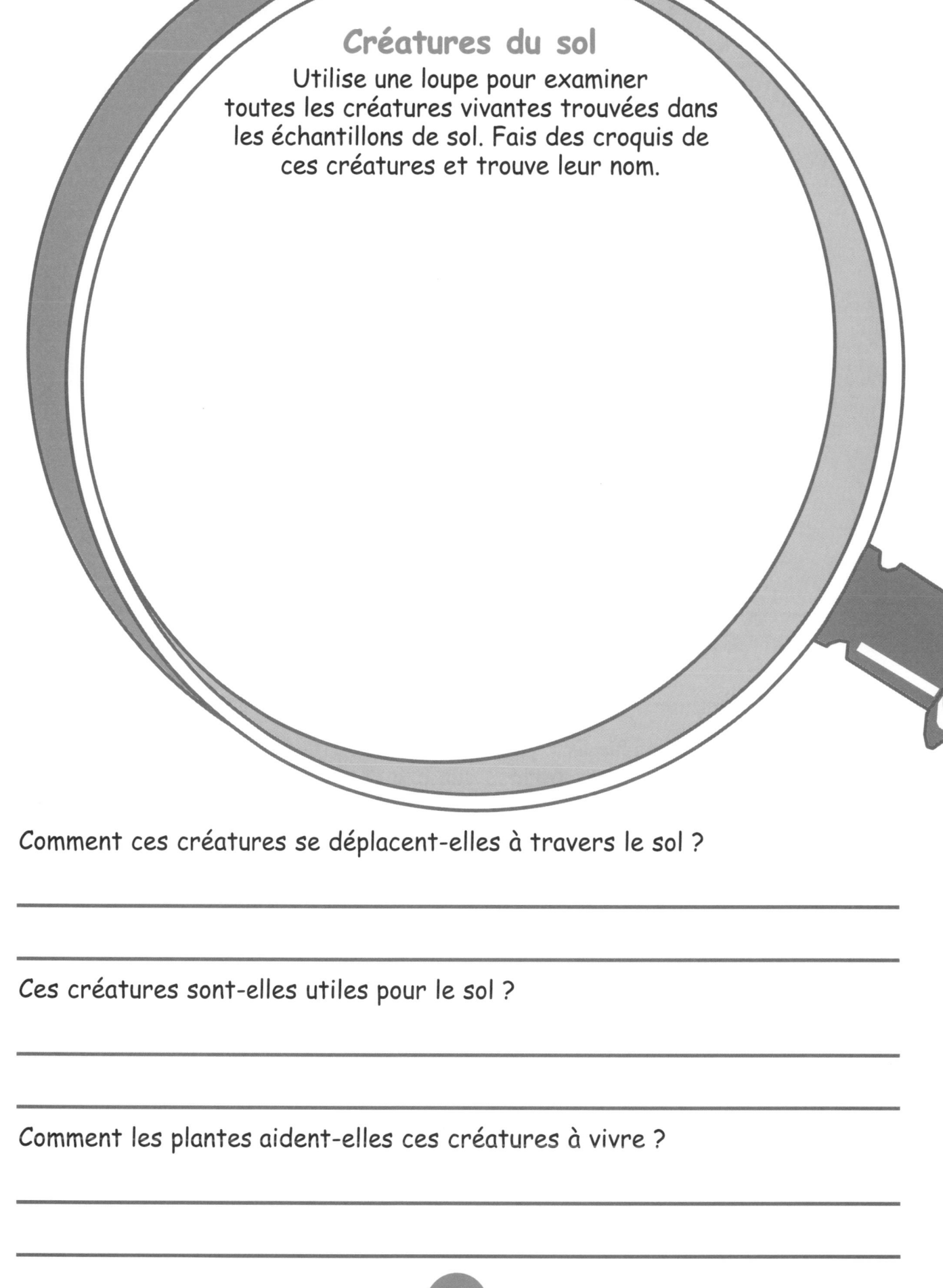

Créatures du sol

Utilise une loupe pour examiner
toutes les créatures vivantes trouvées dans
les échantillons de sol. Fais des croquis de
ces créatures et trouve leur nom.

Comment ces créatures se déplacent-elles à travers le sol ?

_____

_____

Ces créatures sont-elles utiles pour le sol ?

_____

_____

Comment les plantes aident-elles ces créatures à vivre ?

_____

_____

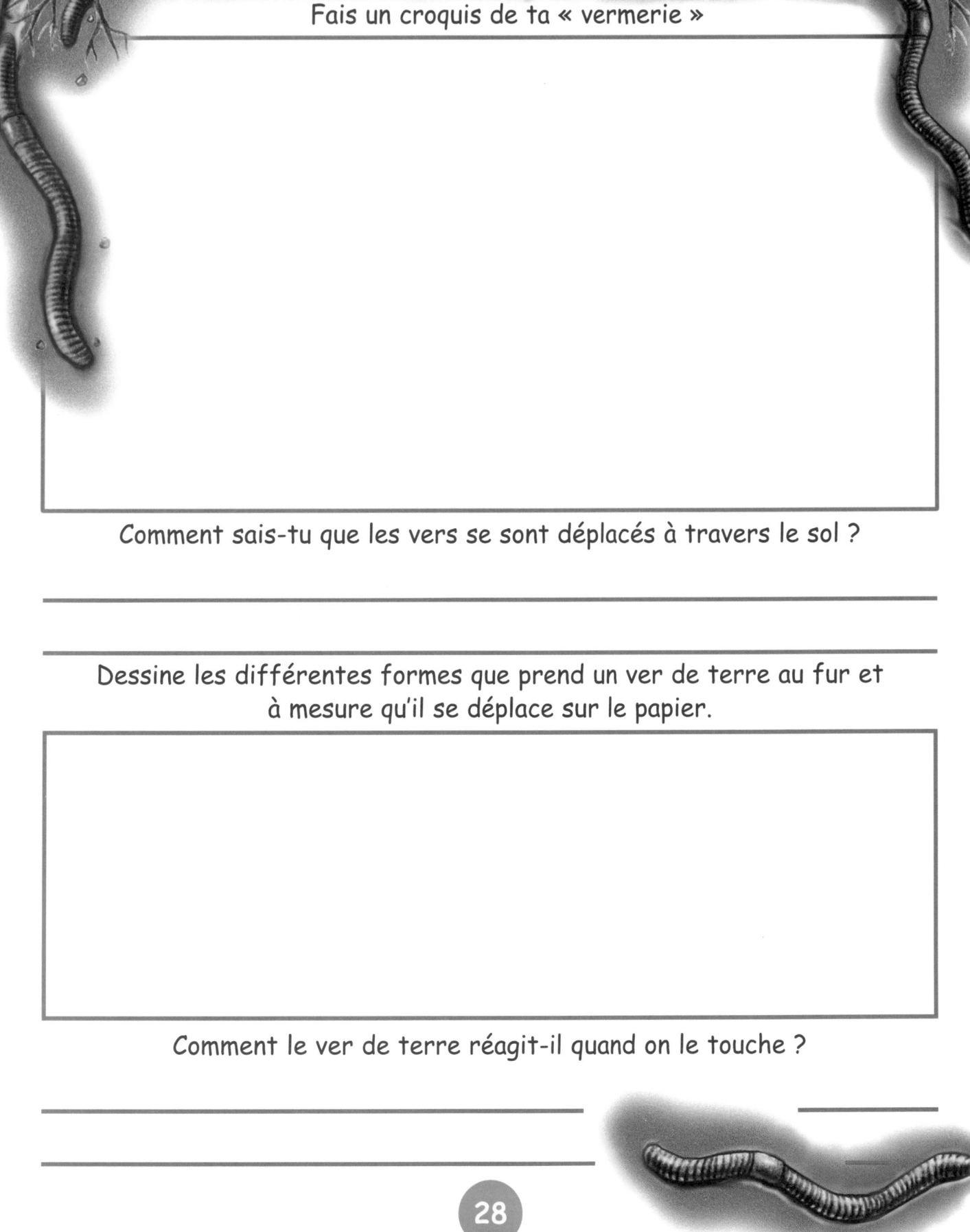

Un élevage de vers de terre

Fais un croquis de ta « vermerie »

Comment sais-tu que les vers se sont déplacés à travers le sol ?

Dessine les différentes formes que prend un ver de terre au fur et à mesure qu'il se déplace sur le papier.

Comment le ver de terre réagit-il quand on le touche ?

À propos... d'êtres vivants

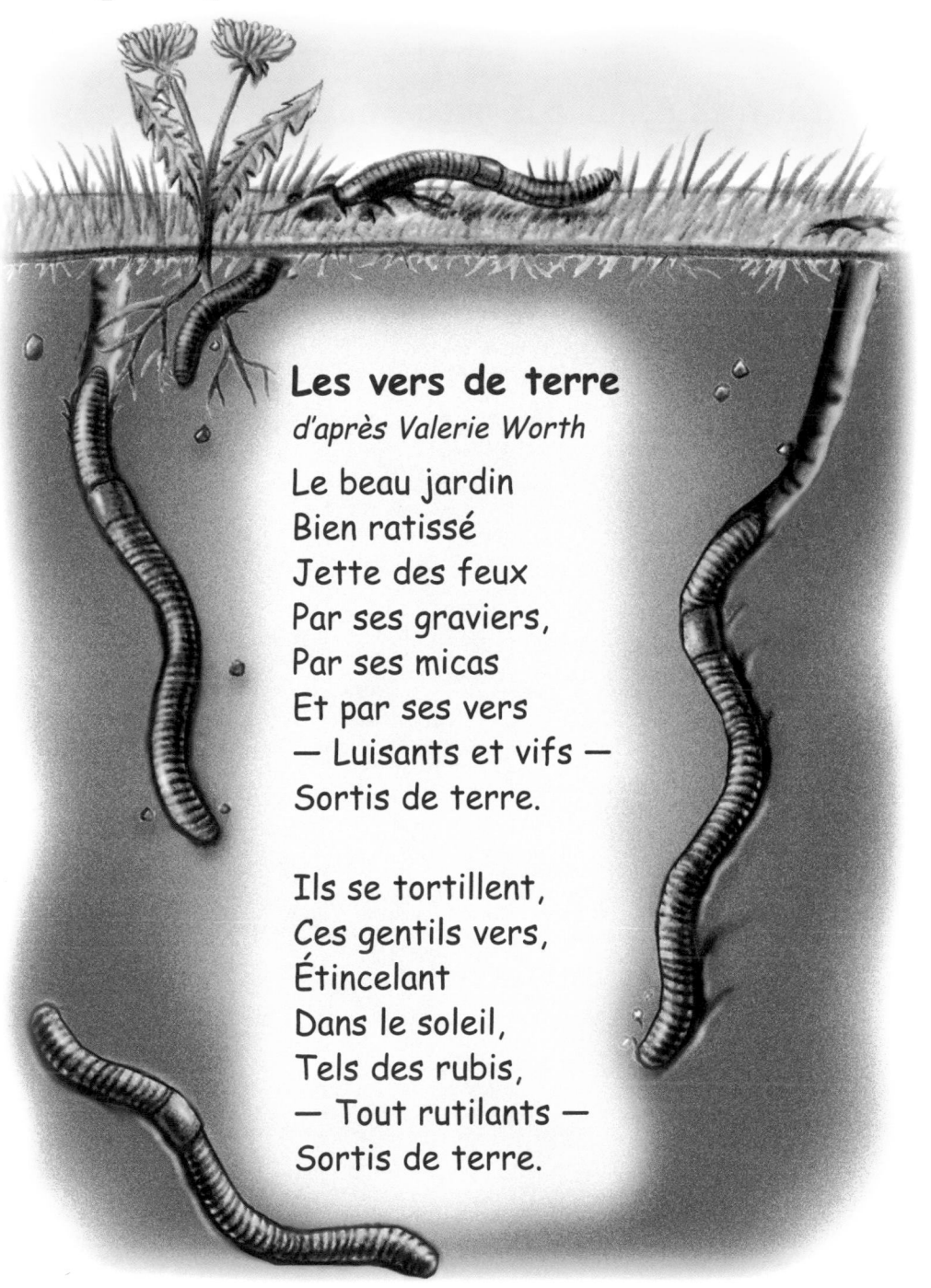

Les vers de terre
d'après Valerie Worth

Le beau jardin
Bien ratissé
Jette des feux
Par ses graviers,
Par ses micas
Et par ses vers
— Luisants et vifs —
Sortis de terre.

Ils se tortillent,
Ces gentils vers,
Étincelant
Dans le soleil,
Tels des rubis,
— Tout rutilants —
Sortis de terre.

Le sol abrite de nombreux types d'ÊTRES VIVANTS, dont certains se nourrissent de matière organique en décomposition qu'ils transforment alors en sol — un sol qui est excellent pour faire pousser les plantes. Les VERS DE TERRE participent activement à cette utile entreprise.

De très nombreux organismes végétaux et
animaux vivent dans le sol,
y compris des millions de micro-organismes
qui ne peuvent être vus qu'au microscope.
Quand les plantes et les animaux meurent,
tous ces êtres qui vivent dans le sol travaillent
à les réduire en petits éléments.

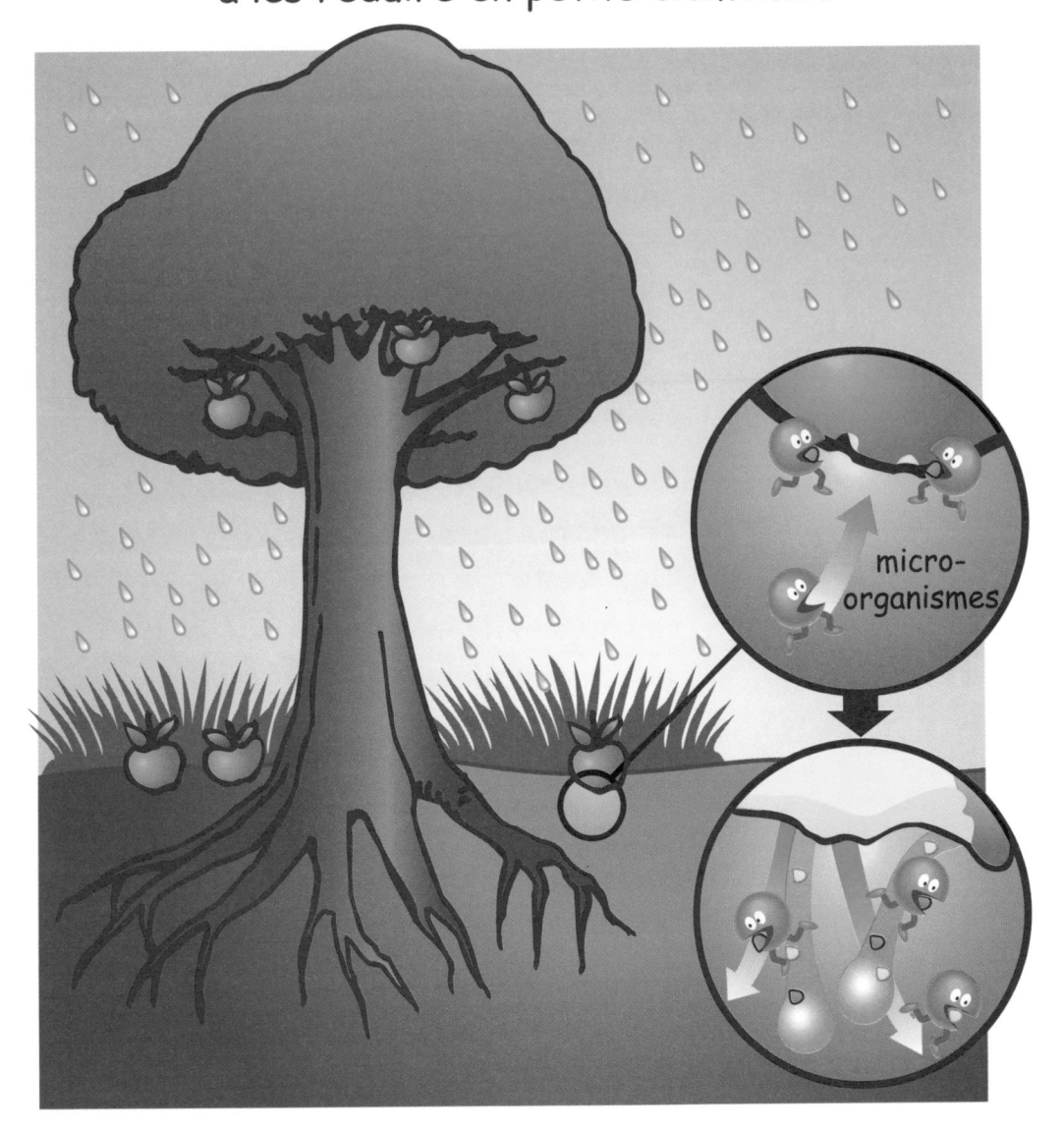

micro-
organismes

Cela s'appelle la décomposition.

Que se passe-t-il dans la décomposition ?

Observe des feuilles de laitue pendant quelques semaines et note tes observations.

Ajouté à la laitue :	après une semaine	après deux semaines
du limon sec		
du limon humide		
rien du tout		

Dans quel sac, les feuilles de laitue se sont-elles le mieux décomposées ? _____
Explique pourquoi.

_____

Dans quel(s) sac(s), les feuilles semblent ne pas s'être décomposées ? _____
Explique pourquoi.

_____

Qu'est-ce qui se décompose ?

D'après toi, quelles sont les matières qui se décomposent et quelles sont celles qui ne se décomposent pas ? Note tes prévisions.

se décomposent	✓	ne se décomposent pas	✓

Après quelques semaines, observe les matières qui sont dans ton seau. Coche « ✓ » celles qui semblent se décomposer.

Quelles sortes de matières se sont décomposées ?

_____

_____

_____

Quelles sortes de matières ne se sont pas décomposées ?

_____

_____

_____

Tes prévisions étaient-elles justes ? Explique pourquoi elles l'étaient ou ne l'étaient pas.

_____

À propos... de décomposition

Des objets qui ont été des êtres vivants, comme les plantes et les animaux, **SE DÉCOMPOSENT** (ou pourrissent) dans le sol.

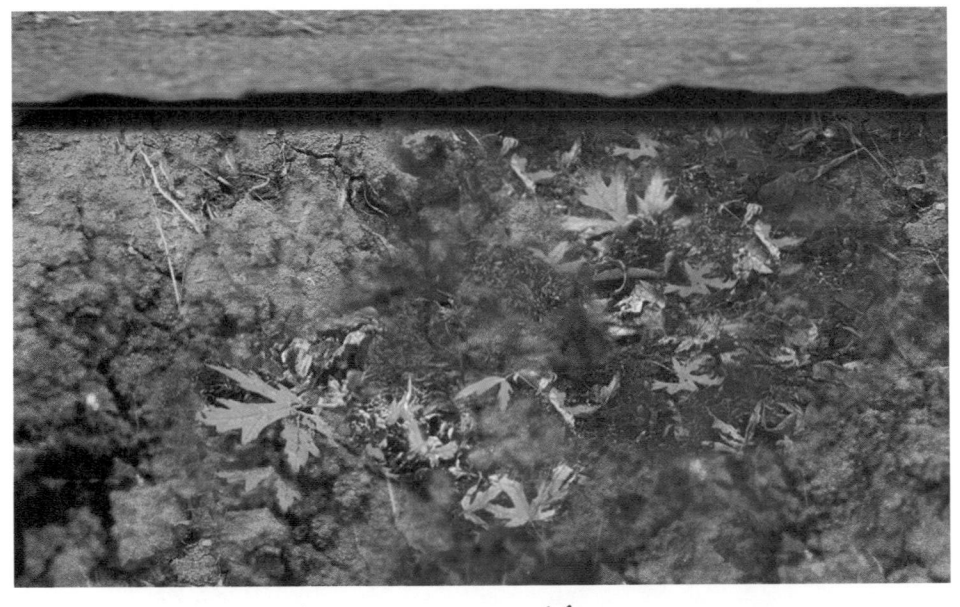

D'autres objets ne se décomposent pas,
même après de nombreuses années.

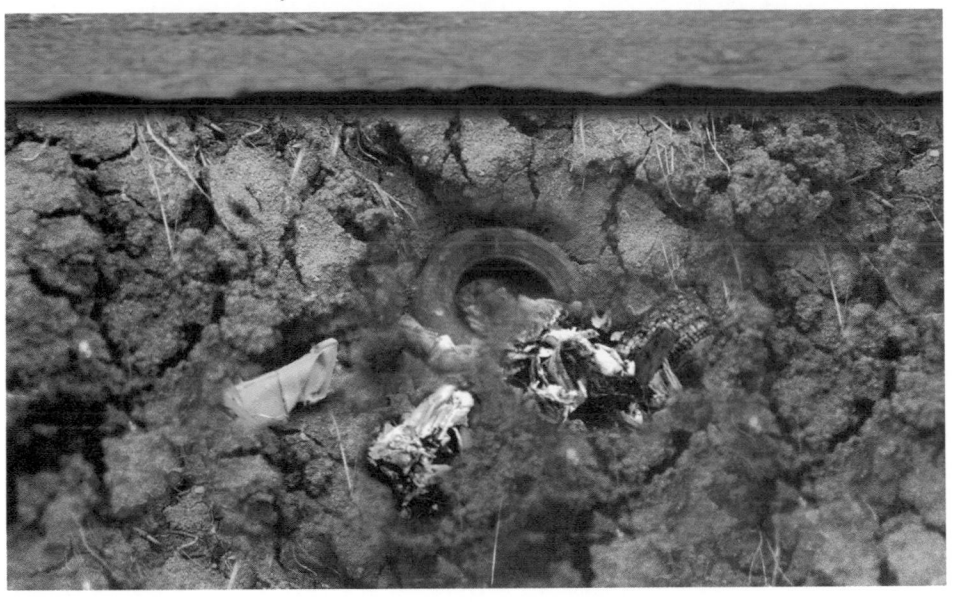

Les objets qui ne se décomposent pas
devraient être réutilisés ou recyclés.

De nombreux « déchets » produits dans nos maisons, comme le gazon tondu, les épluchures et autres rebuts provenant de la cuisine, peuvent être réutilisés comme engrais pour les pelouses et les fleurs.

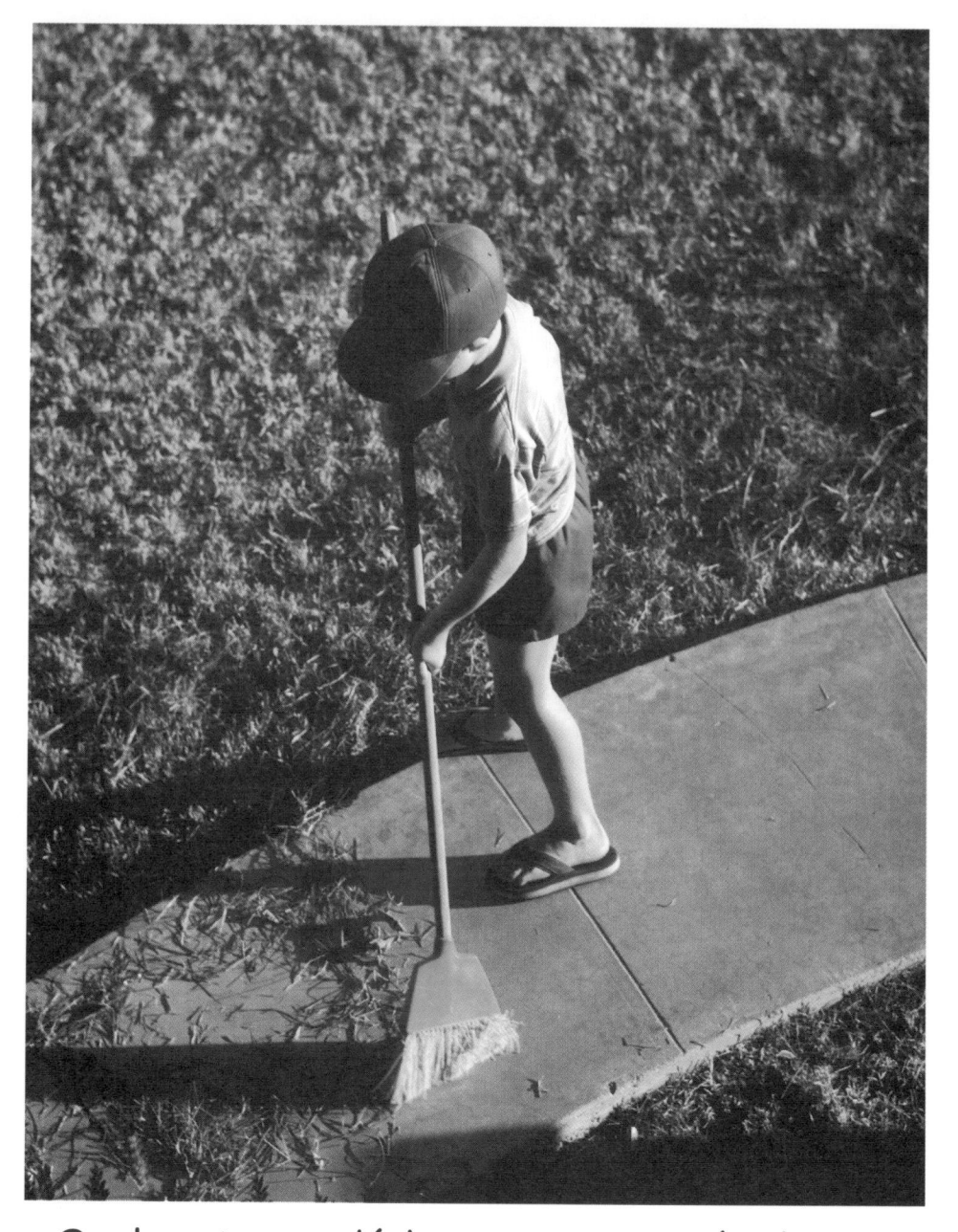

Quels autres « déchets » peut-on réutiliser ?

Les matières compostables

1. Fais deux listes : une pour les matières compostables (qui peuvent être transformées en compost) et une autre pour les matières non compostables.

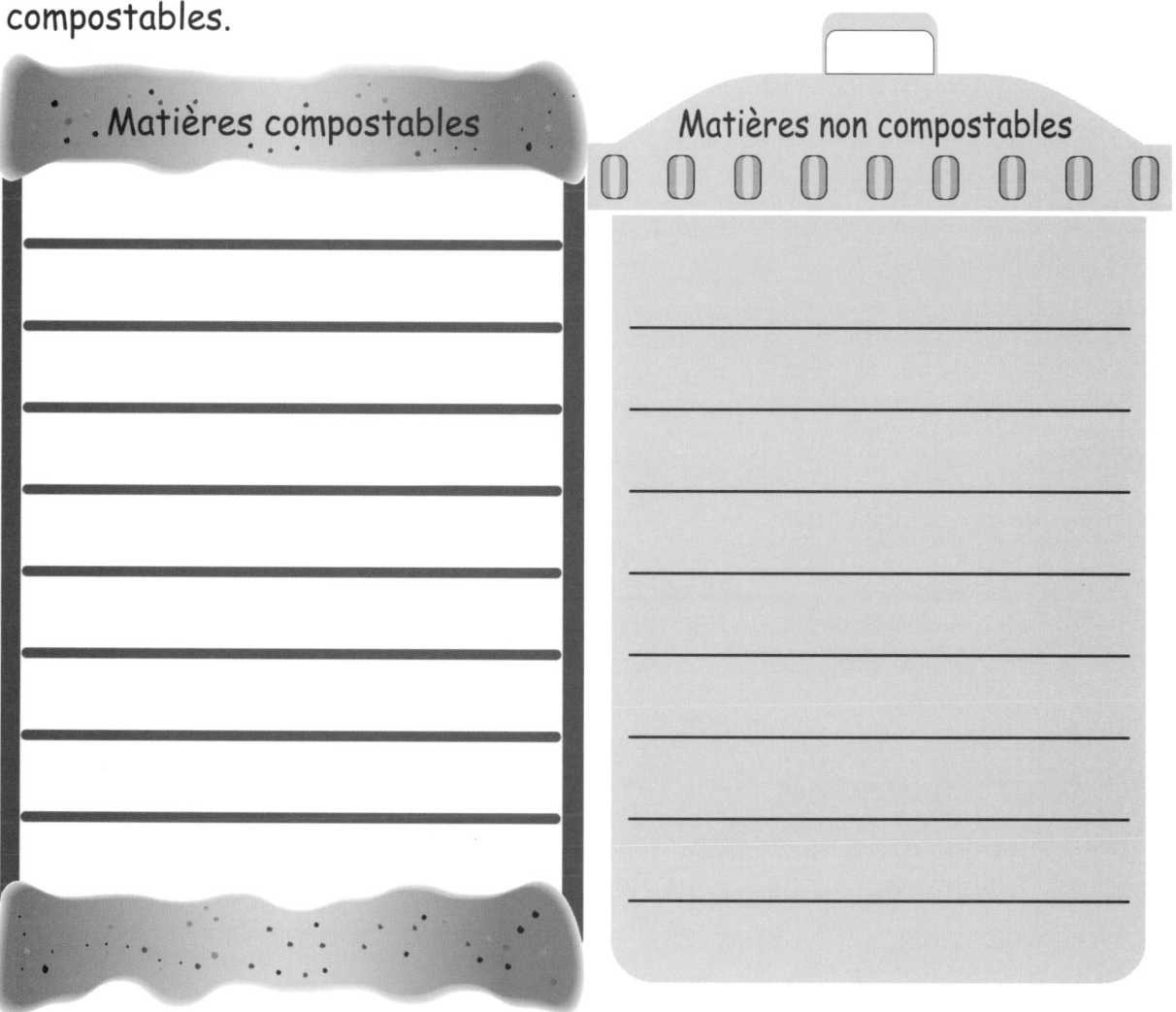

Matières compostables

Matières non compostables

2. Pourquoi la viande et les produits laitiers ne doivent-ils pas être compostés ?

_____

_____

_____

_____

Fabrique un composteur

1. Dessine le plan du composteur.

2. Fais la liste des matériaux et des outils qui te sont nécessaires pour fabriquer le composteur.

_____   _____

_____   _____

_____   _____

3. Maintenant, fabrique-le.

4. Quels changements as-tu apportés à ton plan ?

_____

_____

5. Dessine le composteur que tu as fabriqué.

À propos... de compost

La valeur du COMPOST

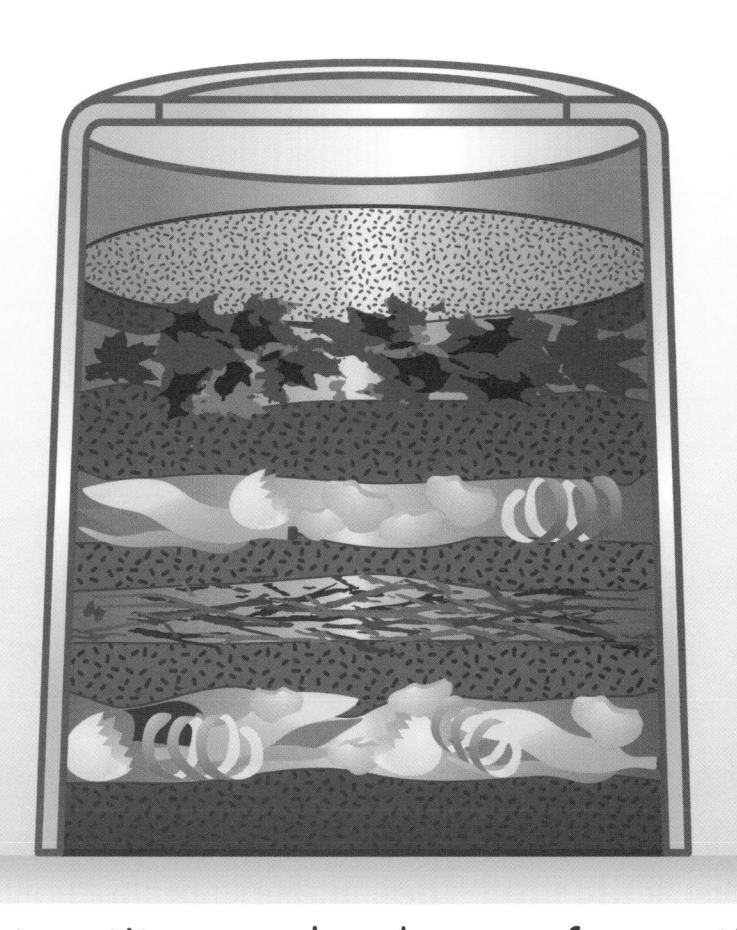

Le compost restitue au sol — dans une forme utilisable — la matière organique.

Cela aide la croissance des plantes de plusieurs manières :

☺ Le compost « scarifie » le sol, c'est-à-dire qu'il brise sa croûte d'argile durcie pour que l'air et l'eau puissent y pénétrer.

☺ Le compost aide le sol sableux à retenir l'eau et les substances nutritives.

☺ Le compost enrichit le sol de substances nutritives essentielles.

Pour construire leurs maisons, les pionniers utilisaient des briques qu'ils fabriquaient avec des matériaux provenant du sol.

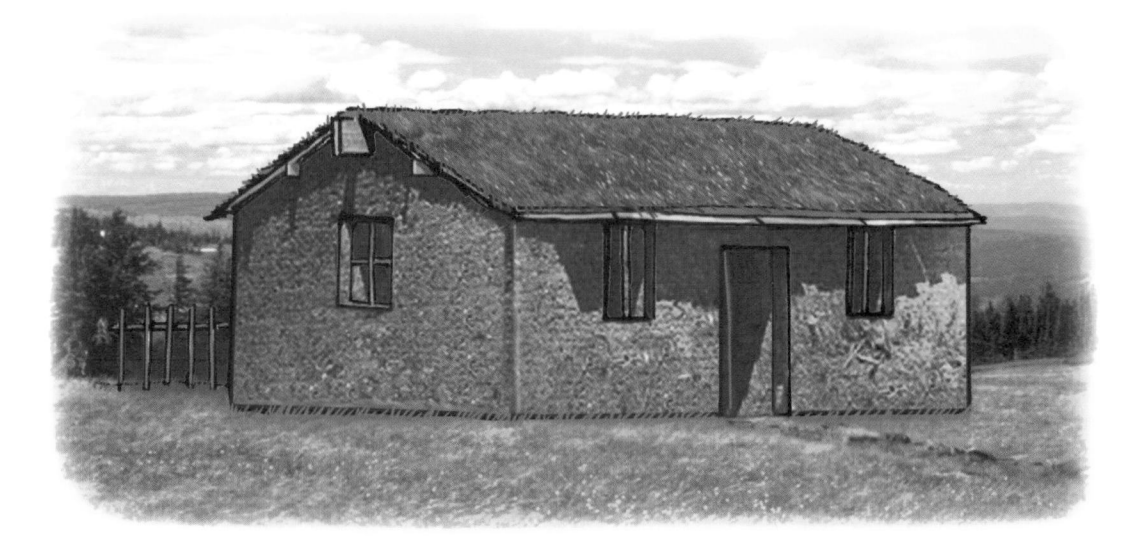

Aujourd'hui, beaucoup de maisons ont
leurs murs extérieurs en briques.
Les briques sont faites avec des matériaux qui proviennent du sol.

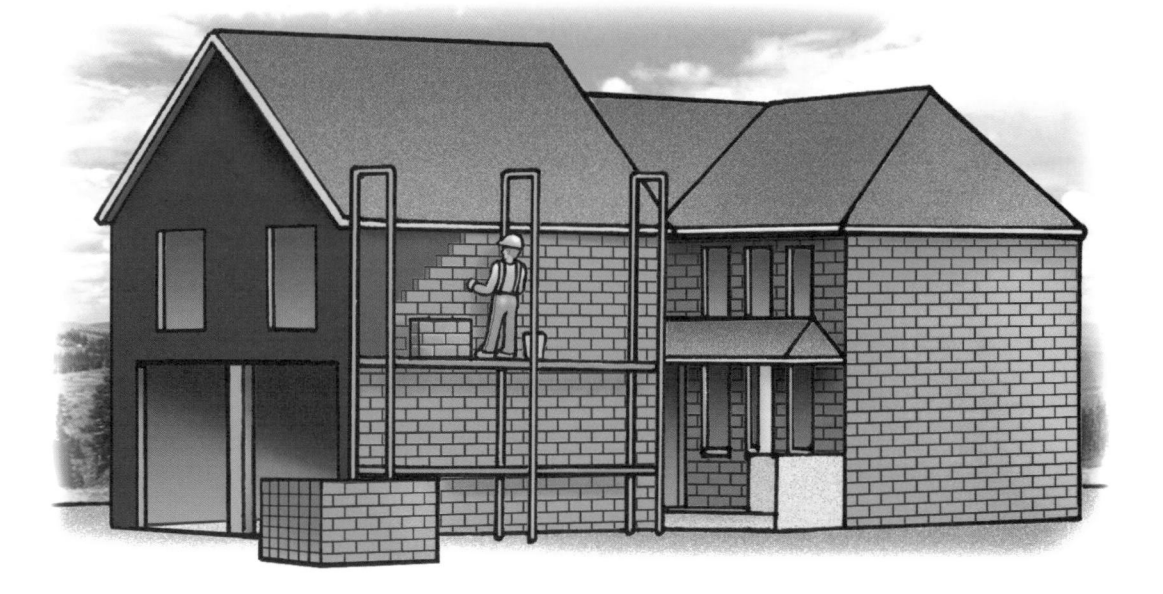

Le grès calcaire

1. Donne la « recette maison » du grès calcaire.

Recette du grès calcaire

_____

_____

_____

_____

_____

_____

_____

2. Fais une sculpture en grès calcaire ; peins-la.

3. Maintenant, dessine ta sculpture vue sous différents angles : devant, derrière et profil.

Du papier sablé

1. Note les étapes à suivre pour fabriquer du papier sablé.

_____

_____

_____

2. Ci-dessous, colle des échantillons de différents grains utilisés dans la fabrication du papier sablé.

| grains fins | grains moyens | gros grains |

Un moulage à l'argile

Dessine la structure à mouler.

Dessine le produit fini après qu'il a été décoré.

À propos... d'objets utiles

De nombreux **OBJETS UTILES** sont faits
avec des matériaux provenant du sol.

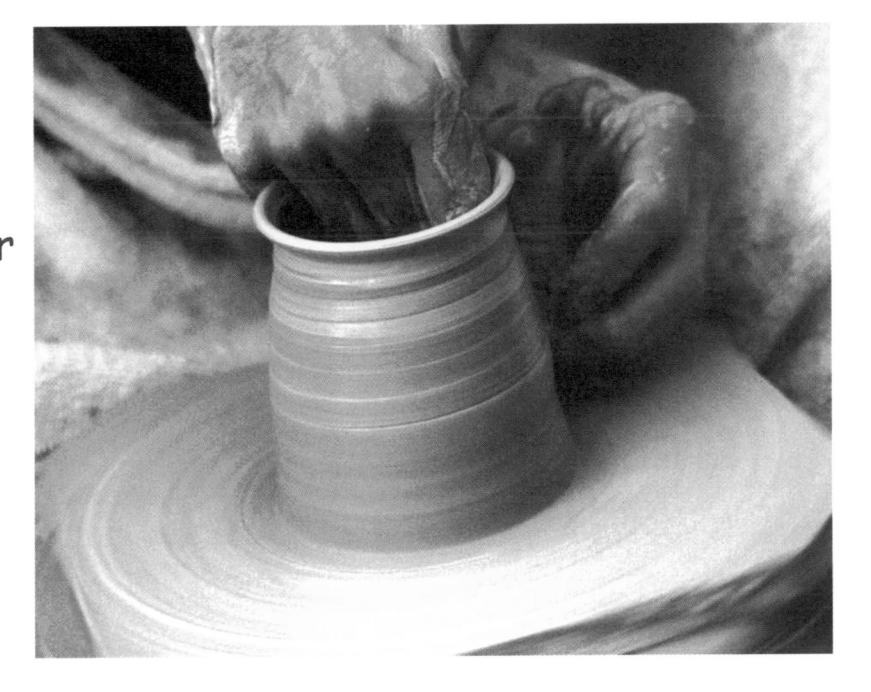

L'argile est utilisée pour
fabriquer des objets
utiles et décoratifs.

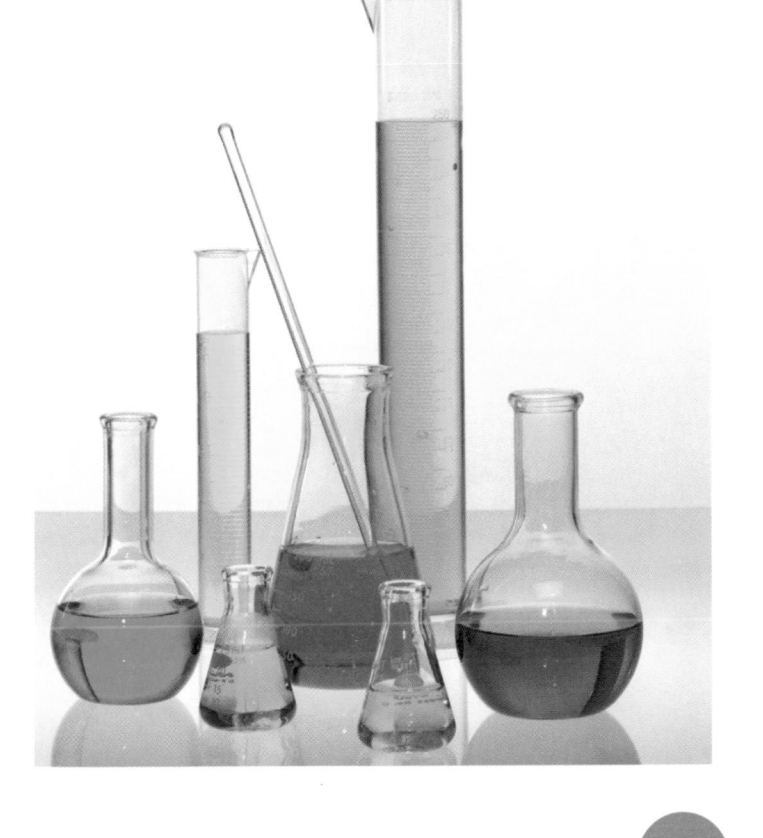

Le quartz, qui est un des
composants du sable,
est utilisé pour
fabriquer le verre.

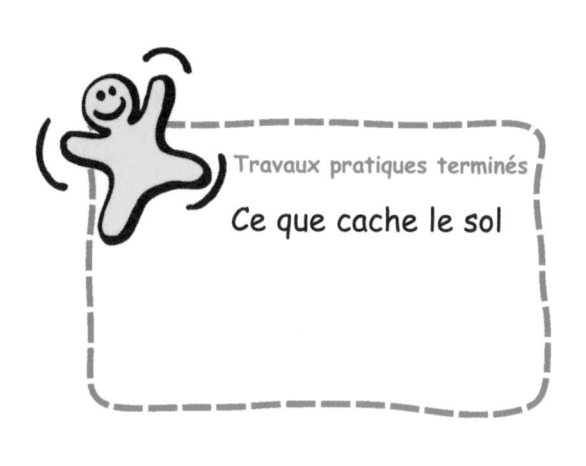

Travaux pratiques terminés

Ce que cache le sol

Commentaires de
ton enseignant/e

_____

_____

_____

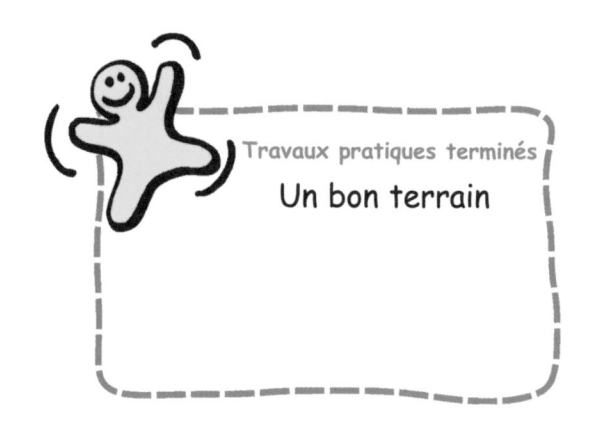

Travaux pratiques terminés

Un bon terrain

Commentaires de
ton enseignant/e

_____

_____

_____

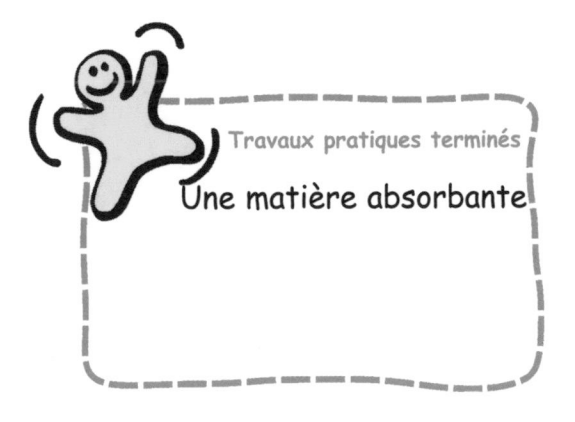

Travaux pratiques terminés

Une matière absorbante

 Commentaires de ton enseignant/e

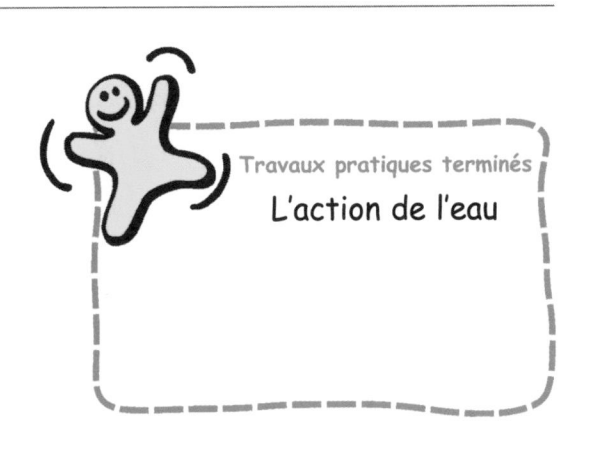

Travaux pratiques terminés

L'action de l'eau

 Commentaires de ton enseignant/e

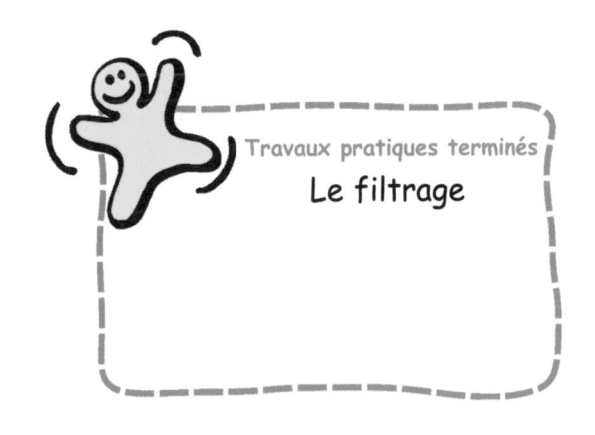

Travaux pratiques terminés

Le filtrage

 Commentaires de ton enseignant/e

Tu es super !!

DATE

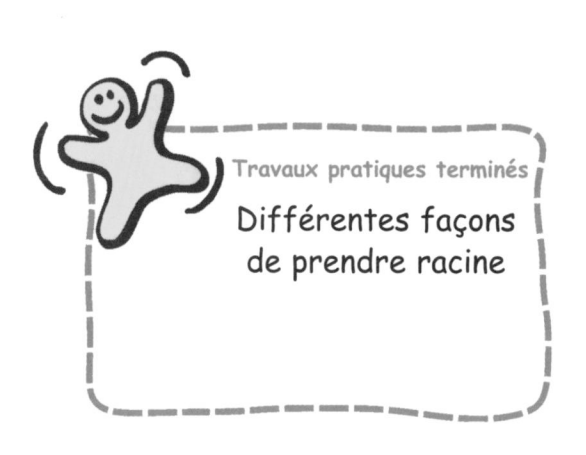

Travaux pratiques terminés

Différentes façons de prendre racine

 **Commentaires de ton enseignant/e**

_____

_____

DATE

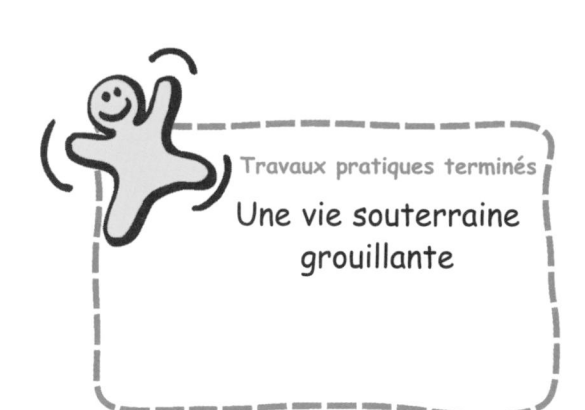

Travaux pratiques terminés

Une vie souterraine grouillante

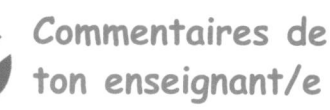 **Commentaires de ton enseignant/e**

_____

_____

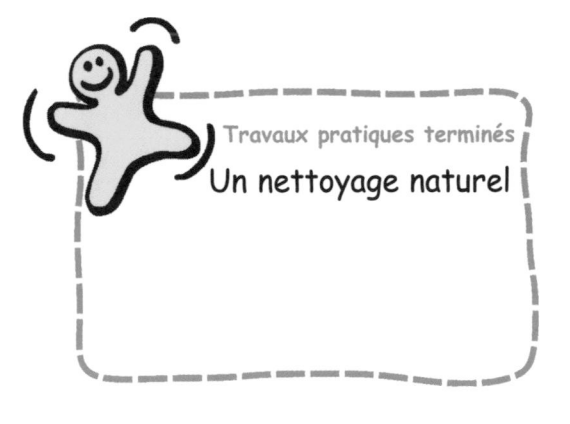

Travaux pratiques terminés

Un nettoyage naturel

 Commentaires de ton enseignant/e

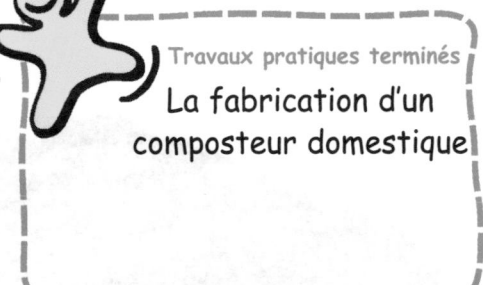

Travaux pratiques terminés

La fabrication d'un composteur domestique

 Commentaires de ton enseignant/e

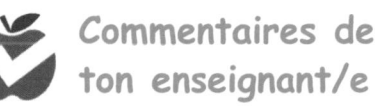

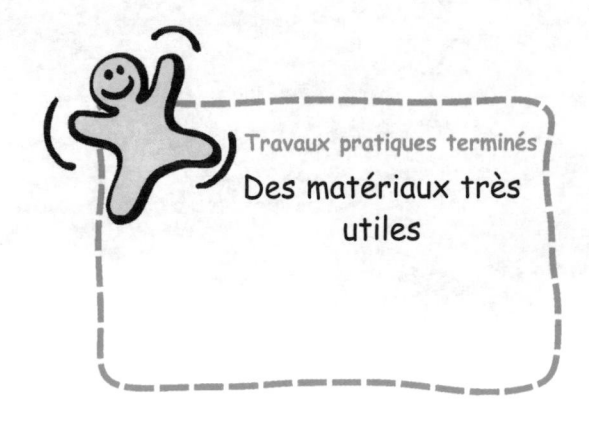

Travaux pratiques terminés

Des matériaux très utiles

 Commentaires de ton enseignant/e